The Massachusetts General Hospital Handbook of Pain Management

The Massachusetts General Hospital Handbook of Pain Management

Edited by

David Borsook, M.D., Ph.D.
Assistant Professor of Anesthesia (Neurology), Department of Anesthesia and Neurology, Harvard Medical School; Director, Massachusetts General Hospital Pain Center, Department of Anesthesia, Massachusetts General Hospital, Boston

Alyssa A. LeBel, M.D.
Instructor of Anesthesia (Neurology), Department of Anesthesia and Neurology, Harvard Medical School; Co-Director, Massachusetts General Hospital Pain Center, Department of Anesthesia, Massachusetts General Hospital, Boston

Bucknam McPeek, M.D.
Associate Professor of Anesthesia, Department of Anesthesia, Harvard Medical School; Massachusetts General Hospital, Boston

Foreword by

Howard L. Fields, M.D., Ph.D.
Professor of Neurology and Physiology, University of California, San Francisco, School of Medicine, San Francisco

Little, Brown and Company
Boston   New York   Toronto   London

Library of Congress Cataloging-in-Publication Data

The Massachusetts General Hospital handbook of pain management /
  edited by David Borsook, Alyssa LeBel, Bucknam McPeek ; foreword by
  Howard L. Fields.
       p.   cm.
  Includes bibliographical references and index.
  ISBN 0-316-54946-0
  1. Pain—Treatment. 2. Analgesia. I. Borsook, David.
II. LeBel, Alyssa. III. McPeek, Bucknam, 1933–
IV. Massachusetts General Hospital.
  [DNLM: 1. Pain—therapy—handbooks.   WB 39 M414 1995]
RB127.M389   1995
616'.0472—dc20
DNLM/DLC
for Library of Congress   95-23369
                                                                    CIP

Printed in the United States of America

ICP

Second Printing

Editorial: Nancy Megley, Richard L. Wilcox
Production Editor: Katharine S. Mascaro
Copyeditor: Tracey Solon
Indexer: Nanette Cardon, IRIS
Production Supervisor: Mike Burggren

To our patients and especially to Melvin Fisher, who suffers from severe chronic pain and who has managed to deal with this affliction with superhuman courage and conviction. He is an inspiration to all of us involved in the treatment and research of pain at MGH and also to numerous fellow beings suffering from pain.

Contents

Foreword

After three decades of progress in unravelling the neural mechanisms of pain, a revolution is underway in the clinical practice of pain management. Simply stated, increasing numbers of physicians are taking responsibility for the relief of their patients' pain. *The Massachusetts General Hospital Handbook of Pain Management* provides an introduction to the knowledge base required for optimal treatment of pain.

Several factors have contributed to this revolution. Perhaps the most important is the evolution of attitude in individuals with pain who are no longer willing to suffer in silence. Pain has, if you will, moved progressively from the realm of the moral to that of the medical. Scientific discoveries that explain some of the most puzzling features of pain have facilitated this change in attitude. For example, the nerve cells that confer pain sensitivity have been found and described, as have the central nervous system pathways that transmit the information to higher centers. Remarkably, we can now visualize the metabolic changes in the brain produced by painful stimuli. In addition, as Chapter 2 of this handbook describes, there are well-described pathways that selectively amplify or suppress pain signals, a finding that has done much to explain the tremendous variability of pain severity reported by different patients with similar injuries. The public at large is familiar with the idea that endogenous opioid substances (endorphins) in the brain can produce bliss and pain relief. The objective description of pathways and mechanisms helps remove pain from the realm of the purely personal, making it less of a burden that one is expected to bear with resignation, like fear of death, and more of a sign of disease, like fever or bleeding. Clearly, the latter are matters of shared concern for both patient and physician.

This growth in our knowledge of neural mechanisms has been paralleled by increased interest on the part of physicians in actively treating pain. Although relief of suffering is accepted as a major goal for physicians, many doctors traditionally assume that pain relief per se is a simple task for which no special training is required. In fact, although acute pain is generally managed in an adequate manner, many health care professionals continue to manage acute and cancer pain inadequately, and chronic pain remains a major challenge. Fortunately, there has been increasing recognition among physicians that persistent pain is a serious and complex problem that often requires the skills of a variety of health care professionals for optimal assessment and treatment. Multidisciplinary pain clinics, a concept originated by the late John J. Bonica at the University of Washington, have now spread around the world, and it is unusual to find an academic medical center that does not have a pain management service. Appendix II of this handbook provides a useful list of pain centers across the country.

Despite the challenge presented by the complexity of pain, it is imperative that all physicians be experienced in its assessment and treatment. There are some simple guidelines; the most important is to ask the patient to tell you how severe his or her pain is and what things make it worse. It is also essential to quickly establish the efficacy (or lack of efficacy) of the treatment given. In chronic pain, psychosocial factors loom large and must be assessed in the initial clinical encounter. This aspect of pain management is described in Chapter 24 of this handbook. The bottom line is that current practice standards make it unacceptable to allow a patient to suffer unnecessary pain.

The Massachusetts General Hospital Handbook of Pain Management both reflects and supports the revolution in pain management by providing a broad introduction to the diagnostic complexities, assessment tools, and multiple treatment modalities that are now available. Master its contents and you will have gone far toward the goal of optimal care for pain patients.

Howard L. Fields, M.D., Ph.D.

Preface

"Pain is not just a symptom demanding our compassion; it can be an aggressive disease that damages the nervous system."

GARY BENNETT

Pain is a significant problem in many medical and surgical disorders. Some clinicians find its treatment difficult and frequently unrewarding. This handbook represents the work of fellows and staff at the Massachusetts General Hospital Pain Center who participated in the treatment of patients with various pain problems. We realize that different approaches are used elsewhere which we have not included here.

Our program—which is a multidisciplinary one with input from anesthesiology, neurology, neurosurgery, psychiatry, psychology, physical therapy, surgery, nursing, and pediatrics—by its nature includes the treatment of patients with a wide spectrum of painful conditions. This book is really a summary of what we do with patients at the MGH. We hope it will prove useful for health workers at every level in approaching and treating patients with pain.

The editors would like to thank Jeanette Cohan and Anne B. Greene.

D.B.
A.A.L.
B.M.

Contributing Authors

David K. Ahern, Ph.D.
Assistant Professor of Psychology, Department of Psychiatry, Harvard Medical School; Director, Behavioral Medicine Unit, Massachusetts General Hospital, Boston

Zahid H. Bajwa, M.D.
Associate Professor of Neurology, Department of Anesthesia, Harvard Medical School; Director, Education and Training, Beth Israel Pain Management Center, Department of Anesthesia, Beth Israel Hospital, Boston

Jane Ballantyne, M.D.
Clinical Fellow of Anesthesia, Harvard Medical School; Assistant in Anesthesia, Massachusetts General Hospital, Boston

David Borsook, M.D., Ph.D.
Assistant Professor of Anesthesia (Neurology), Department of Anesthesia and Neurology, Harvard Medical School; Director, Massachusetts General Hospital Pain Center, Department of Anesthesia, Massachusetts General Hospital, Boston

Daniel B. Carr, M.D.
Saltonstall Professor of Pain Research, Departments of Anesthesia and Medicine, Tufts University School of Medicine; Anesthesiologist and Medical Director, Pain Management Program, Department of Anesthesia, New England Medical Center, Boston

G. Rees Cosgrove, M.D.
Assistant Professor of Surgery, Harvard Medical School; Neurosurgeon, Department of Neurological Surgery, Massachusetts General Hospital, Boston

Juliet M. Cowin, M.D.
Clinical Fellow of Anesthesia, Harvard Medical School; Resident, Department of Anesthesia, Massachusetts General Hospital, Boston

Michael Cutrer, M.D.
Instructor of Neurology, Harvard Medical School; Assistant in Neurology, Massachusetts General Hospital, Department of Neurology, Massachusetts General Hospital, Boston

Andreas Dauber, M.D.

John F. DiCapua, M.D.
Clinical Instructor, Department of Anesthesia, New York University School of Medicine, New York; Staff Anesthesiologist, Northshore University Hospital, Manhasset, New York

Annabel Edwards, R.N., M.S.N.
Clinic Manager, Massachusetts General Hospital Pain Center, Department of Anesthesia, Massachusetts General Hospital, Boston

Elon Eisenberg, M.D.
Director, Pain Management, Department of Anesthesia, Rambam Hospital, Haifa, Israel

Roberto Feliz, M.D.
Instructor of Anesthesia, Harvard Medical School; Assistant in Anesthesia, New England Deaconess, Boston

Scott M. Fishman, M.D.
Instructor of Psychiatry, Department of Anesthesia, Harvard Medical School; Co-Director, Massachusetts General Hospital Pain Center, Department of Anesthesia, Massachusetts General Hospital, Boston

David M. Frim, M.D., Ph.D.
Clinical Fellow of Surgery, Harvard Medical School; Assistant in Neurosurgery, Department of Neurological Surgery, Massachusetts General Hospital, Boston

Donna B. Greenberg M.D.
Assistant Professor of Psychiatry, Harvard Medical School; Psychiatrist, Massachusetts General Hospital, Boston

Asteghik Hacobian, M.D.
Clinical Fellow of Anesthesia, Harvard Medical School; Assistant in Anesthesia, Massachusetts General Hospital, Boston

Janet C. Hsieh, M.D.
Instructor of Anesthesia, Harvard Medical School; Assistant in Anesthesia, Massachusetts General Hospital, Boston

Keith P. Kittelberger, M.D.
Staff Anesthesiologist, Raleigh Anesthesia Associates, Inc., Carolina Pain Consultants, Rex Hospital and Raleigh Community Hospital, Raleigh, North Carolina

Suzanne LaCross, M.D.
Acting Program Director, Pain Rehabilitation Program, Spaulding Rehabilitation Hospital, Boston

Alyssa A. LeBel, M.D.
Instructor of Anesthesia (Neurology), Department of Anesthesia and Neurology, Harvard Medical School; Co-Director, Massachusetts General Hospital Pain Center, Department of Anesthesia, Massachusetts General Hospital, Boston

Paolo L. Manfredi, M.D.
Clinical Fellow of Anesthesia, Harvard Medical School; Assistant in Neurology, Department of Anesthesia, Massachusetts General Hospital, Boston

Bucknam McPeek, M.D.
Associate Professor of Anesthesia, Department of Anesthesia, Harvard Medical School; Co-Director, Massachusetts General Hospital Pain Center, Department of Anesthesia, Massachusetts General Hospital, Boston

Terry Hoskins Michel, P.T., M.S.
Assistant Professor, Institute of Health Professions, Massachusetts General Hospital, Boston

Khyati Mohamed, R.Ph.

Shaffin A. Mohamed, M.D.
Clinical Assistant Professor of Anesthesiology, University of Texas Medical Branch, Galveston, Texas; Director, Center for Functional Restoration, Houston

Ervant Nishanian, M.D.
Clinical Fellow of Anesthesia, Harvard Medical School; Resident, Department of Anesthesia, Massachusetts General Hospital, Boston

Robert O. Ong, M.D.
Clinical Instructor of Anesthesia, Harvard Medical School; Assistant in Anesthesia, Massachusetts General Hospital, Boston

Terry Rabinowitz, M.D., D.D.S.
Instructor of Psychiatry, Harvard Medical School; Staff Psychiatrist, Massachusetts General Hospital and Spaulding Rehabilitation Hospital, Boston

Sharona Soumekh, M.D.
Instructor of Neurology, Harvard Medical School; Medical Director, Pain Rehabilitation Program, Spaulding Rehabilitation Hospital, Boston

Milan Stojanovic, M.D.
Clinical Fellow of Anesthesia, Harvard Medical School; Assistant in Anesthesia, Massachusetts General Hospital, Boston

Jacqueline A. Tejeda, M.D.
Clinical Fellow of Anesthesia, Harvard Medical School; Assistant in Anesthesia, Massachusetts General Hospital, Boston

Donald P. Todd, M.D.
Associate Professor of Anesthesia, Harvard Medical School; Anesthetist, Massachusetts General Hospital, Boston

Cassandra L. Tribble, M.D.
Clinical Fellow of Anesthesia, Harvard Medical School; Assistant in Anesthesia, Massachusetts General Hospital, Boston

Seth A. Waldman, M.D.
Clinical Assistant Professor of Anesthesiology and Pain Management, Cornell University Medical College; Attending, Department of Anesthesiology, Hospital for Special Surgery, New York

Ursula Wesselmann, M.D., Ph.D.
Senior Clinical Fellow of Neurology and Neurosurgery, The Johns Hopkins Medical School, Baltimore

Nicolas A. Wieder, D.O.
Instructor, Department of Facial Pain, University of California Los Angeles Dental School, Los Angeles; Staff, Los Robles Regional Medical Center, Thousand Oaks, California

Harriet Wittink, P.T., H.S.
Physical Therapist, Department of Anesthesia, New England Medical Center, Boston

Melissa Wolff, M.S., P.T.
Senior Physical Therapist, Department of Rehabilitation Services, University of Tennessee Medical Center, Knoxville, Tennessee

Tina U. Wolter, Ph.D.
Instructor and Clinical Associate of Psychology, Department of Psychiatry, Harvard Medical School; Clinical Psychologist, Behavioral Medicine Unit, Massachusetts General Hospital, Boston

I

General Issues

The Pain Management Imperative

Zahid H. Bajwa and David Borsook

> *"Pain is the most urgent of symptoms."*
>
> H. K. BEECHER

The word "pain" is derived from the Latin word "poena" meaning punishment. Pain and its treatment have preoccupied society since antiquity (Fig. 1-1). Recent scientific and clinical advances have revolutionized the field of pain management. Progress has been based on recognizing that unrelieved pain has consequences well beyond temporary suffering. These consequences include delayed healing, an altered immune system, an altered stress response, vegetative symptoms, and the possibility of producing permanent alterations in the peripheral and central nervous systems resulting in chronic pain syndromes. These effects, in turn, are not only detrimental to the individuals but also to their families and society as a whole. It is estimated that individuals suffering from chronic pain syndromes cost the United States several billion dollars in days missed from work, workers' compensation, and legal suits.

Managing pain and relieving suffering are at the core of a health care professional's commitment. Evidence supporting the benefit of aggressive pain management continues to mount from both laboratory and clinical investigations. When considered together with the ethical and socioeconomic benefits of aggressive pain control, an even clearer mandate emerges.

The Challenges

EDUCATION

In first-world countries there has been an explosion in the number of pain clinics. Nevertheless it is estimated that approximately 40% of acute pain is not managed properly (see Chap. 14) and an even greater number of cancer patients suffer from pain (see Chaps. 18 and 19). The problem is even more apparent in many third-world countries, where opioids are not available for a variety of reasons. Nevertheless providing pain relief to all patients has become a universal goal. For example, one of the aims of the World Health Organization is to provide appropriate pain treatment for all cancer patients by the year 2000.

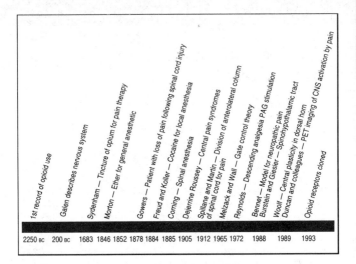

Fig. 1-1. Some major milestones in pain management and scientific advances in the field of pain. PAG ≡ periaqueductal gray matter.

If a patient spikes a temperature the physician intervenes on an urgent basis, providing the appropriate diagnostic evaluation and therapy. When a patient has severe pain, it is not considered a medical emergency. Why?

The lack of understanding on the part of many clinicians is not the only reason for undertreatment of pain. For instance, it is still not widely appreciated that even simple operations can result in severe pain syndromes. Recent research has shown that even a small incision in the skin may produce alterations in the dorsal horn of the spinal cord. These alterations may be the harbinger of more permanent changes in neuronal connectivity within the dorsal horn that are known to take place following nerve injury (see Chap. 13).

Although pain is the most common symptom for which a patient seeks a physician, medical education offers little formal training in this area. At most medical schools in the United States very little time is spent teaching about pain and pain syndromes. The inevitable result is that many patients with pain syndromes are misdiagnosed and are not seen early in the course of their disease, when treatment is often most beneficial.

Many pain management procedures are currently performed that have not undergone the scrutiny of well-controlled clinical trials. Outcome studies for pain treatment are greatly needed.

PREEMPTIVE ANALGESIA

Preemptive analgesia is a concept based on basic science experiments that suggest that analgesic intervention prior to a noxious stimulus can reduce or even prevent subsequent pain and may simplify subsequent pain management. The concept of nervous system plasticity is critical to understanding preemptive analgesia. Nervous system plasticity is a process of structural and functional changes in response to developmental and traumatic events and other stimuli and experiences. Plasticity is possible because the nervous system is neither hard-wired nor preprogrammed. Profound anatomic and biochemical changes are thought to occur in the nervous system in response to noxious stimuli. For example, following peripheral nerve injury, dramatic changes have been demonstrated at the molecular level in the dorsal horn of the spinal cord in various peptide and receptor systems. Similar changes may take place elsewhere along pain pathways, also in response to trauma or noxious stimuli. The exact significance of these changes in biologic terms is not fully understood. However, such plasticity probably underlies the "memory" of noxious stimuli and renders the spinal cord hyperexcitable by subsequent stimuli—a phenomenon that may lead to increased pain in the postoperative period. If such changes in pain pathways can be prevented by proper use of analgesic agents prior to surgical incision, preemptive analgesia may prevent or reduce "pain memory" and lead to reduced postoperative analgesic requirements.

Although controversial, evidence for the effectiveness of preemptive analgesia has emerged from basic animal research. In the 1980s, Woolf and colleagues showed in animal studies that noxious impulses from deep tissues can trigger prolonged, widespread changes of spinal-cord excitability. Once the hyperexcitable state is established, very large doses of opioids are needed to suppress it. However, if relatively small doses of opioids (or other analgesics, such as local anesthetics) are administered to the spinal cord before the arrival of noxious impulses, the hyperexcitable state is prevented.

Further controlled clinical trials are needed to establish appropriate treatment strategies. In some studies the appropriate use of opioids in the preoperative period may decrease postoperative pain and drug requirements. Table 1-1 summarizes some recent trials of effective preemptive analgesia.

UNIVERSAL ANALGESIA

A universal truth of medicine in the 1990s is that **no human should ever suffer unnecessary pain**. Our utmost commitment as health care professionals is not only to treat the disease but also to relieve pain and suffering. While it is not always possible or even advisable to eradicate all pain, since pain often serves as a protective signal for vital body organs, it remains our ethical responsibility to minimize it or at least make it bearable.

Still there are social, cultural, political, and scientific barriers to achieving pain relief for all patients. Even in the United States recent studies demonstrate that women, children, and the elderly receive poor pain treatment. In third-world coun-

Table 1-1. Benefits of preemptive analgesia: Clinical studies

Reference	Comments
Bach et al (1988)	Phantom pain may be inhibited when epidural analgesia given prior to amputation
Katz et al (1992)	Improved postoperative analgesia when epidural fentanyl given before surgical incision
Woolf and Chong (1993)	Review of basic science considerations in preemptive analgesia
Viel et al (1993)	Preemptive analgesia and sympathetically maintained pain

tries, though basic facilities may not be available, the use of opioids that are relatively inexpensive is limited by governments, by lack of education on the part of health care providers, and by social stigma related to the use of such agents.

Basic scientific advances in pain management have undergone rapid progress in the last decade. We now know that neural plasticity results in altered connections and activity within the nervous system. Nevertheless we do not fully understand, nor can we effectively treat, many chronic pain syndromes once they are established. These are the challenges of pain management in the future.

Consequences of Undertreated Pain

Undertreated pain is never benign. In Ronald Melzack's words, "Pain can have a major impact on morbidity and mortality—it can mean the difference between life and death." Pain is frequently accompanied by vegetative features such as depression, which can disrupt the lives of patients and their families and, under certain circumstances, can even lead to suicide. Pain may produce other effects. For example, some reports indicate that chronic pain alters the stress response, especially in the elderly, and that chronic pain may produce suppression of the immune system.

Conclusions

Major developments have reshaped our understanding of the pathophysiology of pain over the last two decades, leading to the development of new analgesic drugs, management strategies, and analgesic technology. Pain management is a rapidly evolving multidisciplinary field now recognized by the U.S. Accreditation Council for Graduate Medical Education as a legitimate academic subspecialty.

As a result of our new understanding of pain physiology and pharmacologic and technical advances, acute and cancer pain is controllable in almost all patients. Important advances have also been made in the management of chronic, nonmalignant pain owing to a multidisciplinary approach, with hopes for improved outcome.

It is almost inconceivable, were it not a fact, that the problem of undertreatment of pain persists, causing patients and their families to suffer. While new advances in analgesia surely lie ahead, every clinician should hold firmly in mind that there is presently every medical and ethical reason to treat pain aggressively with all available resources.

Selected Readings

Bach S, Noreng MF, and Tjellden NU. Phantom limb pain in amputees during the first 12 months following limb amputation after preoperative lumbar epidural blockade. *Pain* 33:297–301, 1988.

Cleeland CS, et al. Pain and its treatment in outpatients with metastatic cancer. *N Engl J Med* 330:592–596, 1994.

Foley KM. The treatment of cancer pain. *N Engl J Med* 313:84–95, 1985.

Katz J, et al. Preemptive analgesia. Clinical evidence of neuroplasticity contributing to postoperative pain. *Anesthesiology* 77:439–446, 1992.

McQuay HJ, Carroll D, and Moore RA. Postoperative orthopaedic pain: the effect of opiate premedication and local anaesthetic blocks. *Pain* 33:291–295, 1988.

Viel E, et al. Les algodystrophies des membres: physiopathologie, aspects préventifs. *Cah Anesthesiol* 41:163–168, 1993.

Woolf CJ and Chong MS. Preemptive analgesia—treating postoperative pain by preventing the establishment of central sensitization. *Anesth Analg* 77:362–379, 1993.

World Health Organization. *Cancer Pain Relief and Palliative Care*. Geneva: World Health Organization, 1990.

Neural Basis of Pain

Keith P. Kittelberger and David Borsook

> *". . . in any path of study*
> *knowledge never comes entirely at*
> *once but piecemeal. Truth presents*
> *herself in fragmentary form, and*
> *we put pieces together . . ."*
>
> R. ABBE

One of the most important functions of the body's nervous system is to provide information on the threat of bodily injury. **Pain** is defined by the International Association for the Study of Pain as **"an unpleasant sensory and emotional experience associated with actual or potential tissue damage."** The body's response to and perception of pain is called **nociception**. The pain system may be divided into the following useful categories:

1. Specialized receptors, called **nociceptors**, in the peripheral nervous system detect and filter the intensity and type of noxious stimuli
2. **Primary afferent fibers** (A-delta and C fibers) transmit noxious impulses to the CNS
3. **Ascending nociceptive tracts** (e.g., spinothalamic tract, spinohypothalamic tract) convey noxious stimuli to higher centers in the CNS
4. **Higher centers**, which are involved in pain discrimination, affective components of pain, memory components of pain, and motor control related to painful stimuli (i.e., withdrawal responses)
5. A means to process and modify incoming impulses and information, called **pain modulation**, which includes **descending systems**

Nociceptors

Nociceptors are **free nerve terminals of primary afferent fibers** that can detect painful stimuli. Nociceptors may be divided according to the type of stimulation that evokes their response and the response characteristics. There are two basic categories of nociceptors: mechano-heat receptors and mechanically insensitive receptors.

Mechano-heat receptors respond to heat and are categorized into the C-fiber and A-fiber groups. C-fiber mechano-heat receptors respond to intermediate heat thresholds (41–49°C), have a slow conduction velocity, and constitute the majority of nociceptive afferent fibers. It is worth noting that itch is also transduced at C-fiber mechano-heat receptors. A-fiber mechano-heat receptors are divided into two types. Type I receptors have a high heat threshold (>53°C) and conduct at relatively fast velocities (30–55 m/sec). These receptors detect pain sensation during high-intensity heat response. Type II receptors have a low heat threshold and conduct at 15 m/sec.

Mechanically insensitive receptors respond to cold and various chemicals (e.g., bradykinin, H^+ ions, serotonin, histamine, arachidonic acid) and may only become responsive after inflammation (e.g., painful bladder inflammation).

RESPONSE CHARACTERISTICS

Response characteristics of nociceptors allow for coding in spatial and temporal information. The various nociceptors' type of response allows for differences in sensitivity (low- and high-threshold nociceptors) and temporal nature (rate of firing) of afferent input to the dorsal horn. Some nociceptors are called **wide dynamic range** (WDR) nociceptors and respond to warmth and also to thermal pain. Others are **nociceptive specific** (NS), which may also be thermoreceptors, but they only respond to stimuli that are in the noxious range. Furthermore, as described above, some nociceptors may be polymodal (C fiber) and respond to a wide range of noxious stimuli (i.e., mechanical, thermal, and chemical) or to specific noxious stimuli.

LOCATION

Nociceptors are found in cutaneous and noncutaneous tissue. In the skin, pain fibers lose their myelin sheath in the epidermal basal lamina. Outside of the skin, nociceptors are present in the cornea, tooth pulp, muscles, joints, respiratory system, cardiovascular system, digestive system, urogenital system, and brain and meninges.

HYPERALGESIA

Tissue damage results in activation of nociceptors and primary hyperalgesia. **Hyperalgesia is the phenomenon in which, following tissue damage, there is a lowered threshold to painful stimuli. Primary hyperalgesia** is hyperalgesia at the site of injury. **Secondary hyperalgesia** is hyperalgesia in the surrounding skin. Interestingly, heat and mechanical stimuli produce pain in primary hyperalgesia, but only mechanical stimuli produce pain in secondary hyperalgesia.

With hyperalgesia there is an alteration in both subjective response and fiber response to stimuli. The subjective response is seen as a lowered pain threshold, an increase in pain to suprathreshold stimuli, and the presence of spontaneous pain. The correlating fiber response is seen as a decreased threshold for response and also an increased response to suprathreshold stimuli. There are also spontaneous fiber discharges. Therefore, in hyperalgesia there is **plastic-**

ity of nociceptor response, and this may be related to the level of noxious stimuli.

As tissue damage occurs, a number of chemical substances and mediators that elicit excitatory postsynaptic potentials and potentiate the nociceptive response are released—serotonin, histamine, potassium, adenosine triphosphate, platelet-activating factor, free radicals, acetylcholine, catecholamines, bradykinin, and arachidonic acid metabolites (prostaglandins, leukotrienes). A number of these substances cause pain on injection.

Inflammation

Inflammation consists of a series of biochemical and cellular events that are activated in response to injury and result in the classic findings of **rubor, calor, dolor, tumor,** and **functio laesa**.

With inflammation there is increased pain when the area is moved or touched and less pain at rest. There are a number of sources for the mediators of inflammation, including substance P (SP) and calcitonin gene related peptide (CGRP) release from the nerve endings (nociceptors). These sources include circulating leukocytes, platelets, vascular endothelial cells, and peripheral nerves, including the primary afferent neuron. The mediators of inflammation include adenosine, bradykinin, complement (C5a), interleukins (1 and 8), leukotrienes, nerve growth factor, prostaglandins (E_2, I_2), serotonin, and substance P.

Primary Afferent Fibers

The neural impulses originating from nociceptors are transmitted via peripheral nerves to the spinal cord, or via cranial nerves to cranial nerve ganglia if from the head. They are classified according to size, degree of myelination, and conduction velocity (Table 2-1).

Primary afferent fibers below the head have cell bodies located in the **dorsal root ganglion** (DRG) of spinal nerves. Primary afferent fibers of the head have cell bodies in the sensory ganglia of cranial nerves V, VII, IX, and X.

The primary afferent axons activated by nociceptors are the free endings of myelinated A-delta and unmyelinated C fibers. The majority of nociceptor afferent fibers are in the C-fiber velocity range and respond maximally to polymodal noxious stimuli applied to receptive fields. Eighty to ninety percent of C fibers respond to nociceptive input. A-delta fibers respond to noxious mechanical stimuli. These two types of fibers, with their differences in conduction velocities and stimulus properties, may explain the pain sensation commonly experienced after a noxious stimulus: a first pain (so-called epicritic pain) that is rapid and pricking in character con-

Table 2-1. Classification of fibers in peripheral nerves

Fiber group	Innervation	Mean diameter (μm)	Mean conduction velocity (m/sec)
A-alpha	Primary muscle spindle motor to skeletal muscle	15	100
A-beta	Cutaneous touch and pressure afferent fibers	8	50
A-gamma	Motor to muscle spindle	6	20
A-delta	Mechanoreceptors, **nociceptors**, thermoreceptors	<3	15
B	Sympathetic preganglionic	3	7
C	Mechanoreceptors, **nociceptors**, thermoreceptors, sympathetic postganglionic	1	1

Source: From JJ Bonica. Anatomic and Physiologic Basis of Nociception and Pain. In: JJ Bonica (ed.), *The Management of Pain* (2nd ed.). Philadelphia: Lea & Febiger, 1990. P 31. Used with permission.

ducted by A-delta fibers (velocity = 5–30 m/sec), followed by a second pain (so-called protopathic pain) that is burning and conducted by C fibers (velocity = 0.5–2.0 m/sec).

Visceral afferent nociceptive fibers (C and A-delta) travel with sympathetic and parasympathetic fibers. Their somata are found in the DRG.

There are numerous neuromodulators in the dorsal root ganglion, and receptors for many of these are present in the dorsal horn. For example, there are high concentrations of opioid receptors (based on specific in situ hybridization studies of receptor mRNA) in the DRG and lower concentrations in the dorsal horn. Therefore, endogenous opioids may be modulated at this level.

The Dorsal Horn

Figure 2-1A illustrates the dorsal horn. The synapse between the primary afferent fibers and neurons within the dorsal horn is an important location for further processing and integration of incoming nociceptive information. The dorsal horn may be a point at which nociceptive information is conducted to higher centers or at which nociceptive information is inhibited by descending systems (see below). Furthermore, just as in the case of sensitization of nociceptors, neurons in the dorsal horn, including projection neurons (i.e., spinothalamic tract neurons), may have altered states depending on the prior history of noxious afferent input.

LISSAUER'S TRACT

Lissauer's tract is a bundle of predominately (80%) primary afferent fibers, consisting mainly of A-delta and C fibers that run longitudinally between the surface of the spinal cord and dorsal horn. A-delta and C fibers access the spinal cord and run up or down one or two segments prior to synapsing with second-order neurons in the dorsal horn (i.e., spinothalamic tract neurons).

REXED'S LAMINAE

Figure 2-1B illustrates Rexed's laminae. The gray matter of the spinal cord can be divided into laminae (I–X) named after Rexed and based on the histologic organization of the numerous types of cell bodies and dendrites. With respect to connections made by afferent fibers conveying nociceptive information, the most important include lamina I (marginal zone), lamina II (substantia gelatinosa), and lamina V. This is a simplistic view of nociceptive information, since primary visceral and somatic nociceptive afferent fibers are known to synapse in other laminae. Thus cutaneous mechanoreceptor A-delta afferent fibers synapse in laminae I, II, and V; visceral mechanoreceptor A-delta fibers synapse in laminae I and V; cutaneous nociceptor C fibers synapse in lamina I

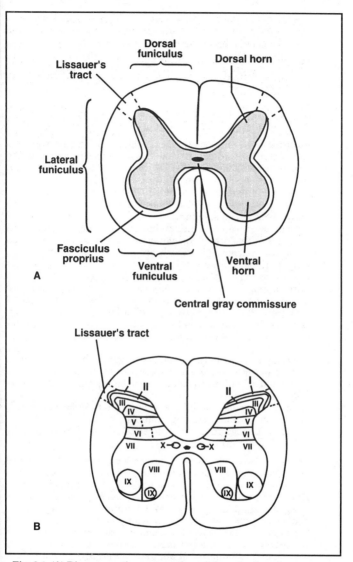

Fig. 2-1. (A) Diagrammatic cross section of the spinal cord.
(B) Rexed's laminae I–X of the spinal cord.

and II; and visceral nociceptive C fibers synapse in many laminae including I, II, IV, V, and X. There are two broad generalizations about central termination of peripheral nociceptive afferent fibers in the dorsal horn: (1) Afferent nociceptive fibers terminate predominantly in Rexed's laminae I, II, and V. (2) In the case of visceral nociceptors, deeper Rexed's laminae are also involved.

Laminae I–VI make up the dorsal horn. Six laminae are thought to be most involved in nociceptive processing.

Lamina I is called the marginal layer and is the most superficial lamina. It consists of many nerve bundles, giving it a reticular appearance. In addition to the NS and WDR neurons, the most abundant cell type in lamina I is projection cells, some of which make up the ascending pathways, and others synapse with interneurons.

Lamina II is the substantia gelatinosa because of its gelatinous appearance. Like lamina I, there are NS and WDR neurons. Two other types of cells are the stalked cells and central or islet cells, which are excitatory and inhibitory, respectively. These are important in relaying inputs from other primary afferent fibers to the projection cells found in lamina I. Still other cells contribute to the ascending tracts. In contrast to primary afferent fibers, no visceral afferent fibers terminate in lamina II.

Lamina III is made up of many myelinated axons and dendrites from deeper laminae. It also contains central or islet cells.

In **lamina IV** the most common cell type is the low-threshold mechanoreceptor, which responds to innocuous tactile and thermal stimuli to the skin. These cells are activated by A-beta fibers.

Lamina V consists mainly of WDR neurons and axons, which give rise to the ascending systems.

Lamina X surrounds the central canal and has some cells that are nociceptive.

There are two major types of projection neurons in the dorsal horn that respond to nociceptive stimuli. **NS neurons** respond only to a specific type of noxious stimuli. Their **receptive fields are small** and organized somatotopically and are most abundant in lamina I. **WDR neurons** are nociceptive nonspecific; they respond to a wide range of stimuli, from light touch or low heat to noxious stimuli. They have **larger receptive fields**, are the most prevalent cells in the dorsal horn, and are found in all laminae, especially lamina V.

BIOCHEMICAL MEDIATORS

Numerous neurotransmitters and neuromodulators are present in the dorsal horn. They are derived from three sources: (1) primary afferent fibers, (2) interneurons, and (3) descending fiber systems. Although the neurochemistry of the dorsal horn is very complicated, it is useful to think in terms of whether the neuroactive substances are neuropeptides or the more classic neurotransmitters. The latter generally have rapid actions that are of a short duration, while the former have a slower onset of action and may have more prolonged effects. Further, each group can be classified by its functional effects—excitatory or inhibitory. Examples are listed below:

Excitatory Neurochemical Mediators

The excitatory amino acids glutamate and aspartate
Substance P
Substance K (neurokinin A)
Calcitonin gene–related peptide (CGRP)
Vasoactive intestinal peptide (VIP)
Cholecystokinin (CCK)

Inhibitory Neuromediators

The endogenous opioids, such as enkephalin, dynorphin, and
    endorphin
Somatostatin
Serotonin (5-HT)
Norepinephrine
Gamma-aminobutyric acid (GABA)
Galanin

There are specific receptors for many of these neuromodulators in the dorsal horn. For example, high levels of N-methyl-D-aspartate receptors are present in the dorsal horn; these are the receptors for the excitatory amino acids such as glutamate and aspartate. There are also specific neuropeptide receptors.

Ascending Tracts: Pathways to Brain Areas Involved in Nociception

The ascending pathways involved with nociceptive transmission (Fig. 2-2) arise mainly from laminae I, II, and V, but the other laminae do contribute. These pathways include the spinothalamic tract, spinohypothalamic tract, spinoreticular tract, and spinopontoamygdala tract.

SPINOTHALAMIC TRACT

The spinothalamic tract is the most important of the ascending pathways for the transmission of nociceptive stimuli and is located in the anterolateral quadrant of the spinal cord. Most of the axons originating in the dorsal horn cross in the ventral white commissure of the spinal cord to ascend in the opposite anterolateral quadrant; however, some do remain ipsilateral. Neurons from more distal regions of the body (i.e., the sacral region) are found more laterally and neurons from more proximal regions (i.e., the cervical region) are found more medially within the spinothalamic tract as it ascends. Spinothalamic tract neurons segregate into **medial and lateral projections** to the thalamus (see Limbic System below).

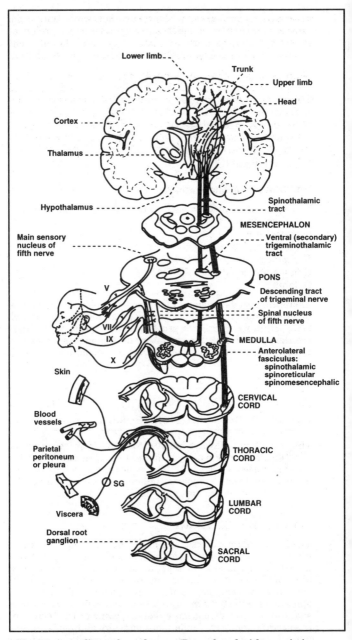

Fig. 2-2. Ascending pain pathways. (Reproduced with permission from Bonica JJ, *The Management of Pain* (vol I). Philadelphia: Lea & Febiger, 1990. P. 29.)

Neurons that project to the **lateral thalamus** arise from laminae I, II, and V, and from there synapse with fibers that project to the somatosensory cortex. The fibers are thought to be involved in sensory and discriminative aspects of pain.

Neurons projecting to the **medial thalamus** originate from the deeper laminae VI and IX. The neurons send collateral projections to the reticular formation of the brain stem and midbrain, the periaqueductal gray matter and the hypothalamus, or directly to other areas of the basal forebrain and somatosensory cortex. They are thought to be involved with autonomic reflex responses, state-of-arousal, and emotional aspects of pain.

SPINOHYPOTHALAMIC TRACT (SHT)

Nociceptive and non-nociceptive information from neurons within the dorsal horn is conveyed to diencephalic structures, such as the hypothalamus, directly by a recently discovered pathway—the spinohypothalamic tract. This pathway projects to the region of the brain (the hypothalamus) that is involved in autonomic functions such as sleep, appetite, temperature regulation, stress-response, etc. Therefore it forms the anatomic substrate that allows reflex autonomic reactions to painful stimuli. Some of these connections (e.g., to the suprachiasmatic nucleus, which partly controls the sleep/wake pattern) may account for behaviors such as difficulty in sleeping with painful conditions, particularly chronic pain. The majority of these neurons respond preferentially to mechanical nociceptive stimulation, and a smaller number to noxious thermal stimulation.

The pathway ascends in the spinal cord and the majority (60%) of neurons project to the contralateral medial or lateral hypothalamus and therefore are presumed to have a significant role in autonomic and neuroendocrine response to painful stimuli. The fibers have been shown to cross in the supraoptic decussation.

OTHER TRACTS

These tracts, like the medial STT, are likely involved with state of arousal and emotional aspects of pain:

Spinoreticular tract (SRT)
Spinopontoamygdala tract

CRANIAL NERVES

The transmission of pain in the head has many of the same characteristics of the nociceptive system as for the rest of the body, as discussed thus far. The face and oral cavity are richly innervated with nociceptors. The primary nociceptive afferent fibers for the head originate mainly from cranial nerve V, and also from cranial nerves VII, IX, and X. The upper cervical nerves can also contribute. The primary afferent fibers of these cranial nerves project to the trigeminal nuclei system, whereas the upper cervical nerves project to the dorsal horn of the spinal cord. From here, stimuli project to the supraspinal system.

The **trigeminal system** consists of three sensory nuclei, all of which have cell bodies located within the trigeminal ganglion, a structure similar to DRG. The three nuclei are the trigeminal mesencephalic nucleus, the main sensory nucleus, and the spinal trigeminal nucleus, which is further subdivided into the subnucleus oralis, the subnucleus interpolaris, and the subnucleus caudalis.

The subnucleus caudalis, also known as the **medullary dorsal horn**, extends caudally from the medulla to the upper cervical segments of the spinal cord. The trigeminal nucleus receives afferent input from the three divisions of the trigeminal nerve of the face (ophthalmic, maxillary, and mandibular) as well as from the dura and the vessels from a large portion of the anterior two thirds of the brain.

The various trigeminal nuclei give rise to several ascending pathways. The axons of cell bodies in the main sensory nucleus and subnucleus oralis project either ipsilaterally, forming the dorsal trigeminothalamic tract, or contralaterally, in the ventral trigeminothalamic tract. Both tracts terminate in the thalamus. The subnucleus caudalis contributes as well to the trigeminothalamic tracts, but also has direct projections to the thalamus, reticular formation, and hypothalamus.

OTHER CRANIAL NERVES

These nerves may also contribute input to the spinal nucleus and tract of lamina V.

Glossopharyngeal nerve (IX) conveys impulses concerned with tactile sense, thermal sense, and pain from the mucous membranes of the posterior third of the tongue, tonsil, posterior pharyngeal wall, and eustachian tube.

Vagus nerve (X) conveys impulses concerned with tactile sense from the posterior auricular skin and external auditory meatus, visceral sensation from the pharynx, larynx, trachea, esophagus, and thoracic and abdominal viscera via the spinal trigeminal tract and fasciculus solitarius.

The Supraspinal System: Integration and Higher Processing of Painful Stimuli

Integration of pain in higher centers is a complex issue. At a basic level the integration and processing of painful stimuli may fall into the following broad categories:

Discriminative component: This is somatotopically specific and involves primary (SI) and secondary (SII) sensory cortex. This level of integration allows the brain to define the location of the painful stimulus. Integration of somatic pain, as opposed to visceral pain, takes place at this level. The primary and secondary cortices receive input predominantly from the ventrobasal complex of the thalamus, which is also somatotopically organized.

Affective component: The integration of the effective component of pain is very complex and involves various limbic structures. In particular, the cingulate cortex, which receives input from the parafascicular thalamic nuclei and which projects to various limbic regions, is involved in the affective components of pain. The amygdala is also involved in the integration of noxious stimuli.

Memory components of pain: Recent evidence has demonstrated that painful stimuli activate CNS regions such as the anterior insula.

Motor control and pain: The supplemental motor area is thought to be involved in the integration of the motor response to pain.

THALAMUS

The thalamus is a complex structure that acts as the relaying center for incoming nociceptive stimuli. With respect to nociceptive processing, there are two important divisions of the thalamus that receive nociceptive input. First is the **lateral division** formed by the ventrobasal complex to which nociceptive specific input from NS and WDR neurons synapse. It is somatotopically organized and projects to the somatosensory cortex. Second is the **medial division**, which consists of the posterior nucleus and the centrolateral nucleus. It is thought that these nuclei project to limbic structures involved in the affective component of pain, since there is no nociceptive-specific information conveyed by them to higher cortical regions.

Medial and Intralaminar Nuclei

These receive input from the many ascending tracts, in particular the spinothalamic tract, and the reticular formation. There is little evidence for somatotopic organization of these nuclei.

Ventrobasal Thalamus

This portion of the thalamus is organized somatotopically and can be further subdivided into (1) the **ventral posterior lateral nucleus**, which receives input mainly from the spinothalamic tract but also from the dorsal column system and somatosensory cortex, to which it projects, and (2) the **ventral posterior medial nucleus**, which receives input from the face via the trigeminothalamic tract and projects to the somatosensory cortical regions of the face.

Posterior Thalamus

Input to the posterior thalamus comes mainly from the spinothalamic tract, spinocortical tract, and dorsal column nuclei. The receptive fields are large and bilateral and lack somatotopic organization. The posterior nuclei project to the somatosensory cortex and appear to have a role in the sensory experience of pain.

Centrolateral Nucleus

The spinothalamic tract also sends projections to this nucleus, which is involved in motor activity (e.g., cerebellum and cerebral cortex).

HYPOTHALAMUS

The hypothalamus receives innocuous and noxious stimuli from all over the body, including deep tissues such as the viscera (see Spinohypothalamic Tract above). These neurons are not somatotopically organized and therefore do not provide discriminatory aspects and localization of pain. Some hypothalamic nuclei send projections to the pituitary gland via the hypophyseal stalk, brain stem, and spinal cord. The gland regulates both the autonomic nervous system and neuroendocrine response to stress, including pain.

THE LIMBIC SYSTEM

The limbic system consists of subcortical parts of the telencephalon, mesencephalon, and diencephalon. It receives input from the spinothalamic tract, the thalamus, and reticular formation, and it projects to various parts of the cerebral cortex, particularly the frontal and temporal cortex. Its role involves the motivational and emotional aspects of pain, including mood and experience.

CEREBRAL CORTEX

The **somatosensory cortex** and **cingulate cortex** are regions of the cerebral cortex involved in pain. The somatosensory cortex is the most important area of the cerebral cortex involved with nociception and is located posterior to the central sulcus of the brain. It receives input from the various nuclei of the thalamus, particularly the ventral posterior lateral and medial nuclei and posterior thalamus. The somatosensory cortex is cytoarchitecturally organized and therefore has an important role in the discriminatory aspect and localization of pain. Efferent fibers from the somatosensory cortex travel back to the thalamus and contribute to the descending system.

THE CINGULATE CORTEX

This cortical area is part of the larger limbic system that receives sensory system and cortical impulses and activates visceral and somatic effectors that contribute to the physiologic expression of behavior and emotion. The limbic system includes the subcallosal, cingulate, and parahippocampal gyri and hippocampal formation as well as the following subcortical nuclei: amygdala, septal nuclei, hypothalamus, anterior thalamic nuclei, and nuclei in the basal ganglia. Recent work has demonstrated that the cingulate gyrus is activated in humans by painful stimuli. Cingulate cortex lesions have been used in an attempt to alleviate pain and suffering.

Endogenous Mechanisms of Pain Modulation

Figures 2-3 and 2-4 illustrate the endogenous mechanisms of pain modulation. The evidence for descending controls came from two basic observations. The first observation, in the late 1960s, was that neurons in the dorsal horn of decerebrate animals are more responsive to painful stimuli with spinal cord blockade. The second observation, in the late 1980s, was that electrical stimulation of the periaqueductal gray matter profoundly relieved pain in animals. So great was the **stimulation-produced analgesia** that surgery could be performed on these animals without apparent pain. Furthermore, the animals behaved normally in every other way and there was no observed effect on other sensory modalities. These studies were pivotal in demonstrating an anatomic basis for the "natural equivalent" of stimulation-produced analgesia (i.e., stress-induced analgesia). Furthermore, subsequent studies demonstrated that small concentrations of morphine, when injected into regions such as the periaqueductal gray matter, produced significant analgesia. Interestingly, both stress-induced analgesia and stimulation-induced analgesia can be reversed by opioid antagonists.

There are a number of regions of the brain that are involved in the intrinsic modulation of noxious stimuli. These include the somatosensory cortex, the hypothalamus (paraventricular nucleus, lateral hypothalamus), the midbrain periaqueductal gray matter, areas in the pons including the lateral tegmental area, and the raphe magnus. Electrical stimulation of these regions in humans (some cases) and in animals produces analgesia.

Fibers from these central structures descend directly or indirectly (e.g., periaqueductal gray matter to raphe magnus) via the dorsolateral funiculus to the spinal cord and send projections to laminae I and V.

Activation of the descending analgesic system has a direct effect on the integration and passage of nociceptive information at the level of the dorsal horn. Blockade of the dorsolateral funiculus (with cold or sectioning) increases the response of nociceptive neurons activated by painful stimuli. The descending system has three major components, which are functionally interrelated.

The **opioid system** is involved in descending analgesia. Opioid precursors (pro-opiomelanocortin, proenkephalin, and prodynorphin) and their respective peptides (beta-endorphin,

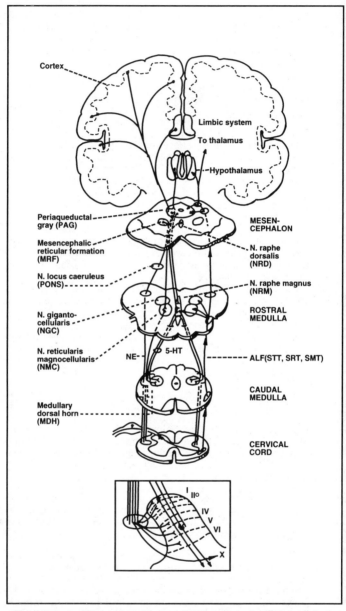

Fig. 2-3. Descending pain pathways. 5-HT = serotonin; NE = noradre-nergic input; ALF = anterolateral fasciculus; STT = spinothalamic tract; SRT = spinoreticular tract; SMT = spinomesencephalic tract. (Reproduced with permission from Bonica JJ, *The Management of Pain* (vol I). Philadelphia: Lea & Febiger, 1990. P. 108.

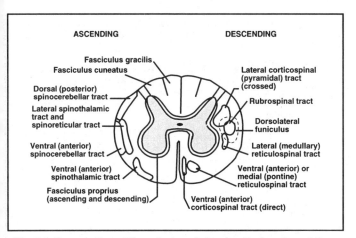

ASCENDING   DESCENDING

Fasciculus gracilis
Fasciculus cuneatus
Dorsal (posterior)
spinocerebellar tract
Lateral spinothalamic
tract and
spinoreticular tract
Ventral (anterior)
spinocerebellar tract
Ventral (anterior)
spinothalamic tract
Fasciculus proprius
(ascending and descending)

Lateral corticospinal
(pyramidal) tract
(crossed)
Rubrospinal tract
Dorsolateral
funiculus
Lateral (medullary)
reticulospinal tract
Ventral (anterior) or
medial (pontine)
reticulospinal tract
Ventral (anterior)
corticospinal tract (direct)

Fig. 2-4. Cross section of the spinal cord showing the location of the ascending (e.g., spinothalamic tract) pain pathways. The descending pain pathways are in the dorsolateral funiculus (not shown) of the spinal cord.

Met- and Leu-enkephalin, and prodynorphin) are present in the amygdala, the hypothalamus, the periaqueductal gray matter, the raphe magnus, and the dorsal horn. With the recent advent of opioid receptor cloning, knowledge is steadily increasing about the action sites of the various opioids (i.e., on mu, delta, and kappa receptors).

In the **noradrenergic system,** noradrenergic neurons project from the locus caeruleus and other noradrenergic cell groups in the medulla and pons. These projections are found in the dorsolateral funiculus. Stimulation of these areas produces analgesia, as does the administration (direct or intrathecal) of an alpha$_2$-receptor agonist such as clonidine.

In the **serotonergic (5-hydroxytryptamine [5-HT]) system**, many neurons in the raphe magnus are known to contain 5-HT, and they send projections to the spinal cord via the dorsolateral funiculus. Pharmacologic blockade, or lesioning, of the raphe magnus can reduce the effects of morphine and administration of 5-HT to the spinal cord produces analgesia.

"ON" AND "OFF" CELLS: A MODEL OF DESCENDING ANALGESIA

Neurons in the dorsal horn can be stimulated or inhibited by stimulation of the periaqueductal gray matter (PAG). Therefore a mechanism that describes facilitative and inhibitory descending controls is necessary to explain this observation (Fields, 1987). A model can be demonstrated in the raphe magnus, and in other areas known to be involved in descending modulation (e.g., PAG). Different types of neurons have been found in the raphe magnus, including "on" cells, "off" cells, and neutral cells.

"On" cells are active prior to a nocifensive withdrawal reflex (e.g., tailflick). These cells are stimulated by noxious stimuli; they are excited by stimulation and are inhibited by morphine. "On" cells facilitate nociceptive transmission in the dorsal horn.

"Off" cells shut off prior to a nocifensive withdrawal reflex. These cells are inhibited by noxious stimuli; they are excited by electrical stimulation and by morphine. It has been postulated that opioids act to inhibit inhibitory interneurons (GABAergic) that act on "off" cells and, in this way, produce a net excitatory effect on these cells. These cells inhibit nociceptive transmission in the dorsal horn.

"Neutral" cells do not respond to noxious stimuli.

PROJECTIONS TO THE DORSAL HORN

The nerve fibers that originate in nuclei that are involved in pain modulation terminate in the dorsal horn predominately in laminae I and II but also in other laminae, including IV, V, VI, and X. Thus there is a circuitry of projecting neurons acting directly or indirectly via interneurons on afferent fibers as well as projecting neurons such as the spinothalamic tract neurons.

Conclusions

The neuroanatomy of the pain system is extremely complex. Neuroanatomic techniques have taught us a great deal about the "connectivity" of the system. Newer techniques such as markers of neural activity (the immediate early gene c-*fos*) have enabled the study of populations of cells in the study of both ascending and descending systems. More recently, sophisticated imaging modalities have allowed us to demonstrate activity that is evoked by noxious stimuli in the whole brain and in chronic pain.

Selected Readings

Besson JM and Chaouch H. Peripheral and spinal mechanisms of pain. *Physio Rev* 67:67–184, 1987.

Bonica JJ. Anatomic and Physiologic Basis of Nociception and Pain. In: JJ Bonica (ed), *The Management of Pain* (2nd ed). Philadelphia: Lea & Febiger, 1990. Pp. 28–94.

Bonica JJ. Biochemistry and Modulation of Nociception and Pain. In JJ Bonica (ed), *The Management of Pain* (2nd ed). Philadelphia: Lea & Febiger, 1990. Pp. 95–121.

Coghill RC, et al. Distributed processing of pain and vibration by the human brain. *J Neurosci* 14:4095–4108, 1994.

Craig AD, et al. A thalamic nucleus specific for pain and temperature sensation. *Nature* 372:770–773, 1994.

Fields HL. *Pain*. New York: McGraw-Hill, 1987.

Giesler GJ Jr., Katter JT, and Dado RJ. Direct spinal pathways to the limbic system for nociceptive information. *Trends Neurosci* 17:244–250, 1994.

Hunt SP, Pini A, and Evan G. Induction of CFOs like protein in spinal cord neurons following sensory stimulation. *Nature* 328:632–634, 1987.

Levine JD, Fields HL, and Basbaum AI. Peptides and the primary afferent nociceptor. *J Neurosci* 13:2273–2286, 1993.

3

Assessment of Pain

Keith P. Kittelberger, Alyssa A. LeBel,
and David Borsook

> *"When you can measure what you
> are speaking about, and express it
> in numbers, you know something
> about it; but when you cannot
> express it in numbers, your
> knowledge is of a meager and
> unsatisfactory kind: it may be the
> beginning of knowledge, but you
> have scarcely, in your thoughts,
> advanced to the stage of science."*
>
> WILLIAM THOMPSON LORD KELVIN

Pain is the most common reason a patient seeks a physician. It is a complex, multidimensional symptom determined not only by tissue injury and nociception but also by personal beliefs, previous pain experience, the psyche, affect, motivation, environment, and pending litigation. **There is no objective measurement of pain**. This presents a problem for both the patient and the physician. How does the patient feel when a complaint of pain cannot be seen, defined, or felt by the physician? How are the true quality of pain, and its intensity, described?

The clinician is often asked to examine a patient whose diagnosis has been elusive and whose history may be ambiguous. Physical pathology may not be identifiable using current methods. These patients may have undergone extensive radiologic studies and even surgical intervention. The patient's motivation or effort may be questionable. Reports of pain may not correlate with the degree of disability or findings on physical examination. To our patients and their families, distress, suffering, and pain behaviors often are not distinguished from the pain itself. Pain is often viewed as a problem only when there is associated distress.

The assessment of pain requires a **complete history and comprehensive physical examination**. Important questions in obtaining a pain history address the location, intensity, timing, and quality of pain as well as ameliorating and exacerbating conditions.

An understanding of pain pathophysiology guides rational and appropriate treatment. Ongoing assessment to monitor the patient's progress and to modify therapy is necessary. It is essential to employ a systematic approach to the assessment of a patient who complains of pain.

Pain History

A complete and detailed pain history includes three main issues—intensity, location, and pathophysiology—that need to be elucidated. The following questions will help define these issues.

1. What is the time course of the pain?
2. Where is the pain?
3. What are the possible mechanisms of the pain?
4. What is the intensity of the pain?
5. What factors relieve or exacerbate the pain?

WHAT IS THE INTENSITY OF THE PAIN?

As stated above, pain cannot be objectively measured. The intensity of pain is one of the most difficult and perhaps frustrating characteristics of pain to pinpoint. Several tests and scales or scores have been developed to help measure pain. Assessing a single dimension such as intensity, however, will inevitably fail to capture the many qualities of pain and the pain experience. There are many competing instruments and scales to evaluate pain. Below are some of the more commonly used methods to measure pain.

Unidimensional Self-Report Scales

In practice, self-report scales serve as very simple, useful, and valid methods for assessing and monitoring a patient's painful condition.

Verbal Descriptor Scales

The patient is asked to describe his or her pain by choosing from a list of adjectives that reflect gradations of pain intensity. The five-word scale consists of mild, discomforting, distressing, horrible, and excruciating. Disadvantages of this scale include limited selection and the fact that patients tend to select moderate descriptors, rather than the extremes.

Numeric Rating Scale (NRS)

This is the most simple and frequently used scale to evaluate pain. On a scale of 0 to 10, with 0 being "no pain" and 10 "the worst pain imaginable," the patient picks a number to describe the pain. Advantages of this scale are its simplicity, reproducibility, and the facts that it is easily understood by the patient and that small changes in pain can be indicated. A major disadvantage is that it does not provide a good reflection of either psychologic or physical disruption caused by a specific disorder.

Visual Analog Scale (VAS)

This is very similar to the NRS, except that the patient marks on a 10-cm line, one end of which is labeled "no pain" and the other end "worst pain imaginable," where the pain falls. The advantages and disadvantages are the same as those of the NRS.

Faces Pain Rating Scale

Evaluating pain in children can be very difficult because of the child's inability to describe pain or understand pain assessment forms. This scale depicts five sketches of facial features, each with a numeric value, ranging from a happy, smiling face to a sad, teary face. To extrapolate this scale to the VAS, multiply the value chosen by two. This scale may also be beneficial for mentally impaired patients.

Multiple Dimension Instruments

These instruments provide much more information about the patient's pain than just intensity. They are especially useful in complaints of complex pain. As such, they are more difficult and time-consuming and reserved for the outpatient and research setting.

McGill Pain Questionnaire (MPQ)

This is the most frequently used multidimensional test. Descriptive words from three major dimensions of pain (sensory, affective, and evaluative) are further subdivided into 20 subclasses, each containing words of varying degrees. Three scores are obtained, one for each dimension, as well as a total score. Studies have shown the MPQ to be a reliable instrument in clinical research.

Brief Pain Inventory (BPI)

In this inventory patients are asked to rate the severity of their pain at its "worst," "least," or "average," and at the time the rating is made. It also asks patients to represent the location of their pain on a schematic diagram of the body. The BPI correlates with scores of activity, sleep, and social interactions. It is cross-cultural and a useful method for performing studies (Fig. 3-1).

The Massachusetts General Hospital (MGH) Pain Center's Pain Assessment Form

This form (Fig. 3.2) combines many of the above assessment instruments and is given to all patients on initial consultation at the MGH Pain Center. It elicits information about pain, its location (body diagram), quality of pain, therapies tried, and past and present medications. It takes 10 to 15 minutes to fill out and is an extremely valuable assessment. Disadvantages are the same as for other multidimensional instruments.

Pain Diary

A diary of a patient's pain is useful in evaluting the relationship between pain and daily activity. Pain is described using the NRS, from 0 to 10, during activities such as walking, standing, sitting, and chores. Blocks of time are usually hourly. Medication use, alcohol use, emotional responses, and family response may also be helpful information to record. Pain diaries may reflect a patient's pain more accurately,

STUDY ID# ________ HOSPITAL# ____________

DO NOT WRITE ABOVE THIS LINE

Brief Pain Inventory (Short Form)

Date: __/__/__ Time: ________

Name: ____________ ____________ ____________
Last First Middle Initial

1) Throughout our lives, most of us have had pain from time to time (such as minor headaches, sprains, and toothaches). Have you had pain other than these everyday kinds of pain today?

1. Yes 2. No

2) On the diagram, shade in the areas where you feel pain. Put an X on the area that hurts the most.

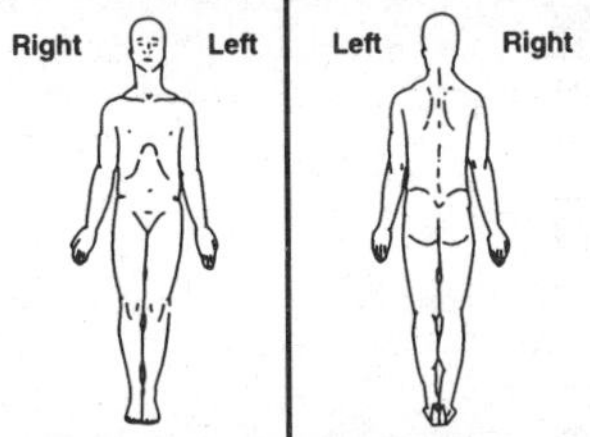

3) Please rate your pain by circling the one number that best describes your pain at its worst in the last 24 hours.

0	1	2	3	4	5	6	7	8	9	10
No Pain										Pain as bad as you can imagine

4) Please rate your pain by circling the one number that best describes your pain at its least in the last 24 hours.

0	1	2	3	4	5	6	7	8	9	10
No Pain										Pain as bad as you can imagine

5) Please rate your pain by circling the one number that best describes your pain on the average.

0	1	2	3	4	5	6	7	8	9	10
No Pain										Pain as bad as you can imagine

6) Please rate your pain by circling the one number that tells how much pain you have right now.

0	1	2	3	4	5	6	7	8	9	10
No Pain										Pain as bad as you can imagine

Fig. 3-1. Brief pain inventory (see text). Reprinted with permission from the University of Wisconsin-Madison, Department of Neurology, Pain Research Group.

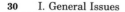

7) What treatments or medications are you receiving for your pain?

8) In the last 24 hours, how much relief have pain treatments or medications provided? Please circle the one percentage that most shows how much relief you have received.

0%	10%	20%	30%	40%	50%	60%	70%	80%	90%	100%
No Relief										Complete Relief

9) Circle the one number that describes how, during the past 24 hours, pain has interfered with your:

A. General activity

0	1	2	3	4	5	6	7	8	9	10
Does not interfere										Completely Interferes

B. Mood

0	1	2	3	4	5	6	7	8	9	10
Does not interfere										Completely Interferes

C. Walking ability

0	1	2	3	4	5	6	7	8	9	10
Does not interfere										Completely Interferes

D. Normal work (includes both work outside the home and housework)

0	1	2	3	4	5	6	7	8	9	10
Does not interfere										Completely Interferes

E. Relations with other people

0	1	2	3	4	5	6	7	8	9	10
Does not interfere										Completely Interferes

F. Sleep

0	1	2	3	4	5	6	7	8	9	10
Does not interfere										Completely Interferes

G. Enjoyment of life

0	1	2	3	4	5	6	7	8	9	10
Does not interfere										Completely Interferes

Pain Research Group • Department of Neurology • University of Wisconsin-Madison

Fig. 3-1. (continued)

compared to a retrospective description that may significantly over- or underestimate pain.

WHERE IS THE PAIN?

The **location** and **distribution** of pain are extremely important characteristics that help in understanding the pathophysiology of the pain complaint. Body diagrams, found in some of the assessment instruments, can prove very useful. Not only can the clinician view the patient's perception of the topographic area of pain, but the patient may show distress

M.G.H. PAIN CENTER
PAIN ASSESSMENT FORM

Information About the Pain

1. What is the problem you would like us to help you with?

2. Please mark the event or events that led to your present pain: (If you experience more than one kind of pain, please write in separate sets of answers for each type of pain you have.)

___ Accident   ___ Cancer

___ Other injury _____   ___ No obvious cause

___ Following an operation   ___ Other disease _____

___ Other _____

3. For how long have you had this pain?

4. How often does the pain occur?
___ Continuously (nonstop)

___ Several times a day

___ Once or twice a day

___ Several times a week

___ Less than 3 or 4 times per month

5. How has the *intensity* of the pain changed throughout the time you have had it?

___ Increased ___ Decreased ___ Stayed the same

6. The following five words represent pain of increasing intensity:

1	2	3
Mild	Discomforting	Distressing

4	5
Horrible	Excruciating

To answer each question below, write the *number* of the most appropriate word in the space beside the question.

a. Which word describes your pain at its worst? ___
b. Which word describes your pain at its least? ___
c. Which word describes your pain right now? ___
d. Which word describes how your pain is most of the time? ___

7. Location of the Pain
(please shadow in the affected areas).

8. Quality of the Pain

Below is list of words that are often used to describe pain. After each descriptive word, indicate with a checkmark whether this word describes a particular quality of your pain and, if it does, the intensity of that quality.

	None (not at all)	Mild	Moderate	Severe
Throbbing	0)	1)	2)	3)
Shooting	0)	1)	2)	3)
Stabbing	0)	1)	2)	3)
Sharp	0)	1)	2)	3)
Cramping	0)	1)	2)	3)
Gnawing	0)	1)	2)	3)
Hot-Burning	0)	1)	2)	3)
Aching	0)	1)	2)	3)
Heavy	0)	1)	2)	3)
Tender	0)	1)	2)	3)
Splitting	0)	1)	2)	3)
Tiring/Exhausting	0)	1)	2)	3)
Sickening	0)	1)	2)	3)
Fearful	0)	1)	2)	3)
Punishing/Cruel	0)	1)	2)	3)

9. Which of the following have an effect on your pain? Please indicate whether it makes the pain better, worse, or has *no effect.*

___ Heat ___ Cold ___ Noise
___ Sitting ___ Standing ___ Lying down
___ Walking ___ Fatigue ___ Particular position
___ Coughing ___ Anxiety/emotions   or movement
___ Vibration ___ Massage/rubbing   explain: _____
___ Climate ___ Alcoholic beverages ___ Caffeinated drinks (coffee, tea, colas)

10. How does the pain affect your activity in these different areas:
Work-school–
Household chores–
Social interactions–
Leisure–
Sexual activity–

11. What is your current employment status?

12. Do you have pending a settlement about disability, workers' compensation, or a legal matter?

___ yes ___ no

If yes, briefly explain: _____

13. What treatments have you tried for your pain?

___ Surgery ___ TENS unit
___ Nerve block ___ Exercise program
___ Brace ___ Trigger point injection
___ Physical therapy ___ Acupuncture
___ Relaxation training ___ Chiropractic therapy
___ Biofeedback ___ Psychotherapy/counseling
Other _____ ___ Hypnosis
___ Massage

14. What specialists have you seen for your pain (e.g., orthopedic surgeon, neurologist, neurosurgeon, psychiatrist)?

15. Pain Medications and Other Treatments

A. What are the medications you are currently taking for pain?

	Drug	Dose	Frequency
1.			
2.			
3.			
4.			

B. What other medications have you taken in the past for pain?

	Drug	Effect on Pain
1.		
2.		
3.		
4.		

Fig. 3-2. The Massachusetts General Hospital (MGH) Pain Center's pain assessment form.

C. Are you allergic to any medications (including local anesthetics)?

          Drug   *Type of Reaction*

D. What other medications are you currently taking?

16. Name, address, and phone number of your primary care physician:

17. Name, address, and phone number of the physician who referred you to us:

Fig. 3-2. (continued)

through poorly localizing the pain or magnifying the pain to other areas of the body.

Is the pain localized or referred? Localized pain is pain confined to its site of origin without radiation or migration. Referred pain usually arises from visceral or deep structures and radiates to other areas of the body. A classic example of referred pain is shoulder pain from phrenic nerve irritation, such as with liver metastases from pancreatic cancer (Table 3-1).

Is the pain superficial/peripheral or visceral? Superficial pain, arising from tissues rich in nociceptors such as skin, teeth, and mucous membranes, is easily localized and limited to that part of the body the nerve innervates. Visceral pain arises from viscera, which contain relatively few nociceptors. The pain is diffuse and often poorly localized. In addition, it has a significant autonomic component.

WHAT IS THE PATHOPHYSIOLOGY OF THE PAIN?

By taking a complete history and answering the above two questions, the clinician can begin to formulate the etiology of the pain complaint. By doing so, the rest of the history, as well as the physical examination, can be tailored to systematically explore aspects of pain, such as symptoms and physical signs, common to the particular pain in question.

Types of Pain (Definitions)

nociceptive—pain arising from activation of nociceptors; nociceptors are found in all tissues except the CNS. The pain is clinically proportionate to the degree of chemical, thermal, or mechanical activation of afferent nerve fibers in the skin or viscera and can be acute or chronic (somatic, cancer pain, postoperative pain).

Table 3-1. Examples of referred pain

Origin of pain	Region of pain referral
Head (dura mater or vessels)	
Anterior cranial fossa	Ipsilateral forehead
Middle cranial fossa	Ipsilateral supraorbital region, temples
Posterior cranial fossa	Ipsilateral ear, postauricular region, occiput
Pharynx	Ipsilateral ear
Chest	
Esophagus	Substernal region
Heart	Left arm, epigastric
Abdomen	
Visceral pain	Segmental muscle spasms
Cholecystitis	Upper abdominal muscles
Appendicitis	Lower abdominal muscles
Renal colic	L2–L3 segments
Subphrenic region	Shoulder pain
Liver	Right phrenic region
Kidney	Lower thorax and back
Ureter	
Upper (renal pelvis)	Groin, testis or ovary
Terminal	Scrotum/labia
Pelvis	
Prostate	Lower back
Uterus	Lower back
Ovary	Anterior thigh
Lower extremity	
Peroneal entrapment at fibula	Dorsum of foot
Other	
Unilateral cordotomy	Pain applied to analgesic side produces pain in symmetrical contralateral body part

Adapted from Brass LM and Stys K. *Handbook of Neurological Lists*. New York: Churchill Livingstone, 1991.

neuropathic—pain arising from injury to peripheral or central pain pathways. The pain persists without ongoing disease (i.e., diabetic neuropathy).

causalgia, reflex sympathetic dystrophy, or sympathetically maintained pain—pain arising from a peripheral nerve lesion and often associated with allodynia, hyperpathia, burning, and vasomotor changes and evidence of sympathetic hyperfunction including sweating.

deafferentation—chronic pain resulting from loss of afferent input to the CNS pain pathways (peripheral or central) (i.e., nerve avulsion or spinal cord lesions).

neuralgia—lancinating pain associated with nerve damage or irritation in the distribution of a nerve (i.e., trigeminal neuralgia).

radiculopathy—pain arising from compression or disruption of nerve root (i.e., disk disease).

central—pain arising from a lesion in the CNS usually involving the spinothalamic cortical pathways (i.e., thalamic infarct).

psychogenic—pain inconsistent with the anatomic distribution of the nervous system. It is often extensively evaluated with no organic pathology to account for the pain.

Pain of Central Origin

Central pain arises from lesions, often traumatic or vascular, in or near pain transmission pathways. The pain is usually constant, with a burning, electrical quality, and is exacerbated by activity or changes in the weather. Hyperesthesia and hyperpathia and/or allodynia are invariably present. Therapy can be unsuccessful.

Referred Pain

Referred pain (see Table 3-1) is pain that most often originates from a visceral organ. It may be felt in body regions remote from the site of pathology. The mechanism of such pain may be the spinal convergence of visceral and somatic afferent fibers on spinothalamic neurons. Common manifestations are both cutaneous and deep hyperalgesia, autonomic hyperactivity, tenderness, and muscular contractions.

Examining the Patient

A complete examination is required, including a general physical examination followed by neurologic, musculoskeletal, and mental status assessments. It is important not to limit the examination to just the painful location and surrounding tissues and structures.

GENERAL PHYSICAL EXAMINATION

This physical consists of the usual head-to-toe examination described in detail in numerous medical texts. Important points to note are:

1. Appearance—obese, emaciated, distressed, flat affect
2. Posture—splinting, scoliosis, kyphosis
3. Gait—limp, use of antalgic or assistance devices
4. Expression—pain, tension, diaphoresis, anxiety
5. Vital signs—sympathetic overactivity (tachycardia, hypertension), temperature discrepancies (hot or cold areas)

It is important to watch how a patient undresses. Favoring an extremity or protection of part of the body may not be appreciated unless this is done. This is regularly overlooked by the clincian for fear of invading the patient's privacy.

EVALUATION OF THE PAIN

Following the general examination, the clinician evaluates the painful area(s) of the body. It is important to look for findings that correlate the physical examination with the history.

Inspection of overlying skin may reveal changes in color, flushing, edema, hair loss, presence or absence of sweat, atrophy, or muscle spasm. Inspection of nails may reveal changes commonly seen with sympathetically maintained pain/reflex sympathetic dystrophy. A damaged nerve root may be associated with goose flesh (cutis anserina) in the dermatone.

Palpation allows mapping of the painful area and detection of any change in pain intensity within the area, as well as during the examination, and reveals the presence or absence of any of the aforementioned definitions and any trigger points. How the patient responds both verbally and nonverbally is important. Is the response appropriate for the level of pain? Is the patient overreacting? Does the patient's affect correlate? Factors that reproduce, worsen, or decrease the pain are sought.

NEUROLOGIC EXAMINATION

Subtle physical findings are often found only during the neurologic examination (Table 3-2). It is imperative that this part of the examination not be overlooked. A neurologic examination can be performed in 5 to 10 minutes.

Mental function is assessed by evaluating the patient's orientation to person, place, and time, short- and long-term memory, choice of words used to describe symptoms and answer questions, and educational background.

Evaluation of the cranial nerves is an absolute necessity, especially in patients complaining of head, neck, and shoulder pain symptoms. Table 3-2 lists the functioning of each cranial nerve.

Spinal nerve evaluation can also be done quickly. Spinal nerve sensation is determined by the use of cotton or tissue paper for light touch, and pinprick for proprioception and deep sensation. There is always sensory abnormality in neu-

Table 3-2. Neurological examination of cranial nerves

Cranial nerves	Function
I—Olfactory nerve	Smell
II—Optic	Vision
III—Oculomotor	
Parasympathetic	Sphincter muscle of iris, ciliary muscle
Motor	Superior, inferior, and medial recti muscles; inferior oblique and levator palpebrae superioris muscle
IV—Trochlear	Superior oblique
V—Trigeminal	
Motor	Muscles of mastication
Sensory	Face, mucosa of nose, mouth, dura, and cornea
VI—Abducens	Lateral rectus muscle
VII—Facial	
Motor	Muscles of expression
Parasympathetic	Lacrimal gland, salivary glands and mucous membranes of mouth
Sensory	Sensation to parts of external ear, auditory canal, and tympanic membrane
	Taste to anterior two thirds of tongue
VIII—Vestibulocochlear	Equilibrium and hearing
IX—Glossopharyngeal	
Parasympathetic	Parotid gland
Motor	Stylopharyngeal muscle
Sensory	Sensation to posterior one third of tongue, pharynx, middle ear, and dura
X—Vagus	
Parasympathetic	Viscera of thorax and abdomen
Motor	Muscles of pharynx and larynx
Sensory somatic	Dura and auditory canal
Sensory visceral	Viscera of thorax and abdomen
XI—Accessory	
Motor	Muscles of larynx and sternocleidomastoid and trapezius
XII—Hypoglossal	Intrinsic muscles of tongue, genioglossus, hypoglossus, and styloglossus

ropathic pain. A differential diagnosis of peripheral neuropathies is given in Table 3-3. Spinal nerve motor function is determined by deep tendon reflexes, the presence or absence of the Babinski reflex, and tests of muscle strength.

Coordination is assessed by testing balance, rapid hand movement, finger-to-nose motion, toe-to-heel motion, gait, and Romberg's test. Cerebellar dysfunction can often be detected during these maneuvers. Table 3-4 lists pain disturbances due to various disease processes that can affect gait.

Pain of psychogenic origin will usually result in a neurologic examination that does not correlate with findings typical of organic pathology. Abnormal pain distributions, such as glove or stocking patterns, are common. Table 3-5 lists common painful root syndromes.

Table 3-3. Painful sensory neuropathies

Endocrinologic
Diabetes mellitus
Hypothyroidism

Metabolic
Uremia
Thiamine deficiency
Acute intermittent porphyria

Toxic
Vincristine
Acrylamide
Heavy metals
Organic solvents

Infectious/inflammatory
HIV-related painful neuropathies
Herpes zoster—acute and chronic postherpetic neuralgia
Guillain-Barré syndrome
Chronic inflammatory polyneuropathy

Immunologic
Polyarteritis nodosa
Cryoglobulinemia
Systemic lupus erythematosus

Physical
Brachial plexopathies
Compressive

Neoplastic
Multiple myeloma
Cancer (including nonmetastatic effects and carcinomatosis)

Genetic
Fabry's Disease
Tangier disease
Familial dysautonomias (Riley-Day syndrome, inherited sensory
  neuropathy III)
Amyloidosis

Table 3-4. Pain-induced disturbances of gait

Diagnosis	Symptoms
Intermittent claudication, arterial insufficiency	Pain on walking a specific distance Pain sooner with increasing intensity of work Pain disappears after rest Pain localized to calf
Cauda equina (neurogenic claudication, spinal stenosis)	Pain on walking after varying distances Patient usually elderly Usually bilateral Radicular in character Pain localized to saddle area, upper thigh, and calf Pain in back on sneezing Pain does not usually disappear on cessation of walking Pain improved when leaning forward
Hip disease	Pain worse on first few steps
Inguinal region	Pain increased on prolonged standing Usually status post appendectomy, hernia repair
Meralgia paresthetica	Pain in the lateral aspect of the thigh
Long bones	Localized pain Evidence of tumor/osteoporosis, Paget's disease, pathologic fracture Status post surgical procedure—anterior compartment syndrome

Feet
  Foot deformities
  Calcaneal spur
  Achilles' tendinitis
	Pain after walking or standing

Tarsal tunnel syndrome	Pain in the plantar aspect of foot (prevents walking)

Adapted from Mumenthaler M. *Neurologic Differential Diagnosis.* New York: Thieme-Stratton, 1925. Pp. 118–119.

Table 3-5. Common painful root syndromes

Root	Sensory loss	Motor changes	
		Weakness	Decreased deep tendon reflexes
Upper extremity			
C5	Lateral aspect of upper arm	Deltoid and biceps	None/biceps
C6	Thumb and index finger	Biceps and brachioradialis	Brachioradialis and biceps
C7	Middle finger	Triceps and pronator teres	Triceps
Lower extremity			
L4	Medial calf	Quadriceps	Knee
L5	Medial half of foot and lateral calf	Peroneal, anterior and posterior tibial and toe extension	Internal hamstring
S1	Lower posterior calf and lateral foot	Plantar flexion	Ankle

MUSCULOSKELETAL EXAMINATION

Abnormalities of the musculoskeletal system are often evident on inspection of the patient's posture and muscular symmetry. Muscular atrophy indicates disuse. Flaccidity indicates extreme weakness, usually from paralysis, and abnormal movements indicate neurologic damage or impaired proprioception. Limited range of motion of a major joint can indicate pain, disk disease, or arthritis. Palpation of muscles will help in evaluating range of motion and whether or not trigger points are present. Coordination and strength are tested as well.

SENSORY EXAMINATION

The following are some definitions of physical findings on sensory examination.

analgesia—absence of pain to a painful stimulus
anesthesia—absence of all sensation
allodynia—pain due to a nonpainful stimulus
dysesthesia—unpleasant, abnormal sensation
hyperesthesia—increased sensitivity to stimulus
hypoesthesia—decreased sensitivity to stimulus
hyperalgesia—increased sensation to painful stimulus
hypoalgesia—decreased sensation to painful stimulus
hyperpathia—increased response to repetitive, nonpainful stimulus
pain threshold—minimal stimulus eliciting pain
pain tolerance—maximal pain level the patient can tolerate

Psychology of Pain

Complete assessment of pain includes analysis of the psychological aspects of pain and the effects of pain on behavior and emotional stability. Such assessment is challenging, because many patients are unaware of or reluctant to present psychological issues. It is also more socially acceptable to seek medical rather than psychiatric care. (See also Chap. 24 on Psychosocial Consequences of Pain.)

Initially, the use of a descriptive pain questionnaire, such as the McGill Pain Questionnaire (see IASP Classification of Pain Appendix), may provide some evidence of a patient's affective responses to pain. For example, whereas words such as "aching" and "tingling" refer to sensory aspects of pain, words such as "agonizing" and "dreadful" suggest negative feelings and do not aid in characterizing the pain sensation.

A patient's personality greatly influences his or her response to pain and choice of coping strategy. Some patients may benefit from the use of strategies of control, such as distraction and relaxation. Patients who have an underlying anxiety may be more likely to seek high doses of analgesics. Therefore, inquiry regarding a patient's history of coping with stress is often useful.

As part of the pain history, the clinician should include questions about some of the common symptoms in patients with chronic pain: **depressed mood, sleep disturbance, preoccupation with somatic symptoms, reduced activity, reduced libido, and fatigue**. Standardized questionnaires, such as the Minnesota Multiphasic Personality Inventory (MMPI), may expand the assessment. On this inventory, patients with chronic pain may score very high on the depression, hysteria, and hypochondriasis scales. However, the MMPI may reflect functional limitation secondary to pain as well as psychological abnormality associated with chronic pain, limiting its interpretation for some patients suspected of having psychogenic pain.

A number of psychologic processes and syndromes predispose patients to chronic pain. These disorders are more fully described in Chap. 24. Briefly, these factors are major depression, somatization disorder, conversion disorder, hypochondriasis, and psychogenic pain disorder. Of note regarding assessment of pain, the diagnosis of somatization disorder is quite specific, although many patients with chronic pain may "somatize" (focus on somatic complaints) to the exclusion of psychologic factors. Somatization disorder requires a history of physical symptoms of several years' duration, beginning before the age of 30 years and including complaints of at least 14 specific symptoms for women and 12 for men. These symptoms are not adequately explained by physical disorder, injury, or toxic reaction.

Psychogenic pain—pain not elicited by noxious stimuli and not due to an abnormality in the pain transmission system—may occur in susceptible individuals. In some patients, pain may ameliorate more unpleasant feelings, such as depression, guilt, or anxiety, and distract the patient from environmental stress factors. Historic features that suggest a psychogenic component to chronic pain include **multiple locations of pain at different times; pain problems dating since adolescence; pain without obvious somatic cause (especially in the facial or perineal area); multiple, elective surgical procedures; substance abuse (patient and/or significant other); and social or work failure.**

Psychogenic pain is distinguished from malingering. Malingerers have an obvious, identifiable environmental goal in producing symptoms, such as evading police, avoiding work, or obtaining financial compensation. Patients with psychogenic pain make illness and hospitalization their primary goals. Being a patient is their primary way of life. Such patients are unable to stop symptom production when it is no longer obviously profitable.

The **physical examination** in patients with psychological factors exacerbating pain may be perplexing. Some findings may not correspond to known anatomic or physiologic information. Examples of such findings include give-away weakness of muscles; manual testing inconsistent with patient observation during sitting, turning, and dressing; grasping with three fingers; antagonist muscle contraction on attempted movement; decreased tremor during mental arithmetic exercises; a positive Romberg's sign with one eye closed; vibration absent on one side of midline (skull, sternum) inconsistency of timed vibration when affected side is tested first; patterned miscount of touches; difficulty touching the good limb with the bad; and a slight difference in sensation on one side of the body. Useful neurologic signs are deep-tendon reflexes, motor tone and bulk, and the plantar response. Observation is critical. Pain drawings at multiple time intervals are also useful in following up on a patient with chronic pain of unclear etiology.

Diagnostic Studies

The diagnosis and understanding of a patient's pain complaint can usually be obtained after a thorough history and physical examination. Diagnostic studies are used to confirm a clinician's suspicion, as well as to assist in the diagnosis. Some of the more common studies used for pain assessment are described below.

Conventional radiography is used to diagnose bony abnormalities, such as pathologic fractures seen in bony metastases, spine pathology like spondylolisthesis and spur formation, and bone tumors. Some soft-tissue tumors and bowel abnormalities can also be seen. X-rays of the painful area have usually been obtained by the referring physician.

A **CT scan** is most often used to define bony abnormalities, and **MRI** for soft-tissue pathology. Spinal stenosis, disk herniation or bulge, nerve root compression, and tumors in all tissues can be diagnosed, as well as some causes of central pain, such as CNS infarcts.

Thermography is a noninvasive way of looking at the body's thermal patterns. A normal thermal pattern is symmetric, from one side of the body to the other. Tissue pathology is associated with chemical and metabolic changes that can cause abnormal thermal patterns by altering vascularity. Certain pain syndromes, such as neuropathic, musculoskeletal, vascular, visceral, and cancer disorders, have a specific thermal pattern and can thus be diagnosed thermographically. Sympathetic dysfunction, as in reflex sympathetic dystrophy, is easily diagnosed by thermography, although the authors have not found it to be useful in the evaluation of patients with pain.

Myelography is the injection of radiopaque dye into the subarachnoid space to visualize spinal cord/column abnormalities radiographically, such as disk herniation, nerve root impingement, and spinal stenosis. Major disadvantages of this procedure are postdural-puncture headache and meningeal irritation.

Electromyography is the examination of skeletal muscle by the use of needle electrodes. Abnormal muscle activity, both at rest and with movement, indicates instability of muscle membranes, denervation, muscle disease, or alterations in the motor unit.

Nerve conduction studies are examinations of conduction of peripheral motor and sensory nerves by external stimulation. Myelinated nerve fibers, which are the larger and faster conducting fibers, are most often studied. Abnormalities in conduction are seen with myelin disorders, nerve trauma, nerve disease, and metabolic disorders.

Bone scanning is the use of a radioactive compound to detect a number of bone lesions, including neoplastic, infectious, arthritic, traumatic, Paget's, and reflex sympathetic dystrophy. The radioactive compound accumulates in areas of increased bone growth or turnover. It is a very sensitive test for subtle bone abnormalities that may not show up on conventional radiographs.

Single-unit nerve studies are performed in only a few centers but can define abnormalities of specific fiber types (i.e., C-fiber activity that cannot be defined using conventional nerve conduction studies).

Functional brain imaging such as positron emission tomography and functional-MRI is still experimental but may become useful in the future for the evaluation of patients with pain.

Diagnostic blocks (see also Chap. 9). Diagnostic blocks may differentiate somatic from visceral pain and confirm the anatomic location of peripheral nerve pain and also define possible therapeutic approaches (e.g., the use of neuropathic medications or sympatholytic medications).

Thermal sensory testing. Various machines are now available that can measure the response to heat and cold pain, and determine noxious thresholds to hot and cold stimuli. Although currently at an experimental stage, these analyzers should become more frequently used in the near future as standards for assessing C- and A-delta fiber responses are obtained.

Conclusions

The assessment of pain can be very difficult, frustrating, and time-consuming. It is important to treat the patient as a whole, and not just the painful location. Believing the patient and establishing rapport are of the utmost importance. A systematic approach, as discussed in this chapter, will assist the clinician in determining the pathophysiology of the patient's pain complaint. With this knowledge, a therapeutic modality can be formulated and initiated.

Selected Readings

Beecher HK. *Measurement of Subjective Responses*. New York: Oxford University Press, 1959.

Boivie J, Hansson P, Lindblom U. Touch, temperature, and pain in health and disease: Mechanisms and assessments. Progress in Pain Research and Management. *Int J Assoc Pain* 3:1993.

Carlsson AM. Assessment of chronic pain I: Aspects of the reliability and validity of the visual analogue scale. *Pain* 16:87–101, 1983.

Gracely RH. Evaluation of multidimensional pain scales. *Pain* 48:297–300, 1992.

Katz J. Psychophysical correlates of phantom limb experience. *J Neurol Neurosurg Psychiatry* 55:811–821, 1992.

Lowe NK, Walker SN, and McCallum RC. Confirming the theoretical structure of the McGill pain questionaire in acute clinical pain. *Pain* 46:53–60, 1991.

McGrath PA. *Pain in children: Nature, Assessment and Treatment*. New York: Guilford Press, 1990.

Melzack R. The McGill questionaire: Major properties and scoring methods. *Pain* 1:277–299, 1975.

Melzack R and Katz J. Pain measurement in persons in pain. In: Wall PD and Melzack R (eds). *Textbook of Pain* (3rd ed.). New York: Churchill Livingstone, 1994.

Price DD, et al. A comparison of pain measurement characteristics of mechanical visual analogue and simple numerical rating scales. *Pain* 56:217–226, 1994.

II

Therapeutic Options

4

Choosing a Therapeutic Approach: Opioids

Janet C. Hsieh and Daniel B. Carr

> *". . . there is none more efficacious
> than opium."*
> THOMAS SYDENHAM

Because of their unrivaled ability to relieve pain, opioids are important in the clinician's choice of a therapeutic approach to pain management. Morphine, named after Morpheus, the Greek god of dreams, and prepared from the juice of the unripe seed capsule of the opium poppy (*Papaver somniferum*), was the first opioid used for analgesia.

Opioids are of three functional types: (1) morphine-like opioid agonists (acting primarily at mu and perhaps kappa and delta receptors), (2) opioid antagonists (devoid of agonist activity at any receptor), and (3) opioids with mixed or partial actions, including the agonist-antagonists and partial agonists.

Definitions

An **Opiate** is a drug derived from opium, including morphine, codeine, and the many semisynthetic morphine congeners.

An **Opioid** is any group of drugs, natural or synthetic, that possesses morphine-like properties.

The term **narcotic** is becoming obsolete because it has legal and regulatory meaning that applies not only to morphine-like drugs but also to any substance that can cause dependence.

Endogenous Opioids

Each of the three families of opioid neuropeptides—enkephalins, endorphins, and dynorphins—are derived from a distinct precursor polypeptide and have distinct anatomic distributions. Like peptide hormones, all three opioid precursors are biologically inactive and generate active agents only after enzymatic cleavage. In addition to the above peptides, it now appears that morphine and related morphinans occur naturally in mammalian tissues, possibly originating in intestinal flora.

Classification of Opioids

Opioid compounds are classified as naturally occurring, semisynthetic, or synthetic. Morphine, codeine, and papaverine

Table 4-1. Classification of opioid compounds

Naturally occurring
Morphine
Codeine
Papaverine
Thebaine (e.g., oxycodone, oxymorphone)

Semisynthetic
Heroin
Dihydromorphone/morphinone
Thebaine derivatives (e.g., buprenorphine)

Synthetic
Morphinan series (e.g., levorphanol, butorphanol)
Diphenylpropylamine series (e.g., methadone)
Benzomorphinan series (e.g., pentazocine)
Phenylpiperidine series (e.g., meperidine, fentanyl, sufentanil, alfentanil)

Source: Bailey P and Stanley T. Narcotic Intravenous Anesthetics. In: R (ed), *Anesthesia.* New York: Churchill-Livingstone, 1990. Pp. 281–366. Use permission.

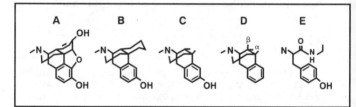

Fig. 4-1. Structure of morphine-like opioids. (A) Morphine, (B) morphinan, (C) benzomorphan, (D) phenylpiperidine, (E) tyramine moeity of endogenous opioids. Note the progressive removal of ring structures—five-ring morphine to 2-ring phenylpiperidine. (Reproduced with permission from Carr DB. Opioids. *Int Anesthesiol Clin* 26:273, 1988.)

are the only natural opioids of clinical importance. Semisynthetic drugs are derivatives of morphine. The synthetic agents resemble morphine but are entirely man-made (Table 4-1). If morphine's starting five-ring alkaloid structure is reduced to four rings, "morphinans" are produced; to three rings, "benzomorphans"; and to two rings, "phenylpiperidines" (Fig. 4-1).

Mechanism of Action

Firm evidence for specific opiate receptors in the central and peripheral nervous systems exists. Table 4-2 lists characteristics of opioid receptors.

Table 4-2. Characteristics of opioid receptors

Receptor	Tissue bioassay	Agonists	Major actions
Mu			
Mu$_1$	Guinea pig ileum	Morphine Meptazinol Phenylpiperidines	Supraspinal analgesia Bradycardia Sedation
Mu$_2$	Guinea pig ileum	Morphine Phenylpiperidines	Respiratory depression Euphoria Physical dependence
Delta	Mouse vas deferens	d-Ala-d-Leu Enkephalin	Spinal analgesia (weak) Respiratory depression
Kappa	Rabbit vas deferens	Ketocyclazocine Dynorphin Nalbuphine Butorphanol	Spinal analgesia (weak) Respiratory depression Sedation Inhibits antidiuretic hormone
Sigma		SKF 10,047 Pentazocine	Dysphoria-delirium, mydriasis Hallucinations Tachycardia Hypertension

Source: Modified from Bailey P and Stanley T. Narcotic Intravenous Anesthetics. In: R Miller (ed), *Anesthesia.* New York: Churchill-Livingstone, 1990. Pp. 281–366.

MU (FOR MORPHINE) RECEPTORS

It is likely that morphine and other morphine-like opioids produce analgesia primarily through interaction with mu receptors. These receptors are present in high concentrations in the midbrain periaqueductal gray matter and the substantia gelatinosa of the spinal cord. Two distinct subtypes of mu receptors are postulated: mu_1 (higher affinity) receptors are thought to mediate supraspinal analgesia, bradycardia, and sedation; mu_2 (lower affinity) receptors are involved in respiratory depression, physical dependence, and euphoria.

KAPPA (FOR KETOCYCLAZOCINE) RECEPTORS

Kappa receptors, which are prevalent in the spinal cord, cause less intense miosis and respiratory depression than do mu receptors. Also, instead of euphoria, kappa agonists can produce dysphoric, psychotomimetic effects.

SIGMA (FOR SKF-10,047, N-ALLYLMETAZOCINE) RECEPTORS

Certain opioid drugs such as pentazocine produce psychotomimetic effects in humans. Although these effects were initially attributed to sigma receptors, the status of these sites is not certain. The sigma receptor may not truly be an opioid receptor, since actions mediated by it are not reversed by naloxone. Evidence suggests that it is also the receptor for phenylcyclidine (also known as PCP or angel dust).

DELTA (FOR DEFERENS) RECEPTORS

These receptors are thought to be preferred by enkephalin. Although spinal analgesic and respiratory depressive effects are proposed, the consequences of stimulating delta receptors in humans are uncertain because of the lack of selective agonists.

EPSILON RECEPTORS

This receptor is postulated as a specific receptor for beta-endorphins, which have been implicated as neuromodulators and which have a role in stress-induced alterations in nociception.

CLONED RECEPTORS

Recently, the mu, delta, and kappa receptors have been cloned. Such advances in the basic sciences will likely have significant implications in the future production of specific opioid agonists.

Opioids may block neuron excitability by a mechanism involving depression of active sodium conductance and increased membrane potassium conductance or by blocking the opening of voltage-sensitive calcium channels. These actions decrease release of excitatory neurotransmitters at presynaptic nerve terminals. In addition, serotonergic pathways and gamma-aminobutyric acid receptors may also have a role in modulating analgesia. Drug action mediated at each of the opioid receptors is reversible by the opioid antagonist naloxone.

Structurally, opioids are complex compounds that exist as two optical isomers, with only the levorotary isomer capable of analgesia. The prototype opioid is morphine; it has a rigid pentacyclic ring that conforms to a T shape, in which the crossbar is piperidine and the vertical bar is a phenyl group. A portion of the structure of all morphine-like compounds resembles the amino acid tyrosine; tyrosine is essential for opioid function.

General Pharmacologic Properties of the Opioid Agonists

The five schedules in Table 4-3 list the narcotic, depressant, stimulant, and hallucinogenic drugs that are covered by the Controlled Substances Act. Examples of substances in each schedule are listed by generic or common name and in some instances by a trade name in parentheses.

CENTRAL NERVOUS SYSTEM

Analgesia

Opioids selectively relieve pain, their primary therapeutic application. An important feature of this analgesic activity is that it occurs without loss of consciousness or impairment of other sensory systems such as vision, hearing, and touch.

Mood Alteration

Drowsiness commonly occurs with administration of opioids, although occasionally patients will experience euphoria or dysphoria. The mechanism of mood alterations is not clear but is thought to involve both dopaminergic and nondopaminergic processes.

Nausea and Vomiting

Nausea is the most common acute adverse effect of opioids. Two actions contribute to this. First, there is a direct stimulation of the central trigger zone of the medulla. Second, there is an increase in vestibular sensitivity so that ambulatory patients experience more frequent nausea and vomiting. In equi-analgesic doses, all opioids are thought to be associated with a comparable incidence of nausea, although some patients may have variable sensitivity to the different opioids. Treatments to reduce nausea and vomiting include:

1. Anticholinergic drugs, especially scopolamine, 0.4–1.0 mg PO or SQ, or 0.5 mg postauricular transdermal disc every

Table 4-3. Schedules of controlled substances (US Department of Justice, Department of Drug Enforcement Administration, Washington, DC)

Schedule	Characteristics	Examples
I	• no accepted medical use in the United States • high abuse potential	fenethylline, heroin, LAAM, LSD, marijuana, MDMA, mescaline, methaqualone, peyote
II	• high abuse potential with severe psychic or physical dependence liability • are generally substances with therapeutic utility	**Narcotics:** morphine, codeine, fentanyl (Innovar, Sublimaze), hydromorphone (Dilaudid), levorphanol (Levo-Dromoran), meperidine (Demerol), methadone (Dolophine), oxycodone (Percodan), oxymorphone (Numorphan), opium, anileridine (Leritine) **Narcotic veterinary products:** etorphine hydrochloride (M 99), diprenorphine (M50-50) **Non-narcotics:** amphetamine (Dexedrine), methamphetamine (Desoxyn), methylphenidate (Ritalin), phenmetrazine (Preludin), amobarbital (Amytal), pentobarbital (Nembutal), secobarbital (Seconal), phencyclidine, dronabinol in sesame oil as gelatin capsules (Marinol), nabilone (Cesamet)
III	• less abuse potential than drugs in Schedules I and II	**Narcotics:** nalorphine (Nalline); mixtures of limited, specified quantities of codeine, dihydrocodeine, hydrocodone, morphine, or opium with noncontrolled active ingredients **Non-narcotics:** mixtures of amobarbital, pentobarbital, or secobarbital with other noncontrolled medicinal ingredients; glutethimide (Doriden), methyprylon (Noludar), benzphetamine (Didrex), phendimetrazine (Plegine) *Barbiturates:* aprobarbital, butabarbital, butalbital, talbutal, thiopental *Veterinary combination product:* tiletamine/zolazepam (Telazol)

IV	• less abuse potential than drugs in Schedule III	**Narcotics:** dextropropoxyphene, pentazocine (Talwin) *Benzodiazepines:* alprazolam (Xanax), chlordiazepoxide (Librium), clonazepam (Klonopin), clorazepate (Tranxene), diazepam (Valium), flurazepam (Dalmane), halazepam (Paxipam), lorazepam (Ativan), midazolam (Versed), oxazepam (Serax), prazepam (Centrax), quazepam (Dormalin), temazepam (Restoril), triazolam (Halcion) **Barbiturates:** *(Long-acting):* barbital, mephobarbital, phenobarbital *(Ultra-short):* methohexital (Brevital) **Other depressants:** chloral hydrate, ethchlorvynol (Placidyl), ethinamate (Valmid), meprobamate (Miltown), paraldehyde **Appetite suppressants:** diethylpropion (Tenuate), fenfluramine (Pondimin), mazindol (Sanorex), phentermine (Tonamin) **Stimulant:** pemoline (Cylert)
V	• less abuse potential than drugs in Schedule IV	**Narcotics:** Buprenorphine (Buprenex); antidiarrheal and cough-suppressant preparations with limited, specified quantities of codeine, dihydrocodeine, diphenoxylate (Lomotil), ethylmorphine, or opium

A complete listing of drugs controlled under CSA may be found in Title 21 Code of Federal Regulations. Part 1300 to end, Sections 1308.11 to 1308.15. This publication may be purchased from the Superintendent of Documents, U.S. Government Printing Office, Washington, DC 20402.

3 days (glycopyrrolate is ineffective because it does not cross the blood-brain barrier).

2. Butyrophenones, especially those with antidopaminergic properties such as droperidol (Inapsine), 1.25–2.5 mg IV or IM.

3. Phenothiazines, such as prochlorperazine (Compazine), 5–10 mg PO or IV or IM, or a 25-mg rectal suppository.

4. Metoclopramide (Reglan), 10–15 mg PO or IV, which acts both at the central trigger zone as a dopamine antagonist and peripherally on the GI tract.

Convulsions

Opioids have been implicated in a variety of neuroexcitatory symptoms ranging from nystagmus and nonspecific eye movements to generalized seizures. The precise mechanism is not understood. Naloxone is more effective in treating seizures produced by some opioid agonists (i.e., morphine, methadone) than by others (i.e., meperidine). Normeperidine, a convulsant metabolite of meperidine, may be partially responsible.

Neuroendocrine Response

Despite great variability in stimuli, the body's stress response is induced by some common denominators, including stimulatory hormones released from the hypothalamus that stimulate pituitary release of corticotropin, growth hormone, prolactin, endorphin, and antidiuretic hormone. Catabolic substances including cortisol, catecholamines, glucagon, and thyroxine are also secreted in greater amounts. This stress response is attenuated effectively by opioid antinociception. However, the hypothesis that inhibition of the neurohumoral response is clinically beneficial in terms of morbidity and mortality is still unproven.

Temperature Alteration

Opioids can change the equilibrium points of the hypothalamic heat-regulatory mechanism, so that the temperature usually falls slightly. Shivering is common following anesthesia, with the physiologic purpose of producing heat; however, its occurrence in opioid anesthesia is not consistent. Nevertheless, shivering can cause extreme increases in oxygen consumption. Meperidine (25–50 mg IV) is unique among the opioids in its ability to attenuate this undesirable side effect in most patients.

Antitussive Activity

Opioids depress the cough reflex at least in part by blocking medullary integration of this reflex. The doses of opioid required to suppress coughing are much less than those needed for pain relief.

Pupils

Most opioids cause pupillary constriction. Miosis is secondary to opioid action on the Edinger-Westphal nucleus, resulting in excitation of the autonomic segment of the oculomotor nerve. Pinpoint pupils are pathognomonic for toxicity of mu agonists; however, marked mydriasis appears when hypoxia is present. This miotic effect can be counteracted by atropine. Even though some tolerance to miotic effects occurs, patients and addicts on high doses of opioids chronically continue to demonstrate constriction of pupils.

RESPIRATORY SYSTEM

Respiratory Depression

In humans, death from opioid overdose is nearly always due to respiratory arrest. The main mechanism involves a direct effect on the brain stem respiratory centers, causing a reduction in the responsiveness of such centers to carbon dioxide. This results in a rightward shift of the carbon dioxide response curve, an increased resting level of carbon dioxide, and a higher apneic threshold. All phases of respiratory activity, including rate, minute volume, and tidal exchange, are depressed. Irregular or periodic breathing, or both, is often seen because opioids interfere with pontine and medullary respiratory centers that regulate respiratory rhythmicity. Most studies have found that when equi-analgesic doses of different opioids are compared, the degree of respiratory depression observed is not significantly different. The respiratory depressant effects are increased and prolonged when administered with other CNS depressants (i.e., benzodiazepines, alcohol, inhaled anesthetics). Natural sleep decreases the medullary center's sensitivity to carbon dioxide; the effects of opioids and sleep are additive. Pain and surgical stimulation counteract respiratory depression. Tolerance to opioid-induced respiratory depression can take months to develop in patients receiving chronic opioid therapy, and is usually incomplete. Maximum respiratory depression occurs within 5 to 10 minutes of an intravenous dose of morphine or within 30 to 90 minutes of intramuscular or subcutaneous administration. Delayed or recurring respiratory depression has been reported with most opioids and is thought to be related to significant secondary peaks and fluctuations in plasma opioid levels during the elimination phase. All components of opioid-produced respiratory depression are effectively reversed by opioid antagonists.

Chest Wall Rigidity

Opioid-induced rigidity is characterized by increased muscle tone progressing to severe stiffness, particularly in the thoracic and abdominal muscles. This phenomenon is not uncommon during rapid infusion of a large-bolus injection during fentanyl, alfentanil, or sufentanil anesthesia, when the rigidity can impair spontaneous ventilation or controlled ventilation in a nonparalyzed patient. Both muscle relaxants and naloxone can resolve the rigidity; however, the manner by which opioids produce muscle rigidity is not clearly understood.

CARDIOVASCULAR SYSTEM

Hypotension and Hypertension

Potential mechanisms underlying morphine-induced hypotension include:

1. Histamine release
2. Centrally mediated decrease in sympathetic tone
3. Vagal-induced bradycardia
4. Direct and indirect venous and arterial vasodilation
5. Splanchnic sequestration of blood

This hypotension can be decreased by histamine antagonists, slow infusion rates, and volume loading. Caution is advised in patients with decreased blood volume, because opioids can aggravate hypovolemic shock. Fentanyl and sufentanil, which are potent mu agonists, are less likely to cause hemodynamic instability, partly because of the lack of histamine release.

Sudden hypertension with intubation or surgical stimuli is commonly associated with high-dose narcotic-based anesthesia, especially in patients with intact left ventricular function. This problem is most often attributed to light anesthesia, sympathetic activation, and cardiogenic reflexes.

Heart Rate and Rhythm

Stimulation of the central vagus nucleus is the primary mechanism of most opioid-induced bradycardia. Morphine is also thought to have direct effects on the sinoatrial node and innervated myocardium in that it depresses atrioventricular conduction. Asystole may subsequently follow opioid bradycardia; this usually responds to atropine and isoproterenol. Because of its vagolytic effect, meperidine administered intravenously is the only opioid known to cause tachycardia. Opioids may have antifibrillatory action, decreasing the incidence of malignant ventricular arrhythmias.

Other Cardiac Effects

The effect of opioids on myocardial contractility, with the exception of meperidine, is not major in most clinical circumstances. Most opioids do not have significant effect on coronary autoregulation. Although opioids alone have limited effects on hemodynamics, drug combinations (i.e., with benzodiazepines) may exert profound changes.

GASTROINTESTINAL TRACT

Delayed Gastric Emptying

This delay is effected by the central vagus nerve and peripheral opiate receptors in the myenteric plexus and cholinergic nerve terminals. Relatively low doses of opioids decrease gastric motility, with the tone of the antral stomach and the first part of the duodenum increased. Passage of gastric contents through the duodenum can be delayed by as long as 12 hours.

Opioids also result in relaxation of the lower esophageal sphincter. Naloxone reverses opioid-induced delays in gastric emptying, but metoclopramide does not.

Slowed Intestinal Transit Time

The resting tone of the bowel is increased and periodic spasms are observed with opioids. The upper part of the small intestine is affected more than the ileum. Propulsive peristaltic waves in the colon are diminished to the point of spasm. The anal sphincter tone is greatly increased and the reflex relaxation response to rectal distention is reduced. Water is absorbed more completely because the passage of bowel contents and intestinal secretions is decreased, thus the viscosity of the bowel contents is increased. All opioids cause constipation in almost all patients with normal bowel function. Constipation should be anticipated in all people and managed prophylactically with stool softeners and cathartics (i.e., senna [Senokot], 2 tablets one or two times a day). Although some tolerance to the effects of opioids on GI motility develops, patients who take opioids chronically usually continue to experience some degree of constipation.

Biliary Tract System

All opioids are thought to increase biliary duct pressure and sphincter of Oddi tone in a dose-dependent manner. The duration of this action seems to be correlated with plasma opioid levels, but the clinical importance of this phenomenon has been minimal. This increase in biliary pressure can be reversed with naloxone and glucagon, and partially prevented with atropine and nitroglycerin. In a few limited studies, meperidine, fentanyl, butorphanol, and nalbuphine show less or no elevation in intrabiliary pressure.

SKIN

Opioids can directly produce vasodilation and release histamine, leading to flushing of the skin. Histamine is also responsible for injection-site urticaria. Pruritus is thought to involve opioid action on neurons, because it is also associated with those opioids that do not increase histamine concentrations and is quickly abolished by small doses of naloxone.

GENITOURINARY SYSTEM

Ureter and Bladder

Urinary retention can result from opioid administration, sometimes requiring catheterization. Ureter contractions are increased in tone and amplitude; inhibition of the urinary voiding reflex, increased tone of the external sphincter, and a rise in bladder volume all contribute to this side effect. The bladder develops tolerance to these effects of opioids.

Uterus

If the uterus has been made hyperactive by oxytocins, morphine tends to reduce tone, frequency, and amplitude of uterine contractions to baseline, possibly prolonging labor.

Precautions for Opioid Use

The Massachusetts General Hospital Pain Center offers guidelines on prescribing controlled substances for patients with nonmalignant chronic disease (Table 4-4).

HEPATIC AND RENAL DISEASES

In these disease processes, because of decreased metabolism and elimination of opioids, some concerns arise:

1. Active metabolites of morphine and codeine, especially morphine-6-glucuronide, may accumulate and lead to opioid toxicity.
2. Meperidine administration can lead to accumulation of normeperidine, causing subsequent CNS excitation with tremors or seizures.
3. Repeated doses of propoxyphene may cause naloxone-insensitive cardiac toxicity secondary to its metabolite norpropoxyphene.

RESPIRATORY DISEASES

One should proceed with caution when using opioids in any situation in which respiratory reserve is decreased (i.e., emphysema, kyphoscoliosis, or severe obesity). Opioids that release histamine may precipitate asthma attacks and bronchoconstriction. A depression of cough reflex and drying of secretions can also occur.

HEAD INJURIES

An increase in P_{CO_2} from respiratory depression can lead to elevated intracerebral pressure. Miosis, vomiting, and mental clouding, which are important clinical signs and symptoms for evaluation of the head injury, can be obscured.

ALLERGIC REACTIONS

Allergies to opioid analgesics are possible but quite rare. Wheals at the injection site are from histamine release. Most patients who say they have opioid allergies usually describe side effects such as nausea or dysphoria rather than true anaphylactic reactions.

DRUG INTERACTIONS

Small doses of amphetamines (i.e., methylphenidate hydrochloride (Ritalin), 20–30 mg daily in 2 or 3 divided doses) substantially enhance analgesia and euphoria and decrease

Table 4-4. MGH Pain Center's guidelines on prescribing controlled substances for patients with nonmalignant chronic disease

1. Controlled substance prescriptions will not be sent by mail.
2. Prescriptions will not be written as "brand name medically necessary" and "no substitution."
3. When chronic opioid therapy is initiated, the primary referring physician must concur with this decision and continue to monitor the patient as well. If, as the patient is observed, there is no demonstrable benefit to the patient's function or quality of life, then the opioid should be tapered. Before chronically maintained opioids can be tapered in a patient, the Pain Center physician should discuss the plan in advance with the primary referring physician, if he or she can be found, and if the patient has been seen by that physician in the last year. The concurrence of the primary referring physician with the decision to start or taper opioids must be documented on the chart.
4. Where there is no primary physician, our unit must provide the patient with the opportunity to secure such a physician. We cannot be the primary source of general medical care for any patient.
5. Discovery that a patient has obtained concurrent prescriptions for controlled substances from multiple medical doctors will result in immediate termination of our Center's relationship with the patient.
6. The second instance of a lost or otherwise early depletion of a prescription will result in no further controlled substances being dispensed to that patient from our unit. This need not necessarily result, however, in cessation of the therapeutic relationship with our unit, nor in our ceasing to prescribe noncontrolled substances.
7. There are to be no prescription refills if a patient arrives without an appointment prior to the time of his or her next scheduled refill. Even when a medical follow-up visit is not necessary, the patient must still inform the Center at least the day before picking up a prescription. Failure to do so disrupts the Center's schedule and needlessly inconveniences those working in it or waiting to be seen.
8. Options for physical therapy, behavioral medicine treatment, or other consultations (e.g., psychiatry, orthopedics), as appropriate, should be offered to patients who are being tapered from chronic opioid use. These options may be offered through an inpatient rehabilitation program providing that insurance is available to cover it, or, if not, then through the MGH outpatient departments.
9. No more than 1 month should elapse between scheduled follow-up appointments during the long-term follow-up of any patient receiving controlled substances in the absence of malignant disease.
10. Apart from the regulatory dimension, our first role is to treat the patient. Thus it is essential that our notes document the history, physical and laboratory findings, diagnosis, and plans for medical and other therapies (including specifics and timing of schedules for tapering opioids). Initiating or tapering controlled substances in the absence of a documented explanation of medical rationale is not acceptable.

sedative side effects of opioids. A number of antihistamines (i.e., hydroxyzine, starting doses of 25–50 mg qid) exhibit modest analgesic actions if given alone and can enhance the analgesic effects of low-dose opioids. Tricyclic antidepressants used in chronic neuropathic pain treatment do not appear to decrease acute pain, but desipramine may enhance morphine analgesia postoperatively. Interactions of opioids with monoamine oxidase inhibitors are of two types. One type is predominantly evidenced by depressive symptoms of respiratory depression, hypotension, and coma; it is due to accumulation of free opioid and can occur with any of the opioids. The other type is associated with fatal excitatory reactions to excitation, delerium, hyperpyrexia, and convulsions; it is seen uniquely with meperidine, which blocks neuronal uptake of 5-hydroxytryptamine (serotonin) and results in central serotonergic overactivity.

WITHDRAWAL, TOLERANCE, AND PHYSICAL DEPENDENCE

These three issues related to opioid use in pain patients demand special consideration. See Chap. 23 for a complete discussion.

Acute Toxicity

Opioids have very high therapeutic indices, and it is difficult to pinpoint the specific blood level of any opioid that is toxic or lethal in humans.

SYMPTOMS AND DIAGNOSIS

Patients are usually stuporous or in a coma. Their respiratory rate is low (sometimes 2–4/min) and cyanosis may be present. The pupils are symmetric and pinpoint, but if hypoxia is severe they may be dilated. Hypotension progresses and urine output is depressed. Body temperature can fall and the skin is usually cold and clammy. Skeletal muscles are flaccid and the jaw and tongue can become relaxed, sometimes causing airway obstruction. Frank convulsions can also occur. When death occurs, it is nearly always attributed to respiratory failure. Noncardiogenic pulmonary edema is possible with opioid poisoning.

TREATMENT

The first steps are the ABCs of resuscitation (Airway, Breathing, and Circulation), especially the establishment of an adequate airway and ventilation. Opioid antagonists can produce dramatic reversal of toxicity. The drug of choice is **naloxone, with titration of intravenous doses of 0.1– 0.2 mg (higher doses of 0.4 mg to 2 mg may be used, depending on urgency) at 2- to 3-minute intervals until the desired effect is seen**. Even when naloxone is effective, subsequent doses or continuous infusion may be needed because of the drug's short duration of action.

Pharmacokinetics

ABSORPTION AND ROUTES OF ADMINISTRATION

New systems and sites for drug delivery have the potential to improve patient care.

ORAL ADMINISTRATION

The effect of a given oral dose is subject to a variable but significant first-pass metabolism in the liver. For example, the bioavailability of morphine is only about 25%. There is wide variability in first-pass metabolism and individual clinical effect, so opioids always need to be titrated to the patient's needs. The duration of action of the oral route is somewhat longer than the parenteral route; controlled, sustained release forms are also available, allowing less frequent dosing intervals.

INTRAVENOUS, INTRAMUSCULAR, AND SUBCUTANEOUS ADMINISTRATIONS

These are the traditional parenteral routes. Recently, patient-controlled analgesia has become a popular method of administration. An apparatus delivers a programmed dose of opioid through an indwelling intravenous line or subcutaneous needle (doses for either route of administration are identical) whenever the patient pushes a button. This approach allows efficient titration of the patient's opioid requirements with fewer peaks and troughs.

RECTAL ADMINISTRATION

First-pass elimination in the liver can be partially avoided with this method. Rectal administration is complicated by interruption of absorption by defecation, mucosal irritation, variable systemic availability, and, at times, poor patient acceptance.

EPIDURAL, INTRATHECAL, AND INTRA-CNS VENTRICULAR ADMINISTRATIONS

The efficacy of opioids placed into the epidural or subarachnoid/ventricular space for providing perioperative analgesia and cancer or chronic pain relief has made this route an important one. Advantages include smaller doses of opioids required, prolonged duration of action, and minimal systemic side effects. Of concern is delayed respiratory depression secondary to rostral spread of morphine in the spinal fluid. This is not a problem with more lipophilic opioid drugs. Catheters can be tunneled through the skin so that the exit site is away from the epidural insertion point; this may theoretically reduce the potential for infection and allow long-term catheter use. Epidural patient-controlled analgesia is a newer option for drug delivery.

TRANSMUCOSAL ADMINISTRATION

More lipophilic opioids are readily absorbed through the nasal or buccal mucosa. Because the oral and nasal cavities are rich in blood vessels and lymphatics, rapid onset of action is possible and the first-pass metabolism of the liver is avoided. Sites for absorption include sublingual, buccal, and gingival surfaces. High-potency drugs need to be used to achieve adequate absorption across the mucosal barrier. Buprenorphine, butorphanol, fentanyl (incorporated into a candy lozenge as a lollipop), and sufentanil have been administered in this manner.

TRANSDERMAL ADMINISTRATION

Fentanyl was the first opioid evaluated in this avenue of delivery because it is highly potent, soluble in both oil and water, and nonirritable to the skin. The rate-limiting step in systemic absorption is passive diffusion of the drug through the keratinous stratum corneum layer of the skin. A typical system consists of a drug reservoir and rate-controlling membrane. Transdermal fentanyl systems are approximately 0.5 mm thick and deliver drug at rates of 25, 50, 75, or 100 μg/hr. With initial placement of the patch, serum fentanyl levels of 1 ng/ml are usually attained by 12–15 hrs. After removal of the transdermal patch, continued absorption from the skin depot contributes to the slow elimination of the drug from the body; continued analgesia can be expected for as long as 12 hours after discontinuation of the patch. Patches are usually changed every 2 or 3 days. Advantages of this system include the elimination of the first-pass effect, convenience and comfort, improved compliance, and consistent analgesia. Disadvantages include the requirement for a relatively stable pain intensity and cumbersome titration. Morphine hydrochloride has been administered for postoperative pain using iontophoresis, a technique that utilizes external electrical current to augment passage of drug through the skin.

Individual Opioid Agonists

All the drugs of the mu agonist type (Fig. 4-2) have similar clinical efficacy, so in general, if an adequate dose of one of these drugs does not work, it is unlikely that an equivalent dose of any other drug will provide relief. However, because patient sensitivities vary and cross-tolerance between opioids is not complete, adverse effects may be seen with one drug and not with equi-analgesic doses of another (Tables 4-5 and 4-6).

MORPHINE

Although morphine was the first opioid analgesic to be introduced into medicine, this drug is still widely used and remains the standard for comparison. In the bloodstream, one third of morphine is bound to plasma protein. Unbound drug is predominantly ionized at physiologic pH and is very hy-

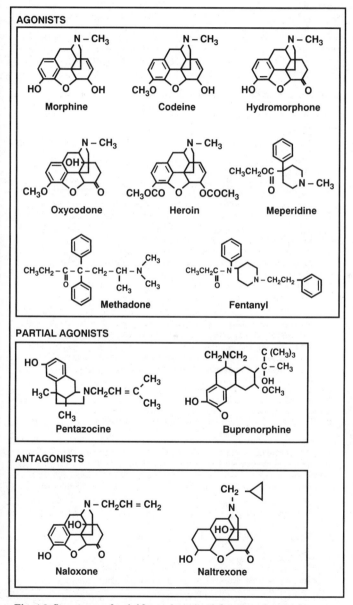

Fig. 4-2. Structures of opioid agonists, partial antagonists, and antagonists.

Table 4-5. Recommendations for specific parenteral and oral opioid conversions

Approximate oral-to-parenteral potency ratio for commonly used opioid agonists

Agonist Drug	Oral-Parenteral Ratio
Morphine	6
Codeine	2
Meperidine	4
Methadone	2
Levorphanol	2
Hydromorphone	5

Approximate multiplication factors for converting other opioids to morphine

Prior PO Opioid	Multiplication Factor
Morphine	1.0
Meperidine	0.10
Methadone	4.0
Levorphanol	7.5
Hydromorphone	4.0

Epidural and intrathecal morphine

Epidural dose of morphine sulfate is approximately one tenth IV morphine dose per 24 hours (starting doses, 1–2 mg q12h).

Intrathecal dose of morphine sulfate is approximately one hundredth IV morphine per 24 hours (starting doses, 0.1–0.5 mg q12h).

Some conversion guidelines for morphine

Oral Morphine Sulfate to MS Contin
   1. Add up patient's total daily dose of morphine.
   2. Divide this dose into two doses to be given PO twice a day.
   3. Titrate as needed.

Parenteral-to-Oral Morphine Sulfate
   1. Add up patient's total daily dose of parenteral morphine.
   2. Look at the conversion of oral-to-parenteral potency ratio chart above (if patient has been on chronic opioids, recommendations are for an oral-to-parenteral ratio of 3 instead of 6).
   3. Give in divided doses, i.e., one sixth of patient's daily dose every 4 hours. (Because of uncertainty and intersubject variability about relative estimates of opioid potency and cross-tolerance, initial dosing regimens should be conservative.)

Example

To convert from other strong opioid analgesics to morphine, i.e., hydromorphone 8 mg PO q4h.
   1. 8 mg times 6 doses = 48 mg/day of hydromorphone.
   2. 48 mg times 4 (from multiplication factor table above) = 192 mg of oral morphine a day.

Example

A patient has been on morphine sulfate 10 mg IM q4h prn. You look at her medication sheets and see that over the last few days she has received about four doses daily. Now that the patient has good oral intake but will probably continue to need pain medications for an extended time period, you would like to switch her to a long-acting oral pain regimen such as MS Contin.
   1. In 24 hours, she has been receiving 40 mg (4 doses of 10 mg) of parenteral morphine.
   2. Because the oral-to-parenteral potency ratio is 6, a total of 240 mg (40 mg × 6) should be given orally in 24 hours.
   3. The dose of MS Contin is 120 mg (240 mg ÷ 2) PO bid. The patient can receive two 60-mg MS Contin tablets orally bid. Remember that the patient will need breakthrough pain supplementation.

Note: Specific recommendations are not possible for other parenteral or oral opioid conversions because of the lack of evidence concerning these specific analgesic substitutions.

drophilic; thus it distributes rapidly to most body tissues but has limited ability to penetrate tissues. The major pathway for metabolism is conjugation with glucuronic acid in the liver, followed by elimination by glomerular filtration. During the first day 90% of the total excretion takes place. Entero-hepatic circulation accounts for small amounts of morphine in the feces. Morphine-3-glucuronide is the major metabolite but is essentially inactive; morphine-6-glucuronide is more potent than morphine and has a longer half-life. Although intravenous injection yields high analgesic plasma levels quickly, there is a relatively slow onset of peak CNS action, with peak spinal fluid concentrations 15 to 30 minutes after IV administration. Plasma half-life is 2 to 3 hours after an intravenous bolus. Morphine, 10 mg per 70 kg SQ or IM, is generally considered to be a good initial dose of morphine; it provides satisfactory analgesia in 70% of patients with mod-erate to severe pain with only minimal side effects. The oral route manifests a marked first-pass effect. Compared to par-enteral administration a sixfold oral dose is required to pro-duce the same level of analgesia. The peak analgesic effect after oral administration is 90 minutes, compared to 30 minutes for intravenous and 45 minutes for intramuscular administration. Small amounts of morphine, either epidur-ally (5–10 mg) or intrathecally (0.2–1.0 mg), can produce profound analgesia that has an onset of 15 to 60 minutes and may last 12 to 24 hours. However, rostral spread of the drug in the cerebral spinal fluid can result in delayed respiratory depression.

Preparations

Morphine sulfate: injections 1, 5, 8, 10, 15, and 30 mg/ml; oral tablets 8, 10, 15, and 30 mg; rectal suppository 5, 10, 20, and 30 mg.

Morphine sulfate controlled release (MS Contin): tab-lets 15, 30, 60, and 100 mg. **(Oramorph SR)**: tablets 30, 60, and 100 mg.

Morphine sulfate immediate release (MSIR, Roxanol, Rescudose, MS/L): oral solution 2 and 4 mg/ml; oral con-centrate 20 mg/ml; tablets and capsules 15 and 30 mg.

Morphine sulfate preservative free solution (Dura-morph and Astramorph) for intravenous, epidural, or in-trathecal use: 0.5 and 1.0 mg/ml.

Morphine sulfate preservative free (Infumorph) for con-tinuous microinfusions for implantable epidural or intra-thecal pumps: 10 and 25 mg/ml.

Formulations containing morphine for treatment of diarrhea include paregoric and laudanum.

CODEINE

A methylation substitution of morphine at the phenolic hy-droxyl group produces codeine. Codeine is less potent than morphine, but its oral-to-parenteral potency ratio is much higher. It is one of the few opioids used therapeutically to suppress cough; its antitussive action probably involves dis-

Table 4-6. Pharmacologic management of acute pain: dosing data for opioids

Drug	Approximate equi-analgesic oral dose	Approximate equi-analgesic parenteral dose	Recommended starting dose (adults more than 50 kg body weight)		Recommended starting dose (children and adults less than 50 kg body weight)[a]	
			Oral	Parenteral	Oral	Parenteral
Opioid agonist[b]						
Morphine[b]	30 mg q3–4h (around-the-clock dosing) 60 mg q3–4h (single dose or intermittent dosing)	10 mg q3–4h	30 mg q3–4h	10 mg q3–4h	0.3 mg/kg q3–4h	0.1 mg/kg q3–4h
Codeine[c]	130 mg q3–4h	75 mg q3–4h	60 mg q3–4h	60 mg q2h (intramuscular/subcutaneous)	1 mg/kg q3–4h[d]	Not recommended
Hydromorphone[b] (Dilaudid)	7.5 mg q3–4h	1.5 mg q3–4h	6 mg q3–4h	1.5 mg q3–4h	0.06 mg/kg q3–4h	0.015 mg/kg q3–4h
Levorphanol (Levo-Dromoran)	4 mg q6–8h	2 mg q6–8h	4 mg q6–8h	2 mg q6–8h	0.04 mg/kg q6–8h	0.02 mg/kg q6–8h
Meperidine (Demerol)	300 mg q2–3h	100 mg q3h	Not recommended	100 mg q3h	Not recommended	0.75 mg/kg q2–3h
Methadone (Dolophine, others)	20 mg q6–8h	10 mg q6–8h	20 mg q6–8h	10 mg q6–8h	0.2 mg/kg q6–8h	0.1 mg/kg q6–8h

Drug						
Oxycodone (Roxicodone, also in Percocet, Percodan, Tylox, others)	30 mg q3–4h	Not available	10 mg q3–4h	Not available	0.2 mg/kg q3–4h[d]	Not available
Oxymorphone[b] (Numorphan)	Not available	1 mg q3–4h	Not available	1 mg q3–4h	Not recommended	Not recommended
Opioid agonist-antagonist and partial agonist						
Buprenorphine (Buprenex)	Not available	0.3–0.4 mg q6–8h	Not available	0.4 mg q6–8h	Not available	0.004 mg/kg q6–8h
Butorphanol (Stadol)	Not available	2 mg q3–4h	Not available	2 mg q3–4h	Not available	Not recommended
Nalbuphine (Nubain)	Not available	10 mg q3–4h	Not available	10 mg q3–4h	Not available	0.1 mg/kg q3–4h
Pentazocine (Talwin, others)	150 mg q3–4h	60 mg q3–4h	50 mg q4–6h	Not recommended	Not recommended	Not recommended

Note: Published tables vary in the suggested doses that are equi-analgesic to morphine. Clinical response is the criterion that must be applied for each patient; titration to clinical response is necessary. Because there is not complete cross-tolerance among these drugs, it is usually necessary to use a lower than equi-analgesic dose when changing drugs and to retitrate to response.

Caution: Recommended doses do not apply to patients with renal or hepatic insufficiency or other conditions affecting drug metabolism and kinetics.

a Caution: Doses listed for patients with body weight <50 kg cannot be used as initial starting doses in babies <6 months of age. Consult the *Clinical Practice Guideline for Acute Pain Management: Operative or Medical Procedures and Trauma* section on management of pain in neonates for recommendations.

b For morphine, hydromorphone, and oxymorphone, rectal administration is an alternate route for patients unable to take oral medications, but equi-analgesic doses may differ from oral and parenteral doses because of pharmacokinetic differences.

c Caution: Codeine doses >65 mg often are not appropriate due to diminishing incremental analgesia with increasing doses but continually increasing constipation and other side effects.

d Caution: Doses of aspirin and acetaminophen in combination opioid/nonsteroidal anti-inflammatory drug preparations must also be adjusted to the patient's body weight.

Source: U.S. Department of Health and Human Services Public Health Service, Agency for Health Care Policy and Research, AHCPR Pub. No. 92-0086, effective March 1992.

tinct receptors that bind codeine itself. In small doses (15–20 mg) it reduces the frequency of pathologic cough, and progressively greater cough suppression is seen as the dose is increased up to 60 mg.

Preparations

Codeine phosphate: injections 15, 30, and 60 mg/ml; tablets 15, 30, and 60 mg; oral solution 3 mg/ml.
Codeine sulfate: tablets 15, 30, and 60 mg.

Codeine is available in various combinations with acetaminophen and aspirin (i.e., codeine, 15 mg in Tylenol #2, 30 mg in Tylenol #3, and 60 mg in Tylenol #4 [each with 300 mg acetaminophen]). Numerous cough suppression preparations with codeine are also manufactured.

HYDROMORPHONE

Hydromorphone, a clinically useful semisynthetic derivative of morphine, is 10 times more potent as an analgesic, with corresponding greater respiratory depressant effect. While intravenous injection yields high plasma levels quickly, there is a relatively slow onset of peak CNS action with peak spinal fluid concentrations 15 to 30 minutes after intravenous dose. Plasma half-life is 2 to 3 hours after an intravenous dose. Its intramuscular analgesic effect is seen within 30 minutes with a duration of action longer than 3 hours. Onset of action is seen within 45 minutes after oral dosing. The typical dosing requirement is 2–6 mg PO or 1.5 mg parenterally every 3 to 4 hours.

Preparations

Hydromorphone hydrochloride (Dilaudid): injections 1, 2, and 4 mg/ml; tablets 1, 2, 3, 4, and 8 mg; suppository 3 mg; cough syrup 1 mg in 5 ml; oral liquid 1 mg/ml.
Hydromorphone hydrochloride (Dilaudid HP) highly concentrated for opioid-tolerant patients: 10 mg/ml.

OXYCODONE

This drug, which has a similar profile to morphine, is popular in combination with other non-narcotic analgesics. As Percocet or Roxicet, its dosing is limited by the nonopioid portion because of possible acetaminophen hepatotoxicity.

Preparations

Oxycodone hydrochloride (Percocet): tablet 5 mg with 325 mg acetaminophen; **(Tylox):** capsule 5 mg with 500 mg acetaminophen.
Oxycodone hydrochloride (Roxicet): oral solution 5 mg with 325 mg acetaminophen per 5 ml.
Oxycodone hydrochloride (Percodan): tablet 5 mg with 325 mg aspirin.
Oxycodone hydrochloride (Roxicodone): tablet 5 mg; oral solution 5 mg in 5 ml; concentrated oral solution (Intensol) 20 mg/ml.

OXYMORPHONE

(Similar to Morphine)

Preparations

Oxymorphone hydrochloride (Numorphan): injections 1.0 and 1.5 mg/ml; rectal suppository 5 mg.

DIACETYLMORPHINE

Also known as **heroin**, this drug has high solubility and produces analgesia rapidly. It appears to be a prodrug; following absorption, heroin is metabolized quickly to acetylmorphine and morphine, both of which have analgesic properties. Heroin is presently not clinically available in the United States.

MEPERIDINE

Meperidine is highly protein bound in plasma (70%); it is less ionized and more lipid soluble than morphine. Average initial dosing is 50–100 mg parenterally or orally every 3 hours. Analgesic effects are detectable 30 to 40 minutes after an oral dose, peak in about 1 to 2 hours, and then gradually subside over several hours. Onset of analgesic effect is within 20 minutes after a subcutaneous or intramuscular dose, and peak effect occurs in about 1 hour. Clinically, duration of effective analgesia is 2 to 4 hours. Meperidine's cardiovascular effects generally resemble those of morphine, including its ability to release histamine. It differs from other opioids in that intravenous administration frequently produces tachycardia secondary to its vagolytic effect. Sometimes it is specifically requested by patients because of its inherent euphoric properties.

Meperidine has a unique toxicity. Normeperidine is the toxic meperidine metabolite excreted through the kidneys. In patients with normal renal function, normeperidine has a half-life of 15 to 20 hours; this time extends greatly in elderly individuals and patients with impaired renal function. Normeperidine is a cerebral irritant that can cause effects ranging from dysphoria to irritable mood through excitatory symptoms of tremors, to muscle twitches, to dilated pupils, to hyperactive reflexes, and to frank convulsions. Extreme caution must accompany use of meperidine in patients with hepatic and especially renal disease in whom normeperidine is likely to accumulate. Cerebral irritation has been observed even in young, otherwise healthy patients given sufficiently high doses of meperidine postoperatively. Therefore, meperidine should be limited to very brief courses in otherwise healthy patients when other options are not available.

Interactions between opioids and monoamine oxidase inhibitors can result in fatal excitatory reactions, as described previously in this chapter.

Preparations

Meperidine hydrochloride (Demerol): injections 25, 50, 75, and 100 mg/ml; tablets 50 and 100 mg; syrup 50 mg in 5 ml; **(Mepergan):** injection 25 mg/ml with 25 mg promethazine.

Congeners of meperidine are **diphenoxylate hydrochloride (Lomotil)** and **loperamide hydrochloride (Imodium)**, which are used to treat diarrhea.

LEVORPHANOL

This is the only commercially available opioid agonist of the morphinan series. Its most important feature is a long duration of action. An average 2-mg SQ or PO dose produces analgesia 6–8 hours longer than morphine. Although its pharmacologic effects closely parallel morphine, some clinical reports suggest it produces less nausea and vomiting. Levorphanol can be crushed and administered effectively through a gastrostomy tube for long-acting analgesia (MS Contin is a sustained-release morphine tablet that must not be broken, since doing so could result in a rapid release of morphine with possible toxicity).

Preparations

Levorphanol tartrate (Levo-Dromoran): injection 2 mg/ml; tablet 2 mg.

METHADONE

Although methadone is a long-acting pain reliever, the side effects of sedation and respiratory depression of this synthetic opioid can outlast the analgesic effects. Thus, when given at 4-hour intervals, accumulation can occur. Because of its long half-life and less severe abstinence symptoms, methadone is often used for detoxification or maintenance treatment of narcotic addiction. Initial doses are 2.5 to 10 mg parenterally or orally every 4 hours for 1 or 2 days, with later dosing intervals changing to 24 hours. A typical maintenance therapy in addicts is 40–100 mg daily. Analgesia occurs 10 to 20 minutes after parenteral administration and 30 to 60 minutes after oral medication. Peak levels are reached 1 to 2 hours after a subcutaneous or intramuscular dose, and 4 hours after an oral dose. Because of its long duration of action, methadone is slow and difficult to titrate.

Preparations

Methadone hydrochloride (Dolophine): injection 10 mg/ml; tablets 5 and 10 mg (40-mg specialized dose for opioid addiction); oral solution 1, 2, and 10 mg/ml.

PROPOXYPHENE

This opioid is usually given in combination with aspirin or acetaminophen. After oral administration, it reaches peak concentration in 1 to 2 hours. The major metabolite, norpropoxyphene, lasts about 30 hours and will accumulate with repeat dosing. The drug is irritating when given intravenously or subcutaneously.

Preparations

Propoxyphene napsylate (Darvon): capsule 65 mg.
Propoxyphene napsylate (Darvocet-N50 and Darvocet-N100): tablet 50 mg with 325 mg acetaminophen, or 100 mg with 650 mg acetaminophen.
Propoxyphene hydrochloride (Wygesic): tablet 65 mg with 650 mg acetaminophen.
Propoxyphene napsylate (Darvon-N): tablet 100 mg; suspension 10 mg/ml.
Propoxyphene hydrochloride (Darvon Compound-65, PC-CAP): 65 mg with 389 mg aspirin and caffeine.

FENTANYL

This phenylpiperidine is 60 to 80 times as potent as morphine. In analgesic (2–10 μg/kg) or anesthetic (20–100 μg/kg) doses, it seldom causes significant hemodynamic changes, even in patients with poor left ventricular function. Hypotension is most likely secondary to bradycardia, which usually is not severe and responds to anticholinergic stimulation. Fentanyl's onset of action after intravenous dosing is very rapid but maximum analgesic and respiratory effects may not be apparent for several minutes and with intramuscular administration onset is delayed for 20 to 30 minutes. Duration of action after intravenous administration is 30 to 60 minutes and 1 to 2 hours after intramuscular injection. Fentanyl is approved for general anesthesia and have been used in both the intrathecal and epidural spaces.

Preparations

Fentanyl citrate (Sublimaze): injection 50 μg/ml.
Fentanyl transdermal system (Duragesic): patches 25, 50, 75, 100 μg/hr.
Fentanyl citrate (Innovar): 50 μg with 2.5 mg droperidol per milliliter for neuroleptanalgesia.
Fentanyl citrate (Fentanyl oralet): oral transmucosal lozenge 200, 300, or 400 μg.

ALFENTANIL

This drug has the most rapid onset time and the shortest duration of action of all the opioids, reflecting its high degree of nonionization at physiologic pH. Unlike other opioids, continuous infusions do not seem to produce cumulative drug effects, and postoperative awakening is usually prompt without persistence of ventilatory depression. Alfentanil is one fifth to one third as potent as fentanyl and less reliable than fentanyl or sufentanil at blocking increases in heart rate and blood pressure. Usual doses of 50–75 μg/kg IV bolus are sometimes followed by continuous infusions of 0.5–3.0 μg/kg per minute.

Preparations

Alfentanil hydrochloride (Alfenta): injection 500 µg/ml.

SUFENTANIL

This opioid is 5 to 10 times more potent than fentanyl. Because it produces minimal changes in cardiovascular dynamics and has the highest safety margin of any opioid, it is popular for cardiac anesthesia where induction doses of 8–30 µg/kg are used. Analgesic doses are as much as 8 µg/kg.

Preparations

Sufentanil citrate (Sufenta): injection 50 µg/ml.

Agonist-Antagonist and Partial Agonist Opioids

We find that agonist-antagonist and partial agonist opioids have a very limited role in pain management, so we almost never use them. These drugs bind to the mu receptor and can therefore compete with other substances for these sites, but they either exert no actions (competitive antagonists) or they exert limited actions (partial agonists) at the mu receptors (see Fig. 4-2). They are less prone to patient abuse because they cause less drug-seeking behavior and less physical dependence. Withdrawal symptoms can be managed by gradual reduction of the drug or by substitution of a mu agonist. Agonist-antagonists may precipitate withdrawal when given to patients who are physically dependent on mu agonists. After an opioid-free interval of 1 or 2 days, it is usually possible to administer these drugs safely.

PENTAZOCINE

This is a benzomorphan derivative with either a weaker antagonist or partial agonist action at the mu receptor and more powerful agonist effect at the kappa receptor. CNS effects include analgesia, respiratory depression, and sedation. Ceiling effects to both analgesia and respiratory depression occur; increasing pentazocine doses beyond 30 mg does not produce proportionate increases in respiratory depression. Although pentazocine at low doses produces sedation similar to that of the morphine-like opioids (60–90 mg), dysphoria and psychotomimetic effects attributed to sigma-receptor activity may occur. The cardiovascular responses differ from those of morphine. The drug elevates blood catecholamine levels that increase blood pressure and heart rate, and it also causes a depression of myocardial contractility. Typical dosing is 25–50 mg orally every 3 to 6 hours. Analgesia is clinically evident after 2 to 3 minutes of intravenous administration, 15 to 20 minutes of intramuscular administration, and 15 to 30 minutes of oral administration. Peak concentrations occur 15 to 60 minutes after intramuscular administration and 1 to 3 hours after oral administration.

Preparations

Pentazocine lactate (Talwin): injection 30 mg/ml.

Pentazocine hydrochloride (Talwin): caplet 12.5 mg base with 325 mg aspirin; **(Talacen):** caplet 25 mg with 650 mg acetaminophen.

Pentazocine hydrochloride (Talwin (Nx)): tablet 50 mg base with 0.5 mg naloxone.

BUTORPHANOL

This agonist-antagonist opioid is a morphinan congener with a profile of action similar to that of pentazocine but with a lower incidence of psychotomimetic side effects. Appropriate doses are 0.5–2.0 mg IV or 1–4 mg IM every 3 to 4 hours. Onset of analgesia is within a few minutes after intravenous administration. Levels peak 30 to 60 minutes after intravenous or intramuscular administration and 1 to 2 hours after nasal spray. Duration of action is 3 to 4 hours after parenteral administration; slightly longer, 4 to 5 hours, after nasal spray.

Preparations

Butorphanol tartrate (Stadol): injection 1.0 and 2.0 mg/ml.

Butorphanol tartrate (Stadol NS): nasal spray 10 mg/ml, each metered spray averages 1 mg.

NALBUPHINE

This is an agonist-antagonist with a spectrum of effects that qualitatively resemble those of pentazocine, but which also has several differences. It is less likely to produce dysphoric side effects, and when given to stable patients with coronary artery disease, it does not significantly change cardiac work. Nalbuphine exhibits a ceiling effect on analgesia and respiratory depression so that doses beyond approximately 30 mg produce no further effect. Other common side effects are sedation, sweating, and headache. The usual adult dose is 10 mg every 3 to 6 hours. Onset of action is 5 to 10 minutes, and the duration of action is 3 to 6 hours.

Preparations

Nalbuphine hydrochloride (Nubain): injections 10 and 20 mg/ml.

BUPRENORPHINE

This semisynthetic, highly lipophilic opioid appears to be a partial mu agonist with relatively insignificant activity at the kappa and sigma receptors. It has high affinity but low intrinsic activity at the mu receptor and has a slow dissociation

time. Analgesic, CNS, and cardiovascular effects are qualitatively similar to those of morphine. Buprenorphine 0.4 mg
is equal to morphine 10 mg IM, although buprenorphine's
duration is usually longer. The analgesic dose is 0.3 mg IM
or IV every 6 hours. After intramuscular administration effects are seen in 15 minutes and peak at 1 hour; intravenous
adminstration involves shorter onset and peak times. Sublingual doses of 0.4 mg produce effective pain relief.

Preparations

Buprenorphine hydrochloride (Buprenex): injection 0.3
  mg/ml.

Opioid Antagonists

Relatively minor changes in the structure of an opioid can
convert a drug that is primarily an agonist into one with an-
tagonistic properties. Naloxone and naltrexone appear to be
devoid of agonistic actions and probably interact with all
types of opioid receptors. Nalmefene is a relatively pure mu
antagonist that is potent and is currently undergoing clinical
trials. Some clinicians have attempted to reverse opioid effects with physostigmine, a tertiary amine anticholinester-
ase. Although the use of physostigmine may result in persistent analgesia, it is unpredictable, has other side effects
(bradycardia, nausea, and vomiting), and is short lived.
Therefore, reliance on more predictable and specific opioid
antagonists is recommended.

NALOXONE

Although active at all the opiate receptors, naloxone has the
greatest affinity for the mu receptor. Careful intravenous titration of naloxone (one 0.4-mg ampule diluted to 10 ml; 1–
2 ml given every 1–2 min) can usually restore adequate spontaneous ventilation without reversal of analgesia. In patients
with respiratory depression from mu agonists, an increase in
respiratory rate is seen within 1 to 2 minutes. The duration
of action is 1 to 4 hours with a plasma half-life of about 1
hour. Abrupt reversal of narcotic depression may result in
nausea and vomiting, tachycardia, sweating, hypertension,
tremulousness, seizures, and cardiac arrest. These are at
least partially attributed to a sudden surge of sympathetic
activity. Hypotension, ventricular tachycardia and fibrilla-
tion, and pulmonary edema have also been reported. Although absorbed readily from the GI tract, naloxone is almost
completely metabolized by the liver before reaching the
systemic circulation and therefore must be administered
parenterally.

Naloxone is administered orally, with no systemic effects, to
treat constipation. It has a localized effect on the opioid receptors in the gut. Generally, doses range from 0.8 to 4.0 mg,
2–10 ampules, q4h for four doses, or until bowel movement
has occurred.

Preparations

Naloxone hydrochloride (Narcan): injections 0.02, 0.4, and 1.0 mg/ml.

NALTREXONE

Unlike naloxone, naltrexone can be given orally; its duration of action approaches 24 hours. It is used as an adjunct to the maintenance of an opioid-free state in detoxified individuals.

Preparations

Naltrexone hydrochloride (Trexan): injection 100 mg/ml; tablet 50 mg.

Selected Readings

Bailey P and Stanley T. Narcotic Intravenous Anesthetics. In: R Miller (ed); *Anesthesia*. New York: Churchill-Livingstone, 1990.

Carr D. Opioids, *Int Anesthesiol Clin* 26:273–287, 1988.

Carr D and Lipkowksi A. Mechanisms of Opioid Analgesic Actions. In: M Rogers, et al (eds), *Principles and Practice of Anesthesiology*. St. Louis: Mosby–Year Book, 1993.

Colasanti B. Narcotic Analgesia and Antagonists. In: C Craig and R Stitzel (eds), *Modern Pharmacology*. Boston: Little, Brown, 1986.

Craig CR and Stitzel RE (eds.). *Modern Pharmacology* (4th ed.). Boston: Little, Brown, 1994.

Edwards W. Optimizing Opioid Treatment of Postoperative Pain. *J Pain Symptom Manage* 5:S24–36, 1990.

Fields HL. *Pain*. New York: McGraw-Hill, 1987. Pp. 251–279.

Jaffe J and Martin W. Opioid Analgesics and Antagonists. In: A Gilman, et al (eds), *Goodman and Gilman's The Pharmacological Basis of Therapeutics*. New York: Pergamon Press, 1990.

Physician's Desk Reference. Oradell, NJ: Medical Economics, [annual].

5

Choosing a Pharmacotherapeutic Approach: Nonopioid and Adjuvant Analgesics

Shaffin A. Mohamed, Khyati Mohamed, and David Borsook

> *"Take an aspirin and call me in the morning."*
>
> TWENTIETH CENTURY PHYSICIAN

We use non-narcotic adjuvant medications to supplement narcotic analgesics in the treatment of acute and chronic pain. However, unlike our long experience with opioids, our experience with adjuvant medications for pain management remains limited. Inter- and intrapatient variability in response to these medications, in part due to psychologic components, also complicates their investigation and use. The successful administration of these medications depends on a practitioner's ability to titrate them to the clinically desired effect, while attempting to avoid undesired side effects. We often start only one drug at a time, to more easily monitor therapeutic and adverse effects.

The four main drug classes that we most often employ in the care of painful conditions are: (1) **nonsteroidal anti-inflammatory drugs** (NSAIDs), (2) **antidepressants**, (3) **anticonvulsants**, and (4) **neuroleptics**. Some medications are more successful in the treatment of specific conditions, and we discuss a rationale for drug selection with each drug group. We also briefly discuss medications that do not fit into these classes but have demonstrated therapeutic benefits.

Nonopioid Analgesics

Nonopioid analgesics primarily consist of the salicylates, the para-aminophenols, and the NSAIDs.

SALICYLATES

Salicylates are a family of analgesics, of which acetylsalicylic acid (aspirin) is the prototypic compound. In addition to being analgesic, these drugs have anti-inflammatory and antipyretic effects (Tables 5-1 and 5-2).

Mechanism of Action

Aspirin and all NSAIDs irreversibly inhibit cyclo-oxygenase in peripheral tissue, and therefore interfere with prostaglan-

Table 5-1. Nonsteroidal anti-inflammatory drugs

Drug	Duration (hr)	Dosage (mg)	Interval (hr)	Maximum daily dose (mg/d)	Half-life (hr)	Time to peak (hr)
Acetylsalicylic acid (aspirin)	4-6	325-1000	q4-6	4000	2-4	2
Choline magnesium trisalicylate (Trilisate)	8-12	1000-1500	q8-12	3000	2-30	0.5-1.0
Diflunisal (Dolobid)	8-12	1000 load, then 500	q8-12	1500	8-20	1-2
Salsalate (Disalcid)	8-12	500-750	q6-8	3000	2-30	0.5-1.0

Table 5-2. Dosing data for nonsteroidal anti-inflammatory drugs

Drug	Dosage (mg)	Dose interval (hr)	Maximum daily dose (mg/d)	Peak effect (hr)	Half-life (hr)
Diclofenac	25–75	6–8	200	2	1–2
Etodolac acid	200–400	6–8	1200	1–2	7
Fenoprofen	200	4–6	3200	1–2	2–3
Flurbiprofen	50–100	6–8	300	1.5–3.0	3–4
Ibuprofen	200–400	6–8	3200	1–2	2
Indomethacin	25–75	6–8	200	0.5–1.0	2–3
Ketoprofen	25–75	6–8	300	1–2	1.5–2.0
Ketorolac*					
Oral	10	6–8	40	0.5–1.0	6
Parenteral	60 load, then 30	6–8	120 (use no longer than 5 d)		
Meclofenamic acid	500 load, then 275	6–8	400	2–4	3–4
Mefenamic acid	500 load, then 250	6	1250	3–5	22–30
Nabumetone	1000–2000	12–24	2000	2–4	12–15
Naproxen	500 load, then 250	6–8	1250	1–2	13
Naproxen sodium	550 load, then 275	6–8	1375	2	3–3.5
Oxaprozin	60–1200	Every day	1800	2	50–100
Phenylbutazone	100	6–8	400	2	
Piroxicam	40 load, then 20	24	20	2–4	36–45
Sulindac	150–200	12	400	1–2	7–18
Tolmetin	200–400	8	1800	4–6	2

*Use no longer than 5 days.

din-induced inflammation and sensitization of primary afferent terminals. New enzyme synthesis overcomes this effect.

Indications

1. Acute pain, mild to severe in nature (e.g., headache, postoperative, and postpartum)
2. Rheumatoid arthritis and osteoarthritis
3. Neuralgia
4. Myalgia
5. Dysmenorrhea
6. Mild to severe bone pain secondary to cancer

Contraindications

1. Hypersensitivity to salicylates (patients with asthma and nasal polyps are at high risk)
2. Bleeding ulcers
3. Hemophilia
4. Vitamin K deficiency
5. Hypoprothrombinemia
6. Liver damage/disease
7. Renal disease

Pharmacology

Salicylate compounds are rapidly absorbed from the stomach and upper small intestine. Peak plasma concentrations occur in 1 to 2 hours. There is a high first-pass effect in the small intestine and liver. The compound remains primarily plasma bound. Metabolism occurs mainly in the liver, and is dose dependent. For salicylate, the elimination half-life is 2 to 3 hours for low doses, and as long as 30 hours for high doses. Excretion is renal and fecal for conjugated forms.

Choline magnesium trisalicylate has a longer half-life than aspirin and can therefore be given twice a day. Diflunisal also has a long half-life that permits twice-a-day administration. However, diflunisal has a slower onset and requires a loading dose to reach effective plasma concentrations.

Dosing Regimen

Clinical Guidelines

Aspirin is an effective analgesic for certain types of mild to moderate pain (see Indications). One must consider its side effects, especially if the plan is to use it for more than a few days. The most significant side effect for those who take aspirin and NSAIDs is gastric problems, ranging from epigastric distress and nausea and vomiting to erosive gastritis, peptic ulcer disease, and gastrointestinal hemorrhage—all of which are results of mucosal cell damage by aspirin. H_2 blockers and sucralfate are ineffective in preventing these problems. Other options include enteric coating, coadministration of misoprostol (Cytotec; a prostaglandin E_1 analog), and judicious use of one of the other salicylate preparations (i.e., diflunisal, choline magnesium trisalicylate, and salsalate).

Coadministration of aspirin and oral anticoagulants may cause severe gastrointestinal bleeding.

Drug Administration

1. Choice of drug: Consider drug effects, side effects, and effectiveness
2. Initial dosing (see Tables 5-1 and 5-2)
3. Maintenance dosing (see Tables 5-1 and 5-2)
4. Combinations: Consider potential drug interactions and maximum dosages
5. Adverse effects (as discussed below)

Apart from gastric effects (discussed above), the other major adverse effect of all salicylates, except for choline magnesium trisalicylate, is their irreversible **inhibitory effect on platelet aggregation**. A single therapeutic dose inhibits platelet function for its 7-day lifetime, inhibits hemostasis, and prolongs bleeding time. Aspirin inhibits the function of cyclic endoperoxides, which are necessary for thromboxane synthesis. This may produce occult GI hemorrhage and iron-deficiency anemia, as well as hemorrhage. GI and platelet function adverse effects appear less frequently after administering nonaspirin salicylate preparations, and more frequently in patients who receive steroids or chemotherapy.

Furthermore, aspirin **hypersensitivity reactions** have been reported, but occur through an unknown mechanism. There are two types of reactions: respiratory effects including rhinitis, asthma, or nasal polyps; and urticaria, wheals, angioneurotic edema, hypotension, shock, and syncope. These reactions occur within 1 hour following ingestion. This sensitivity also extends to NSAID ingestion.

Liver damage in otherwise healthy adults occurs uncommonly, but exacerbation of preexisting liver disease may occur. Renal tubular damage occurs in patients with renal impairment.

CNS toxicity manifests as headaches and ototoxicity. Ototoxicity manifests as reversible deafness, tinnitus, and dizziness.

Mild, chronic salicylate intoxication, where salicylate plasma levels approach or exceed 30 mg/dl, can result in **salicylism**. Symptoms are headaches, tinnitus, diminished hearing, malaise, fatigue, thirst, hyperventilation, GI symptoms, restlessness, cognitive impairment, and visual impairment. Severe salicylism can result in hallucinations, delirium, and convulsions. Salicylism is more common in children and the elderly.

PARA-AMINOPHENOL DERIVATIVES (ACETAMINOPHEN)

These drugs have analgesic and antipyretic properties but are practically devoid of anti-inflammatory activity. Acetaminophen has no antiplatelet effect and is equipotent to aspirin, but without aspirin's adverse effects (see Table 5-2).

Properties and Administration of Acetaminophen

Drug	Dosage (mg)	Interval (hr)	Maximum daily dose (mg/d)	Time to peak (hr)	Half-life (hr)
Acetaminophen (Tylenol)	325–1000	q4–6	4000	0.5–1.0	2–3

Mechanism of Action

Acetaminophen has only minimal anti-inflammatory effects. It is inhibitory to brain, but not to peripheral cyclo-oxygenase. This central action may result in antipyresis, analgesia, and the absence of anti-inflammatory effects.

Indications

1. Mild to moderate acute pain of noninflammatory origin
2. Musculoskeletal pain, nonarthritic
3. Headaches
4. Fever, particularly for patients who are sensitive to aspirin and for children

Contraindications

1. Glucose-6-phosphate dehydrogenase deficiency
2. Alcoholism
3. Active liver disease

Pharmacology

Acetaminophen is rapidly absorbed from the GI tract and reaches peak plasma concentrations in 30 to 60 minutes. Metabolism occurs in the liver, and excretion is renally. The minor metabolites may produce hepatotoxicity, in the event of an overdose. Plasma protein-binding is negligible, and the elimination half-life is 2 to 3 hours.

Dosing Regimen

Clinical Guidelines

In a patient with normal renal and hepatic function, steady-state plasma concentrations can occur in a day, with a fixed dose and dosing interval. Around-the-clock dosing, as opposed to prn dosing, results in better pain control and use of less drug.

Drug Administration

DOSING. 1000 mg q4h for 24 hours, followed by 500–1000 mg q4–6 h, should provide adequate plasma levels. Doses over 1000 mg yield little additional analgesia, owing to a flat dose-response curve.

COMBINATIONS. Acetaminophen is often sold in combination with narcotics for additional analgesic effects.

ADVERSE EFFECTS. In therapeutic doses, acetaminophen produces relatively few side effects. Hematologic, GI, and cardiovascular adverse reactions rarely occur. In excessive doses, alcoholism, and active liver disease, hepatotoxicity can occur, including jaundice and fatal hepatic necrosis. Hypersensitivity to acetaminophen is rare, and there is no cross-sensitivity with aspirin.

NONSTEROIDAL ANTI-INFLAMMATORY DRUGS

NSAIDs are a heterogeneous class of drugs grouped together on the basis of their anti-inflammatory, antipyretic, and analgesic therapeutic effects. We classify them into two main chemical groups: **acidic** and **nonacidic**. The acidic NSAIDs also consist of two main groups: **enolic acids** and **carboxylic acids** (see Table 5-4 for further classification). In addition, there is a new group of nonacidic NSAIDs: the naphthylalkanones. One member, nabumetone, a newly available NSAID, is purported to be less toxic to the GI tract (Tables 5-2 and 5-3).

Table 5-3. The nonsteroidal anti-inflammatory drugs

Acidic NSAIDs
Carboxylic acids
Propionic acids
    Ibuprofen (Motrin, Nuprin)
    Naproxen (Naprosyn)
    Naproxen sodium (Anaprox)
    Fenoprofen (Nalfon)
    Ketoprofen (Orudis)
    Flurbiprofen (Ansaid)
    Oxaprozin (Daypro)
Anthranilic acids
    Mefenamic acid (Ponstel)
    Meclofenamic acid (Meclomen)
Acetic acids
    Indoleacetic acids
        Indomethacin (Indocin)
        Sulindac (Clinoril)
        Etodolac acid (Lodine)
    Pyrroleacetic acids
        Tolmetin (Tolectin)
        Ketorolac (Toradol)
    Phenylacetic acids
        Diclofenac (Voltaren)
Enolic acids
Pyrazolones
    Phenylbutazone (Butazolidin)
Benzothiazines (oxicams)
    Piroxicam (Feldene)
Nonacidic NSAIDs
Naphthylalkanones
Nabumetone (Relafen)

Mechanism of Action

NSAIDs have both peripheral and central effects. The antipyretic effects occur centrally, through the hypothalamus. The analgesic effects occur peripherally. However, emerging evidence suggests a central component, through facilitation of the endogenous inhibitory descending pain pathways. The predominant theory suggests that NSAIDs, like aspirin, act peripherally to prevent prostaglandin synthesis, and thereby reduce inflammation and pain. Prostaglandin synthesis is prevented by inhibiting cyclo-oxygenase. Cyclo-oxygenase converts arachidonic acid from damaged cells into prostaglandins D, E, and F, prostacyclin, and thromboxane.

Indications

1. Pain due to acute inflammation
2. Arthritis
3. Headaches
4. Myalgia
5. Cancer pain, especially associated with (a) bone pain due to periosteal distention, e.g., bony metastases, (b) soft-tissue pain due to compression or distention of tissues, and (c) visceral pain due to irritation of pleura or peritoneum.
6. Mild to moderate pain of noninflammatory origin

Contraindications

1. Active peptic ulcer disease
2. Esophagitis
3. Bleeding disorders
4. Near-term pregnancy

Pharmacology

NSAIDs are usually rapidly absorbed in the small intestine and stomach following oral administration. Over 90% of the drugs bind to serum albumin. This high level of protein-binding results in a low volume of distribution. Peak plasma levels appear in 1 to 2 hours (except with piroxicam). Extensive liver metabolism occurs. Excretion occurs by the kidney, except for a small fecal component. Drug interactions can occur, particularly with respect to protein binding (e.g., concurrent use of warfarin).

Dosing Regimen

Clinical Guidelines

One of the dozen-plus commonly available NSAIDs can be prescribed for mild to moderate chronic pain. Once the indications for NSAID usage have been satisfied, one must decide on the particular drug. Aspirin—in its original formulation, one of its newer derivatives, or one of its coated preparations—is often the initial choice. A failed trial leads to other NSAIDs, but which one? We find significant interpatient variability, even under the same clinical conditions. In addition, we find a paucity of data on clinical efficacy among the NSAIDs. Hence the search for an NSAID for a given patient involves trial and error. An adequate trial should be performed, beginning with a low dosage, then increasing to the maximum dosage for a period of time, and with careful monitoring for response and adverse effects. In addition to efficacy, individual variation, and the nature of the disease, there are a few other factors that might be considered prior to choosing an NSAID. Adverse effects can be significant, and some NSAIDs appear to be more safe than others, with diminished side-effect profiles. In general, the older drugs such as indomethacin and phenylbutazone appear to have very significant adverse effects and should be reserved for conditions where therapeutic benefit justifies the increased risk, for example, in a cancer pain patient who has had adverse reactions to steroids and who has failed prior trials of less potent NSAIDs.

Inflammation appears to contribute strongly to painful conditions. Hence, an NSAID with anti-inflammatory and analgesic actions should be selected over a purely analgesic one, and vice versa.

Once safety has been considered, other issues such as convenient dosing and cost should be considered. Age does not appear to affect dosing; however, pregnancy and hepatorenal function should be considered.

Furthermore, there is no evidence to support the practice of prescribing more than one NSAID at a time, despite the theoretic claim that this practice may reduce side effects. Finally, a number of drug interactions with NSAIDs have been reported. The combination of aspirin and NSAIDs may result in decreased efficacy or increased efficacy, or may be purely additive. As the exact result is not predictable, combination prescriptions are not recommended.

Drug Administration

DOSING (SEE TABLE 5-2)

ADVERSE EFFECTS. Generally, short-term use of NSAIDs results in few adverse effects, except in particularly sensitive patients. In these sensitive patients, NSAIDs can precipitate **asthma** and **anaphylactoid reactions**. This reaction is also seen with aspirin. NSAIDs also inhibit platelet aggregation, but through a reversible effect on prostaglandin synthetase. Platelet function returns with drug elimination. Reversible agranulocytosis is a rare complication.

Prostaglandin production in the GI tract decreases acid production and produces a protective mucosal coat. Prostaglandin inhibition by NSAIDs can result in **peptic ulceration**, gastric bleeding, and perforation, with or without symptoms.

Renal failure syndromes and hepatic dysfunction can occur with use of NSAIDs, particularly in patients with related histories. NSAIDs can also cause mild fluid retention, which is worse in patients with a history of fluid retention. Uricosuria is also a known effect that is used in the treatment of gout. CNS toxicity manifests as cognitive dysfunction and mood alteration, particularly in the elderly. Headaches and dizziness can also occur.

Adjuvant Analgesics

ANTIDEPRESSANTS

Antidepressants are used in the treatment of a variety of chronic pain syndromes. They appear to have an analgesic effect separate from their antidepressant effect. This group includes the tricyclic antidepressants (TCAs), the monoamine oxidase (MAO) inhibitors, as well as the tetracyclics and other nonpolycyclic antidepressants. (Table 5-4).

Mechanism of Action

Tricyclic Antidepressants

It does not appear that pain relief from antidepressants occurs only through the alleviation of depression. TCAs block reuptake of norepinephrine (NE) and serotonin (5-HT). NE and 5-HT are known to be involved in the endorphin-mediated pain modulation pathways at the central (descending) and spinal cord levels. **Note:** Agents with pure 5-HT uptake blocking effects have **not** been shown to clinically produce analgesia in neuropathic pain states.

Monoamine Oxidase Inhibitors

MAO inhibitors inhibit monoamine oxidase, an enzyme present in the CNS, adrenergic nerve endings, liver, and GI tract. Blocking oxidative deamination of synaptic monoamine neurotransmitters results in increased levels of NE and 5-HT in the cytoplasm of the nerve terminals. As with the TCAs, it is unclear how these elevated monoamine levels result in analgesia.

Indications

1. Arthritis
2. Headaches—migraine, tension
3. Cancer pain, particularly nerve injury pain
4. Lower back pain
5. Neuropathic pain (e.g., diabetic neuropathy, trigeminal neuralgia, postherpetic neuralgia, causalgia, phantom limb pain, postoperative scar pain, perineal neuralgia, fibrositis, chest wall pain)
6. Fibromyositis (fibrositis)
7. Myofascial pain

Contraindications

1. Significant cardiac arrhythmias
2. Symptomatic prostatic hypertrophy
3. Narrow-angle glaucoma

Table 5-4. Antidepressants

Drug	Dosage (mg)	Usual daily dose (mg)	Anticholinergic activity	Central action	Hypotension	Sedation
Amitriptyline (Elavil)*	10–300	75–150	Strong	S(N)	Strong	Strong
Amoxapine (Asendin)	50–400	50–200	Minimal	N	Mild	Minimal
Bupropion (Wellbutrin)	50–100	50–300	Minimal	N/A	Minimal	Minimal
Clomipramine (Anafranil)*	25–250	20–150	Moderate	S(N)	Strong	Mild
Desipramine (Norpramin)*	75–300	50–150	Minimal	N	Mild	Minimal
Doxepin (Sinequan)	30–300	30–150	Moderate	S	Strong	Mild
Fluoxetine (Prozac)	5–80	20–40	Minimal	S	Minimal	Minimal
Imipramine (Tofranil)*	20–300	20–150	Moderate	N/S	Moderate	Moderate
Isocarboxazid (Marplan)	10–40	10–40	Minimal	MAOI	Mild	Moderate
Maprotiline (Ludiomil)	75–300	75–150	Mild	N	Mild	Mild
Nortriptyline (Pamelor)*	25–150	50–150	Mild	N/S	Moderate	Mild
Phenelzine (Nardil)	15–90	45–75	Mild	MAOI	Mild	Moderate
Protriptyline (Vivactil)	15–60	15–40	Moderate	N	Minimal	Mild
Sertraline (Zoloft)	50–200	50–100	Mild	S	Minimal	Mild
Tranylcypromine (Parnate)	10–45	10–20	Minimal	MAOI	Moderate	Mild
Trazodone (Desyrel)	50–600	150–300	Minimal	S	Moderate	Minimal
Trimipramine (Surmontil)	50–200	75–150	Moderate	S(N)	Strong	Mild

*Commonly used for neuropathic pain.
S = serotonergic, N = noradrenergic, (N) = weakly noradrenergic, MAOI = monoamine oxidase inhibitor.

Pharmacokinetics

TCAs are well absorbed after oral administration. They undergo rapid first-pass hepatic metabolism and reach peak plasma concentrations 2 to 8 hours after oral intake. Therapeutic plasma concentrations for depression range from 100 to 300 ng/ml, with toxicity occurring at levels above 500 ng/ml. Therapeutic concentrations for pain treatment are not known, and levels are generally monitored to verify compliance or toxicity. TCAs are highly protein bound and very lipophilic, resulting in a large volume of distribution (V_d), up to 50 L/kg. The drugs are oxidized by the hepatic microsomal system and conjugated with glucuronic acid. The extensive metabolism of the TCAs and their active metabolites takes up to a week, with elimination half-lives averaging 1 to 4 days. Elimination is via urine and feces. The long elimination half-life and wide range of therapeutic plasma concentrations permit once a day dosing.

Dose Regimen

Clinical Guidelines

There is little evidence to support choosing one antidepressant over another. Hence, drugs are chosen not for the therapeutic outcome, but by matching the patient's needs to the drug's side-effect profile. For example, if a patient's sleep pattern has been disturbed, then a sedating drug may be more useful.

Baseline blood studies, liver function tests, hemoglobin, and blood count should be obtained. In patients with a cardiac history, or in the elderly, a baseline ECG should be obtained. Doses should be started slowly to avoid alarming side effects, which may decrease compliance, prior to onset of therapeutic action. Daytime sedation may be overcome in 3 to 4 days, or the dose must be altered. This can sometimes be countered by taking the medication earlier in the evening to prevent sedation the next day. Anticholinergic side effects may be persistent, necessitating a change in medications. **Desipramine and nortriptyline are the least sedating TCAs.** However, for these agents **daytime doses** should be used, because insomnia may result from nocturnal administration. Although these drugs are considered nonaddictive, when stopping their usage, they should be tapered to prevent the unlikely possibility of insomnia, agitation, or mood alterations.

MAO inhibitors require similar baseline blood tests, avoidance of certain medications (TCAs, opioids, sympathomimetics), and the institution of a tyramine-free diet. The analgesic effectiveness of MAO inhibitors is not well documented.

Drug Administration

CHOICE OF DRUG. Based on a comparison of patient profile to a drug's side-effect profile.

INITIAL DOSING. Begin with a low dose and increase regularly until therapeutic effects or intolerable side effects are

reached. This regimen decreases adverse effects and increases compliance. For example, amitriptyline is started at
25 mg PO at bedtime and increased every 1 to 3 days until
a therapeutic dosage or 150 mg/d is reached. It may be
started at 10 mg PO at bedtime in the elderly. If adverse
effects occur, a lower dosage should be continued until a therapeutic effect is noted or until 3 weeks pass. After 1 week at
150 mg/d, if there are no side effects and if no contraindications exist, the dose may be increased by 25 mg every 1 to 3
days to the maximal dose, i.e., 300 mg/d for amitriptyline. If
there is no therapeutic effect after another 3 weeks, the drug
should be tapered. Dosages should be decreased with age, and
slower rates of administration should be employed.

MAINTENANCE ADMINISTRATION. Once maximal therapeutic
response has been achieved, for at lease 1 month, the dosage
can be decreased (10–25 mg) slowly (every 1–2 weeks). Relapse of pain should be closely monitored. After 3 to 6 months
of sustained remission, drug therapy should be slowly tapered in small amounts. If this is not possible, attempts
should be made every 6 months.

NONRESPONSE OR RELAPSE. If the first antidepressant is ineffective, five options are available:

1. If the patient is tolerating the drug, blood level should be
   checked and, if nontoxic, the dose can be increased to a
   therapeutic level.
2. If the first drug has a serotonergic effect and fails, a drug
   with a stronger norepinephrine effect may be substituted,
   and a trial initiated.
3. A neuroleptic may be added to the antidepressant, starting at low dosages of the neuroleptic. If the combination
   is successful, the antidepressant can be tapered, since the
   neuroleptic may be effective alone. If the combination remains ineffective, both should be tapered over 7 to 10
   days.
4. An anticonvulsant may be added to the antidepressant or
   the antidepressant–neuroleptic combination. Success or
   failure should be treated as outlined above (3).
5. Taper the tricyclic and institute an MAO inhibitor, particularly in patients with depressive symptoms. A 2-week
   washout period between the two regimens is necessary to
   prevent drug interactions and adverse effects.

ADVERSE EFFECTS OF TCAS. Apart from the rare **hypersensitivity reactions** (cholestatic jaundice, skin reactions,
agranulocytosis), adverse effects fall into three main groups:
CNS effects, cardiovascular effects, and anticholinergic effects. In addition, drug interactions are prominent in patients
receiving sympathomimetics, inhaled anesthetics, anticholin-
ergics, antihypertensives, and opioids.

1. **CNS** effects appear mainly as sedation but may also result
   in tremors, seizures, insomnia, and delirium.
2. **Cardiovascular effects** are seen as dysrhythmias, particularly atrial and ventricular conduction defects. In addition, orthostatic hypotension may be present owing to
   alpha-adrenergic blockade.

3. **Anticholinergic autonomic effects** manifest as xerostomia, palpitations, visual disturbances, constipation, urinary retention, orthostatic hypotension, paralytic ileus, loss of consciousness, and sexual dysfunction.

ADVERSE EFFECTS OF MAO INHIBITORS. The most common side effects in pain patients are nausea, sedation, weight gain, and dizziness. In addition, orthostatic hypotension may be seen. The interaction of opioids and MAO inhibitors, particularly meperidine, can result in hyperpyrexia and hypermetabolism. Tyramine ingestion, sympathomimetics, and TCAs can result in a hypertensive crisis. Rare reactions include peripheral neuropathy and parenchymal hepatotoxic reactions.

ANTICONVULSANTS

This is a heterogeneous group of drugs usually used in the treatment of seizures, some of which have proven analgesic effects in pain patients. Anticonvulsants appear to benefit patients suffering from neurogenic pain, owing to damage or dysfunction of nerves in the peripheral or central nervous systems. There are four anticonvulsants that are useful in neuropathic pain states—namely, carbamazepine, phenytoin, valproic acid, and clonazepam (Table 5-5).

Mechanism of Action

Although the mechanisms of action for the four analgesic anticonvulsants are different, the mechanisms that underlie their anticonvulsant actions must contribute to their analgesic actions (i.e., the pathophysiology of epilepsy and neurogenic pain may be similar).

1. Phenytoin is believed to have a stabilizing effect on neuronal membranes and can alter sodium, calcium, and potassium flux.
2. Carbamazepine is chemically and pharmacologically related to tricyclic antidepressants and inhibits norepinephrine uptake, and also prevents repeated discharges in neurons. This observation is consistent with its ability to relieve lancinating pain in neuralgia states.
3. Valproic acid is believed to increase the inhibitory activity of gamma-aminobutyric acid (GABA) through interference with GABA transaminase.
4. Clonazepam, a benzodiazepine with anticonvulsant activity, appears to act through enhancement of GABA inhibitory activity, which results in decreased firing of neurons.
5. The analgesic effects of newer agents such as Gabapentin and Lamotrigine are not yet known.

Indications

1. Neuralgia—trigeminal, glossopharyngeal, and postherpetic
2. Neuralgia secondary to peripheral nervous and central nervous systems infiltration by cancer
3. Central pain states (e.g., thalamic pain syndrome and poststroke pain)

Table 5-5. Anticonvulsants

Drug	Half-life (hr)	Therapeutic blood levels, seizures (μg/ml)	Toxic concentration (μg/ml)	Maximum daily dose (mg/d)
Carbamazepine (Tegretol)	10–20	4–12	>8–10	1500
Clonazepam (Klonopin)	18–30	0.02–0.08	>0.06	6
Phenytoin (Dilantin)	6–24	10–20	>20	500
Valproic acid (Depakote)	12	50–100	>100–150	1500–2000 (60 mg/kg per day)

 4. Postsympathectomy pain
 5. Posttraumatic neuralgia
 6. Porphyria, Fabry's disease, and others
 7. Painful diabetic neuropathy
 8. Paroxysmal pain in multiple sclerosis
 9. Migraine headaches
10. Phantom limb pain and postamputation stump pain
11. Peripheral neuropathy secondary to a variety of disease states: e.g.: alcoholism, amyloidosis, diabetes mellitus, HIV/AIDS, malabsorption, porphyria, toxic exposure, sarcoidosis, drug induced.)

Pharmacology

Phenytoin

Phenytoin has variable absorption orally. Its peak serum level is reached 3 to 12 hours after the dose, but generally in 4 to 8 hours. It is highly protein bound and has a normal 10% free fraction, which varies with serum protein levels. Low serum protein levels might result in an elevated free fraction and toxicity at otherwise therapeutic levels. Metabolism is hepatic, with a serum half-life of approximately 24 hours.

Carbamazepine

Carbamazepine is absorbed slowly and unpredictably after oral intake. Peak concentrations are seen in 2 to 8 hours. It is moderately protein bound and has active metabolites. Metabolism is hepatic and excretions are urinary. It has a serum half-life of 10 to 20 hours, averaging 14 hours.

Valproic Acid

Valproic acid has a rapid oral absorption, with peak concentrations in 1 to 4 hours. It is highly protein bound; it undergoes hepatic metabolism, and it is renally excreted. Its half-life is 10 to 12 hours in serum.

Clonazepam

Clonazepam has good oral absorption, with a peak serum concentration in 1 to 4 hours. It is moderately protein bound; it undergoes hepatic metabolism to inactive metabolites; and it is renally excreted. It has a serum half-life of approximately 24 hours.

Dosing Regimen

Clinical Guidelines

These drugs are found to be most effective in the management of paroxysmal lancinating dysesthesias associated with neuropathic pain syndromes, and less so with continuous neuropathic pain.

Although carbamazepine is considered the drug of choice for the treatment of trigeminal neuralgia, the significant potential for side effects usually limits the use of these medications to manage painful conditions refractory to other therapy.

In addition to a complete history and physical examination, complete blood count and liver function baseline tests are recommended. In addition, the blood tests should be followed monthly for the first year, and quarterly thereafter. The medications should be tapered prior to cessation to prevent withdrawal symptoms.

Serum levels do not appear to correlate well with pain response, but the potential for many side effects and toxicity mandates periodic evaluation of the serum level. Doses are generally increased until therapeutic effects or limiting adverse effects are observed, or until plasma concentrations approach high anticonvulsant toxic levels.

Drug Administration

CHOICE OF DRUG. A trial of carbamazepine or phenytoin is usually initiated prior to trials of valproic acid or clonazepam.

INITIAL DOSING

Phenytoin:
In average adult patients start 100 mg tid, check the blood level in 3 weeks, and follow clinical response. The toxic blood level is over 20 μg/ml. Phenytoin should be taken after meals to avoid irritation.

Carbamazepine:
Start 200 mg/d and increase by 200 mg every 1 to 3 days to a maximum of 1500 mg/d. If side effects are encountered, the dose is decreased to the previous level for several days, and then gradually increased. Therapeutic doses usually range from 800 to 1200 mg/d. Carbamazepine may depress hematopoiesis; therefore, biweekly CBCs are recommended; later, monthly CBCs should suffice. Carbamazepine is also a gastric irritant, so should be taken with food.

Valproic Acid:
Start 15 mg/kg per day in divided doses. Increase weekly by 5–10 mg/kg per day until it becomes clinically therapeutic or the maximum dose of 60 mg/kg per day is reached. Baseline and periodic liver function tests are recommended, because fatal hepatic failure has been reported. More commonly, though, is the occurrence of reversible liver enzyme dysfunction.

Clonazepam:
Start 0.5 mg tid and increase by 0.5 mg every 3 to 4 days until an adequate response is achieved or a maximum dose of 6 mg/d is attained. The usual therapeutic pain dosage range is 1–4 mg/d. Clonazepam should be taken at bedtime, owing to its sedative effects. Ataxia and dizziness are sometimes noted early in the course of drug therapy, but improve with continued use.

MAINTENANCE. In some patients, attempts at tapering and discontinuation are successful, but often therapy is maintained at initially achieved therapeutic dosages. These medications should not be discontinued abruptly, but should be tapered over a period of time to avoid withdrawal symptoms.

ADVERSE EFFECTS. These medications have great side-effect potential, and their individual side-effect profiles are quite different.

Phenytoin:
Cerebellar-vestibular dysfunction, allergic reactions (skin rash), GI irritation, hepatotoxicity, and fetal hydantoin syndrome can occur with phenytoin. Folic acid deficiency can also occur, resulting in peripheral neuropathy and megaloblastic anemia. Other side effects include fibrocyte stimulation, producing gingival hyperplasia and requiring meticulous oral hygiene; and hyperglycemia and glycosuria, due to phenytoin-induced inhibition of insulin secretion.

Carbamazepine:
Sedation, nausea, diplopia, and vertigo occur most frequently with this drug. Hematologic abnormalities such as aplastic anemia, **agranulocytosis**, pancytopenia and thrombocytopenia can occur, as well as hepatocellular and cholestatic jaundice, oliguria, hypertension, and **acute left ventricular heart failure**. Hence, regular blood work must be performed.

Valproic Acid:
GI symptoms such as nausea, vomiting, anorexia, and diarrhea can occur, but improve with time. Sedation, tremors, and ataxia are occasionally seen, as are platelet aggregation effects. Hepatotoxicity can also occur.

Clonazepam:
Lethargy and **sedation**, which subside with chronic treatment, are often seen. Psychologic disinhibitory changes occur and are manifested as mood disturbances and delirium. A withdrawal syndrome, including seizures, can occur with abrupt discontinuation of therapy.

NEUROLEPTICS (Antipsychotics)

The neuroleptic or antipsychotic medications are considered second-line adjuvant drugs that occasionally are useful for the treatment of adverse effects of opioids such as nausea (Table 5-6).

Mechanism of Action

The exact mechanisms of neuroleptic analgesia have not been eludicated, but several hypotheses have been debated. The antipsychotic actions are not believed to be involved, i.e., pain relief occurs in the absence of psychosis. The antipsychotic actions apparently occur through postsynaptic dopamine receptor blockade. Neuroleptics also block adrenergic and muscarinic effects, as well as serotonin and histamine transmission. None of these appears to contribute to the neuroleptics' analgesic effects, though. The chemical structure of neuroleptics and opiates is similar, and neuroleptics apparently bind to opiate receptors. However, the action of neuroleptics on the endorphin-mediated analgesia system as well as their analgesic actions remains elusive. These medications are most

Table 5-6. Neuroleptic agents

Drug	Initial dose (mg)	Maintenance dose (mg)	ACE	Sedation	Hypotension	EPS
Chlorpromazine (Thorazine)	75–500	25–150	High	High	High	Low
Chlorprothixene (Taractan)	50–200	80–150	High	High	High	Low
Fluphenazine (Prolixin)	1–10	1–3	Low	Low	Low	High
Haloperidol (Haldol)	0.5–30.0	0.5–10.0	Low	Moderate	Low	High
Methotrimeprazine (Levoprome)*	5–100	10–50	High	High	High	Moderate
Perphenazine (Trilafon)	8–64	4–16	Moderate	Moderate	Moderate	Moderate
Thioridazine (Mellaril)	10–200	25–75	High	High	High	Low

*Available in parenteral form only.
ACE = anticholinergic effects; EPS = extrapyramidal side effects.

frequently used to promote sedation and prevent nausea. Haloperidol may be useful in the treatment of drug-induced delirium.

Indications

1. Conscious sedation for terminal cancer pain patients
2. Excruciating pain with anxiety

Pharmacology

These drugs are absorbed well on oral intake. Highly variable blood levels result from a significant enterohepatic "first-pass" effect, however. They are avidly protein bound and lipophilic, crossing the blood-brain barrier easily. Neuroleptics accumulate in brain tissue in disproportionately high amounts. Metabolism is extensive in the liver and is followed by urinary, biliary, and fecal excretion. Half-lives of the neuroleptics generally range from 24 to 40 hours, allowing "at bedtime" dosing and masking sedative effects. Tremendous inter- and intrapatient variability prevents the use of serum drug levels to guide therapy.

Dosing Regimen

Clinical Guidelines

Neuroleptics should be viewed as second-line agents. In light of their potential side effects and the limited supporting clinical data, these drugs should be used following a rigorous risk-benefit analysis, and only when trials with other adjuvant analgesics are contraindicated or have proved unsuccessful.

Preadministration evaluation should consist of a routine history and physical examination, particularly for signs of parkinsonism, movement disorders, and liver disease. Baseline laboratory studies should include liver tests, urinalysis, a CBC, and an ECG in older patients. In addition, written consent should be obtained prior to starting neuroleptic therapy, because of the risk of irreversible tardive dyskinesia.

Antipsychotic drug trials should be started at the lowest possible doses and then titrated up to the lowest dosage that offers relief. Periodic attempts (approximately every 3 months) should be made to taper and stop the medications, so the period of therapy is the shortest possible. Office visits should include thorough examinations for changed motor patterns or new-onset involuntary movements. These medications do not produce addiction or physical dependence, but abrupt discontinuation may result in insomnia and unusual discomfort.

Drug Administration

CHOICE OF DRUG. There is no evidence to support greater effectiveness of one neuroleptic over another. The clinician usually selects one on the basis of experience and side-effect profile. The side effects of major concern include dopaminergic blockade–induced extrapyramidal side effects, sedation, anticholinergic effects, and orthostatic hypotension. The high-potency neuroleptics, such as haloperidol and fluphenazine, produce less sedation and less orthostatic hypotension, but extrapyramidal symptoms occur more acutely and more commonly with these drugs. The low-potency neuroleptics, such as chlorpromazine and thioridazine, exhibit greater sedative and antimuscarinic effects, as well as enhanced alpha$_1$-adrenergic blockade. However, extrapyramidal side effects can occur with all the neuroleptics. Tolerance to the sedating effects may occur with continued use.

INITIAL DOSING. Doses of neuroleptics should be given slowly and at night to avoid daytime sedation. Daytime dosing should be started if nocturnal administration does not adequately control symptoms. The high-potency medications —namely, haloperidol and fluphenazine—should be started with a 1-mg oral test dose, or 0.25–0.5 mg in the elderly. If tolerated, the dosage should be increased by 1 mg/d to 3–5 mg/d, the usual therapeutic dosage for pain. If no response occurs within 1 week, the dosage may be increased by 1 mg/d to 8–10 mg/d and reevaluated in 2 weeks. If no effect is seen at the maximum tolerable dosage, the drug is tapered and discontinued.

The low-potency drugs are also started at bedtime, in lower dosages, and increased to therapeutic dosages, as tolerated by the patient. Chlorpromazine is known to be therapeutic as an analgesic at the antipsychotic levels, as opposed to the high-potency antipsychotics. Chlorpromazine is reportedly effective at about 400 mg/d. Perphenazine is usually effective in the 4–12 mg range and chlorprothixene in the 25–50 mg range, several times a day.

MAINTENANCE DOSING. Owing to the high risk of adverse events, the dose is tailored to suit the patient's needs, and frequent attempts should be made (every 3 months) to lower the dosage and discontinue the medication.

ADVERSE EFFECTS. The neuroleptics display a number of effects that can be understood through their receptor actions, as well as other effects that are less understood. Their anticholinergic effects are manifested as miosis, decreased hydrogen-ion secretion, decreased GI motility, anhidrosis, and xerostomia. Alpha$_1$-adrenergic blockade is seen as orthostatic hypotension, which may or may not improve with continued therapy. Dopamine-blocking effects at the hypothalamus and pituitary may result in excess prolactin secretion. This is seen as gynecomastia in men and as galactorrhea in women. Dopaminergic blockade at the medullary chemoreceptor trigger zone has an antiemetic effect on patients. In addition, extrapyramidal symptoms can occur, both acutely and later in therapy. The most common early manifestations are akathisia (excessive purposeless motor activity) and acute dystonia (facial grimacing and torticollis). Later in the course of therapy, drug-induced parkinsonism may appear. This is characterized by a shuffling gait, bradykinesia, akinesia, mask facies, and cogwheel rigidity. The most significant and usually late-developing neurologic symptom is tardive dyskinesia (TD). This presents as orofacial dyskinesia and choreoathetosis. Neuroleptic medications should be discontinued at the first signs of TD, because the symptoms can worsen and become permanent.

Other adverse effects can occur, including neuroleptic malignant syndrome, obstructive jaundice, sedation, hypothermia, lowered seizure threshold, skeletal muscle relaxation, and cutaneous reactions. Other rare side effects are agranulocytosis and photosensitivity. Thioridazine, more than the other antipsychotic drugs, is known for rare occurrences of retrograde ejaculation and pigmented retinopathy.

Miscellaneous Adjuvant Analgesics

In addition to the major adjuvant drug groups discussed above, there are a few other medications that can be useful in the management of pain, including local anesthetics, steroids, antihistamines, psychostimulants, clonidine, anxiolytics, calcitonin, and the radiopharmaceuticals baclofen and phenoxybenzamine. There are also other medications with potential applications as adjuvant analgesics, including the calcium-channel antagonists, adenosine L-tryptophan, and caffeine. However, their clinical use remains very limited at present.

LOCAL ANESTHETICS

The use of local anesthetics as blocking agents—subcutaneous, along nerve roots, or at the spinal cord—is well known. However, the use of intravenous local anesthetics as adjuvant analgesics is not as common. Intravenous lidocaine has been found to be useful in the treatment of some neuropathic pain conditions, including continuous and lancinating dysesthesias. Some of the conditions include neuropathic pain due to herpes zoster, phantom limb pain, diabetic neuropathy, and various other pain complaints resulting from neuropathies.

The mechanism of the pain relief appears to be the stabilization of nerve membranes. This occurs as a result of the blockade of sodium channels, which prevents the influx of sodium. The rapid influx of sodium is responsible for the initiation and propagation of depolarization in nerve fibers, which may, in turn, be perceived as pain.

Clinical utilization involves obtaining a baseline ECG and liver function tests. An intravenous lidocaine trial is performed in a patient to evaluate the possible efficacy of oral formulations of lidocaine. An intravenous catheter is placed and $1-2$ mg/kg of lidocaine is injected over 10 to 15 minutes while the patient is adequately monitored. The dose is usually 100 mg for most adult patients. Verbal analogue scores are obtained before, during, and after the test. The patients may commonly experience tinnitus, perioral numbness, a metallic taste in their mouth, and dizziness during the trial. A 50% or greater reduction in pain deserves a trial of oral lidocaine.

The oral formulation of lidocaine, mexiletine (Mexitil), provides the best side-effect profile and is the most used oral anesthetic. Mexiletine is started at 150 mg PO at bedtime for about 1 week. If tolerated, it is increased to 150 mg PO tid. If inadequate pain relief is obtained, the dose can be slowly escalated (every 5–7 days) to the maximum of 1200 mg/d. This can result in remarkable pain relief in some patients. Adverse effects include arrhythmias, syncope, hypotension, ataxia, tremors, nervousness, upper GI distress, dizziness, hepatoxicity, skin rash, visual changes, and fever and chills.

CORTICOSTEROIDS

These medications are useful as analgesic adjuvants, either alone or in combination with opioids. The exact mechanism of action remains elusive; however, some hypotheses exist. A peripheral effect is apparently due to the reduction of inflammation by steroids, and a central effect may occur through neurotransmitters. In addition, they are believed to reduce neuronal excitability by affecting cell membranes directly.

Steroids are used primarily in the pain management of many rheumatic diseases and cancer. They may reduce pain due to metastatic bone tumors, spinal cord compression, plexopathies, lymphedema, hepatomegaly, and some types of primary tumors.

High dosages of steroids can be tried for 1 week. The absence of a positive response should result in termination of therapy. Therapeutic responses with the predominantly glucocorticoid steroids should result in their continuation, but with tapering to the lowest dosage that maintains the response. Prednisone (100 mg every day), dexamethasone (100 mg every day), methylprednisolone (100 mg every day), or prednisolone (7.5 mg every day) can be tried for 1 week, and then tapered.

The numerous adverse effects of steroids are well known, ranging from osteoporosis and infections to gastric ulcerations, perforations, and Cushing's disease. Therefore, these are not first-line medications, and an explicit risk-benefit analysis should precede their administration. Steroids should not be combined with NSAIDs.

ANTIHISTAMINES

Hydroxyzine (Atarax, Vistaril) is an antihistamine with antiemetic, anxiolytic, mild sedative, and, apparently, inherent analgesic properties. It is used as an adjunctive medication in the treatment of acute and refractory chronic pain conditions. It can be used either alone or in combination with an NSAID or a narcotic. Cyproheptadine (Periactin) is also occasionally tried in the treatment of refractory chronic pain.

Hydroxyzine is extensively metabolized in the liver. The starting dose is 25–50 mg PO or IM, q4–6h, or prn. There is an apparent ceiling effect above 150 mg, after which no additional analgesic benefit has been found. Adverse effects include sedation, xerostomia, acute hyperexcitability, multifocal myoclonus, ataxia, and seizures.

PSYCHOSTIMULANTS

The amphetamines dominate the psychostimulant group of adjuvant medications. They are usually administered to treat opioid-mediated sedation. However, they appear to possess additional intrinsic properties, including analgesic, antidepressant, and euphoretic effects. Amphetamines may augment the analgesic effects of opioids, particularly when associated with sedation and depression, but they do not appear to be effective as antidepressants or as primary analgesics. Their exact mechanism of action remains unclear, but the psychostimulants are indirect-acting sympathomimetics, with effects on serotonin, norepinephrine, endogenous opioid pathways, and possibly dopamine.

Dextroamphetamine (Dexedrine) and methylphenidate (Ritalin) are the most commonly used amphetamines. Dextroamphetamine, 5–10 mg, is administered every morning, following a 2.5-mg test dose. The dosage can be increased to a maximum of 20 mg/d, or until side effects appear. Dextroamphetamine is administered in divided doses, with none taken after noon, to prevent insomnia. Methylphenidate is started at 10 mg PO every morning and increased to a maximum of 40 mg/d before noon. Cocaine is also occasionally used, but studies of its efficacy are equivocal.

Tolerance to psychostimulant effects may occur, and is treated with upward dose titration. Furthermore, the half-life of methylphenidate (3–6 hr) is shorter than that of dextroamphetamine (34 hr); therefore, if methylphenidate is able to mask respiratory depression and sedation, these effects may appear at night and play havoc with patients. These medications are contraindicated in patients with hyperthyroidism, seizure disorders, cardiac arrhythmias, or uncontrolled hypertension. Baseline studies should include an ECG and a CBC.

Adverse effects include restlessness, insomnia, anxiety, delirium, visual disturbances, seizures, personality changes, exacerbation of preexisting psychological diseases, psychological dependency, and withdrawal syndrome. Cardiovascular effects include headache, palpitations, hypertension, hypotension, angina, cardiac arrhythmias, and circulatory collapse. Hypersensitivity syndromes can occur with arthralgias and skin reactions, as well as thrombocytopenia. GI side effects include anorexia, nausea, vomiting, and abdominal cramps.

CLONIDINE

Clonidine is an alpha$_2$-adrenergic agonist that blocks the release of norepinephrine and nociceptive substance P from preganglionic adrenergic receptors at the spinal cord level (dorsal horn). Hence, it is used as an adjunctive analgesic, usually to potentiate opioid-mediated analgesia and to reduce opioid doses. Analgesic effects have been demonstrated in a variety of acute and chronic pain conditions, using multiple routes of delivery (i.e., oral, topical, spinal, and intramuscular). A trial of clonidine should be conducted on refractory neuropathic pain patients.

The initial oral dose should be low (0.1 mg PO bid or tid). The dosage may be titrated up by 0.1–0.2 mg/d every few days. The escalation should occur over a few weeks, until side effects occur or to the maximum dose of 2.4 mg/d in 2 or 3 divided doses. Transdermal clonidine patches are also available. The patches should be applied to a hairless area, starting with 0.1 mg/d. The patches should be changed every 3 to 7 days, and the sites rotated, including to painful areas for a possible local effect. The dose of the patches can be escalated every week, to a maximum of 0.3 mg/d. Clonidine is also used in combination with opioids for spinal analgesic effects (both intrathecal and epidural).

Clonidine's main adverse effects are bradycardia, hypotension, and sedation, often necessitating discontinuation of therapy. Other side effects include xerostomia, constipation, pruritus, myalgias, nausea, urticaria, insomnia, impotence, and hyperglycemia, due to the inhibition of insulin release.

PHENOXYBENZAMINE

Phenoxybenzamine (Dibenzyline) is an $alpha_1$- and $alpha_2$-adrenergic receptor antagonist. We have found it useful in the treatment of some patients with sympathetically maintained pain, as defined by decreased pain following either a local anesthetic (e.g., stellate) or a phentolamine block.

The mechanism of action of phenoxybenzamine in the treatment of sympathetically maintained pain is not completely understood. Current thinking is that in sympathetically maintained pain there is an upregulation of the sympathetic noradrenergic system as well as an increase in $alpha_1$ receptors on the injured pain fibers (i.e., postsynaptic). Inhibition of release of noradrenaline at the sympathetic synapse therefore inhibits the activation of the $alpha_1$-receptor–mediated changes in damaged peripheral fibers. Thus phenoxybenzamine's main action is on the $alpha_1$ receptors.

Phenoxybenzamine is usually started at 10 mg PO tid. It is increased by 10 mg every 2 days. The dosage is titrated upward to effect, usually to a maximum of 90–120 mg/d, although higher doses may be used if there is a good clinical effect without side effects. However, even small doses may not be tolerated, owing to the drug's major side effect—**orthostatic hypotension**. Other side effects include reflex tachycardia, syncope, shock, miosis, lethargy, nausea, vomiting, diarrhea, nasal congestion, and headaches. Toleration of the drug is variable among patients. It is relatively contraindicated in the elderly. The side effects can be detected early and treated by lowering the dose and slowing the increase of the treatment by carefully monitoring the patient.

ANXIOLYTICS

These agents are **not** routinely used for pain relief (Table 5-7). The anxiolytic medications primarily comprise the ben-

Table 5-7. Benzodiazepines

Drug	Dosage (mg/d)	Average dose (mg/d)	Half-life (hr)	Active metabolite
Alprazolam	0.5–4.0	1.5	12–15	No
Chlorazepate	7.5–60.0	30	30–200	Yes
Chlordiazepoxide	10–100	30	5–45	Yes
Diazepam	5–40	15	20–50	Yes
Lorazepam	1–6	3	10–20	No
Oxazepam	30–120	60	5–15	No

zodiazepines (BZDZs). The BZDZs enhance gamma-amino-butyric acid (GABA) release and inhibitory activity. In addition, they inhibit serotonin and norepinephrine release. **These effects can potentially antagonize opioid-induced analgesic effects, particularly when delivered parenterally or with prolonged use. Furthermore, apart from clonazepam, these drugs are not considered to possess clinically significant sensory analgesic effects.** However, they may reduce the emotional reactivity to pain, which can often be hard to distinguish from true analgesic effects. There are, however, animal models that point toward BZDZ-induced analgesic effects at the spinal level, through GABA receptors in the substantia gelatinosa.

The main CNS effects of BZDZs are anxiolysis, sedation, anticonvulsant activity, amnesia, and muscle relaxation. Some of the BZDZs are used primarily as hypnotics, e.g., flurazepam (Dalmane), temazepam (Restoril), and triazolam (Halcion). Others are used for muscle spasms, e.g., diazepam (Valium), and some for seizures and neuralgias, e.g., clonazepam (Klonopin). The remainder are used primarily for anxiolysis, e.g., chlordiazepoxide (Librium), chlorazepate (Tranxene), lorazepam (Ativan), oxazepam (Serax), and alprazolam (Xanax). Alprazolam also appears to have some antidepressant effects. These medications are used in initial states of anxiety or during acute exacerbations of chronic pain conditions, but usually only for short periods of time (1–2 months, maximum). The drugs are administered according to their respective dosages (see Table 5-8) and then tapered after 3 to 4 weeks, over 1 week.

Adverse effects following short courses of BZDZs, in therapeutic dosages, do not generally occur. The most common side effects are daytime sedation and impaired cognition and coordination. Attention, intellect, judgment, and memory are cognitive functions that may be affected. The potential for drug abuse, addiction, and withdrawal symptoms exists with all the BZDZs. Paradoxical excitement and occasional hostile or aggressive behavior have been noted. Tolerance to anxiolytic effects develop in 4 to 6 weeks, but some anxiolytic effects persist. The BZDZs have minimal hemodynamic or autonomic effects.

CALCITONIN

Calcitonin is a polypeptide hormone that consists of 32 amino acids. It is involved in calcium homeostasis and it inhibits osteoclast activity. Although its analgesic effects in Paget's disease are thought to result from its effects on bone formation and osteoclast function, studies have revealed some intrinsic analgesic properties. Calcitonin is used in cancer patients with intractable pain or bony metastases. It can be administered with opioids, since its actions are not mediated through the opioid system. Its exact mechanism of action is unknown, but it is postulated that calcitonin acts through descending serotonin systems that modulate nociception in the dorsal horn of the spinal cord.

Calcitonin is derived from salmon (Calcimar, Miacalcin) or human (Cibacalcin). Salmon calcitonin may be administered either subcutaneously or intramuscularly. A test done of 1 U (10 U diluted in 1 ml normal saline) is injected intradermally to test for mild erythema or a wheal. The initial dose is 100 U/d, with a maintenance dose of 50–100 U every 1 to 3 days. Cibacalcin is administered subcutaneously at 0.5 mg/d, with a maximum of 1 mg/d, for severe cases. Calcitonin has also been administered epidurally and intrathecally.

Adverse effects include nausea, vomiting, and hypersensitivity to salmon protein or the gelatin diluent. Other less frequent side effects include diarrhea, anorexia, facial flushing, swelling, rash, diuresis, headache, chills, dizziness, nasal congestion, and shortness of breath.

RADIOPHARMACEUTICALS

Treatment of pain in cancer patients with metastatic disease has traditionally been with systemic analgesics or local external beam radiation, or both. Recently, the use of systemic radiopharmaceuticals has increased, although they have been used since the early 1940s. The main ones are phosphorus 32, strontium 89 (Metastron), rhenium 186, and samarium 153. The last two are still under investigation. Phosphorus 32 has been found to be associated with severe hematologic toxicity in about one third of patients. Strontium 89, however, has been found to be as effective as phosphorus 32, but with less hematologic toxicity.

Strontium 89, a pure beta-emitter, is used for the relief of bone pain in patients with painful skeletal metastases, whose pain is not easily controlled with systemic analgesics. Therapy involves a single injection, on an outpatient basis, which may provide up to 6 months of pain relief. This is reflected in decreased pain scores and diminished analgesic use. Pain relief occurs in 7 to 20 days, and therefore should not be used in patients with a very short life expectancy.

Adverse effects include bone marrow toxicity and should be monitored with peripheral blood cell counts every other week. Thrombocytopenia and leukocytopenia are most prominent, with a nadir at 12 to 16 weeks after administration. A transient increase in pain complaints is noted in about 10% to 20% of patients at 36 to 72 hours postinjection. This is usually mild and controlled by additional analgesics.

BACLOFEN

Baclofen (Lioresal) is an antispasmodic drug that is often used in the treatment of spasticity associated with multiple sclerosis and spinal cord lesions. However, it is believed to possess some analgesic properties, which may augment opioid-induced analgesia. This apparently occurs through its GABA–B agonist actions. Baclofen appears to be useful in the treatment of painful spasticity, trigeminal neuralgia, and other forms of neuropathic pain, particularly lancinating pain. It should be avoided in patients with seizure disorders and impaired renal function.

Baclofen is usually started at 5 mg PO tid. Each dose can be increased by 5 mg every 3 days, to a maximum of 80 mg/d. Baclofen is also administered intrathecally, and pump systems are sometimes implanted for continuous infusion therapy in selected patients. Common side effects include drowsiness, fatigue, vertigo, orthostatic hypotension, headaches, hypotonia, psychiatric disturbances, insomnia, slurred speech, ataxia, hypotonia, rash, urinary frequency, and GI distress. These can be avoided through slow titration and avoidance of abrupt discontinuation.

TRAMADOL

Tramadol (Ultram) is an atypical opioid analgesic. It has very weak μ opioid binding but is thought to exert its analgesic effects by inhibition of reuptake of norepinephrine and serotonin. It has been used extensively in Europe since 1977. It has such minimal opioid side effects that it is not schedule II.

Tramadol is usually started at 50–100 mg dose and can be given every 4–6 hours, not to exceed 400 mg/d total dose. Side effects are predominantly sedation, nausea, and vomiting. Most side effects occur when a starting dose of 100 mg is used. Clinical side effects such as respiratory depression, constipation, or withdrawal signs are minimal or nonexistent.

Selected Readings

General

Sunshine A and Olson NZ. Non-narcotic analgesics. In: PD Wall and R Melzack (eds), *Textbook of Pain* (2nd ed). Edinburgh: Churchill-Livingtone, 1994. Pp 923–942.

Nonsteroidal Anti-inflammatory Drugs

Cummings DM and Amadio P Jr. A review of selected newer nonsteroidal anti-inflammatory drugs. *Am Fam Physician* 49: 1197–1202, 1994.

McCormack K. Non-steroidal anti-inflammatory drugs and spinal nociceptive processing. *Pain* 59:9–43, 1994.

Schoenfeld A, Bar Y, Merlob P, and Ovadia Y. NSAIDs: Maternal and fetal considerations. *Am J Reprod Immunol* 28:141–147, 1992.

Urquhart E. Central analgesic activity of nonsteroidal anti-inflammatory drugs in animal and human pain models. *Semin Arthritis Rheum* 23:198–205, 1993.

Membrane Stabilizers and Antiepileptics

Chabal C, et al. The use of oral mexiletine for the treatment of pain after peripheral nerve injury. *Anesthesiology* 76:513–517, 1992.

Espir ML and Millac P. Treatment of paroxysmal disorders in multiple sclerosis with carbamazepine (Tegretol). *J Neurol Neurosur Psychiatry* 33:528–531, 1970.

Fenollosa P, et al. Chronic pain in the spinal cord injured: Statistical approach and pharmacological treatment. *Paraplegia* 31:722–729, 1993.

Green MW and Selman JE. Review article: The medical management of trigeminal neuralgia. *Headache* 31:588–592, 1991.

Guieu R, Mesdjian E, Rochat H, and Roger J. Central analgesic effect of valproate in patients with epilepsy. *Seizure* 2:147–150, 1993.

Reddy SVR, Maderdrut JL, and Yaksh TL. Spinal cord pharmacology of adrenergic agonist-mediated antinociception. *J Pharmacol Exp Ther* 213:525–533, 1980.

Rowbotham MC. Managing post-herpetic neuralgia with opioids and local anesthetics. *Ann Neurol* 35:S46–49, 1994.

Stracke H. Mexiletine in the treatment of diabetic neuropathy. *Diabetes Care* 15:1550–1555, 1992.

Tanelian DL and Browse WG. Neuropathic pain can be relieved by drugs that are use-dependent channel blockers: Lidocaine, carbamazepine, and mexiletine. *Anesthesiology* 74:949–951, 1991.

Antidepressants

Watson CP. Antidepressant drugs as adjuvant analgesics (review). Pain Symp Management 9:392–405, 1994.

Neuroleptics

Patt RB, Propper G, and Reddy S. The neuroleptics as adjuvant analgesics. *J Pain Symptom Manage* 9:446–453, 1994.

Adrenergic Agonists

Ghostine SY, et al. Phenoxybenzamine in the treatment of causalgia. *J Neurosurg* 60:1263–1268, 1984.

Raja SN, Treede RD, Davis KD, and Campbell JN. Systemic alpha-adrenergic blockade with phentolamine: a diagnostic test for sympathetically maintained pain. *Anesthesiology* 74:691–698, 1991.

Nonpharmacologic Treatments for Pain

Annabel Edwards

> "... impatient at being kept awake by pain, I availed myself of the stoical means of concentration upon some indifferent object of thought, such for instance as the name of 'Cicero' with its multifarious associations; in this way I found it possible to divert my attention, so that the pain was soon dulled ..."
>
> IMMANUEL KANT

Important Considerations in the Use of Nonpharmacologic Pain Treatments

Nonpharmacologic treatments for pain appear deceptively simple. Most require little more than common household supplies; very few involve the use of "high-tech" equipment or a special environment. Like all therapies one must learn to use them correctly and safely. In addition, the patient's acceptance of these treatments depends on how they are presented.

When recommending nonpharmacologic means for pain control to patients, a few issues should be considered:

Present the idea of using nonpharmacologic treatments to patients with the conviction that they work well for many people.

Try to select treatments that patients seem comfortable with to increase the likelihood that they will use them.

If possible, teach the techniques to patients when they do not have severe pain.

Tell patients to use the treatment **before** pain becomes severe; intervention tends to be more successful this way.

Teach patients a variety of treatments.

Tailor techniques to patients' specific abilities.

As with all treatments, modify the plan based on patients' responses.

Encourage patience and repetition of therapies.

Allow patients to try their own ideas, as long as such treatments are not harmful.

Remind patients that these techniques are just one aspect of their overall treatment plan.

The specific potential benefits of using nonpharmacologic treatments for pain are many:

Reducing or eliminating nociceptive aspects of pain.

Increasing patients' ability to participate in the activities o daily living, thus improving their self-esteem and sense o control.

Improving patients' ability to participate in physical therapy thus improving their overall health.

Allowing for the involvement of friends and family member in the care of the patients, thus increasing social contacts

Increasing patients' coping skills.

Specific Treatment Techniques

TRANSCUTANEOUS ELECTRICAL NERVE STIMULATION

Transcutaneous electrical nerve stimulation (TENS) is a form of external peripheral nerve stimulation. TENS may reduce pain by acting as a counterirritant; stimulating sensory nerve fibers, thus "closing the gate on" the pain signals; and serving as a distraction. At the Massachusetts General Hospita (MGH), the Physical Therapy Department is responsible for teaching the use of TENS and applying TENS units.

TENS is commonly used to treat postoperative pain, low back pain, neuropathic pain, headache, intercostal or chest pain arthritis, phantom limb pain, and cancer pain.

ACUPUNCTURE

Acupuncture is an ancient, medical–religious Chinese prac tice of unclear physiology; it involves the placement of fine needles at specific treatment points along the body's "merid ians," reportedly to treat patients by "restoring and balancing the flow of the life force, Chi." The study of acupuncture is currently funded by the WIH. In a carefully controlled, ran domized clinical trial acupuncture has not been shown to be more effective than placebo.

MASSAGE

Massage therapy may augment a patient's feeling of comfor and well-being. Aggressive or vigorous forms of massage re quire a trained physical therapist, but gentle massage is a basic skill. Pain need not he localized for massage to provide comfort. Massage is commonly used to treat headache, mus cle aches and tension, and back pain. Contraindications to the use of massage include thrombophlebitis, inflammatory arthritis, local infection, and unstable joints.

TECHNIQUES THAT ENHANCE RELAXATION

Anxiety and a high level of tension may be associated with increased pain. In general, relaxation techniques require that a person focus on a specific image or series of images. In this regard, relaxation techniques also work by distraction. It is best if the patient learns the technique while not in pain. Also, daily use of the technique, whether or not pain is present, helps to reinforce its use and, therefore, improve its effect. In an acute pain setting, one frequently does not have control over the environment, but for chronic pain patients, the environment can almost always be chosen or arranged. The best environment is a quiet, peaceful place where one can be left undisturbed for at least 20 minutes. After which, people often report feeling light, tingly, or rested, or simply say they feel "pleasant sensations."

Deep Breathing

The technique of deep breathing requires that patients focus on their breathing. To help patients slow their respiration, they are instructed to breathe slowly in, hold their breath for a couple of seconds, and then exhale over several seconds. If the patient is anxious, coaching is useful first to slow the rate and then to deepen the respirations.

Uses of deep breathing in pain treatment include: preparation for painful procedures; to decrease anxiety; sudden onset of pain; and preparation of the individual for other follow-up techniques such as imagery.

Progressive Muscle Relaxation

The use of this technique, compared to deep breathing, generally results in a more profound physiologic response from the body. In this exercise, patients focus sequentially on different muscle groups in the body. They tense and hold their muscles, then relax the muscles, and concentrate on how it feels for the muscles to be relaxed versus tense. All the muscle groups are tested in this way. After the exercise is complete, the patient is asked to rise slowly, stretch, and then slowly ambulate. Some people can be light-headed after performing progressive muscle relaxation. The complete process takes about 20 minutes.

Progressive muscle relaxation is commonly used for chronic back pain, headache, preparation for known painful events, general use in chronic pain management, and reduction of postoperative tension. Research results support the contention that progressive muscle relaxation provides more profound physiologic effects compared with other types of relaxation exercises. Tapes and other instructional media are available to help a person learn this technique.

TECHNIQUES THAT ENHANCE DISTRACTION

Distraction techniques divert a person's attention away from their pain experience. Attention is projected to something that is pleasurable or positive to the patient.

Imagery

To practice imagery, a person needs to be relaxed; therefore, a relaxation technique may be used prior to imagery. The patient is then asked to create a mental image that is personally meaningful—an image of a place and time that brings about pleasant feelings. Images that involve all of the senses are most effective for this kind of exercise. Consider the image of the beach, for example. One can think of the smell of low tide, the taste of salt water, the feel of the sun-heated sand, the sound of waves and birds, and the sights of swimmers and boats. The image used should be chosen by the patient. Another type of image that can be used is one related to the treatment of the patient's pain. A good example of this is the use of the image of the hand being cooled to a low temperature. Once the hand feels cool, the patient places it on areas of pain. The cool sensation acts like an analgesic.

Imagery for pain is commonly used in patients receiving cancer therapy, in the chronic pain population generally, during pregnancy and labor, and to augment effects of relaxation.

Biofeedback

Biofeedback is a learning tool in which any number of physiologic responses—of which the patient is usually unaware—can be monitored to cue the patient to the effects of such responses on the physiologic functioning of their body.

The machines used for biofeedback are sensitive to such parameters as the galvanic skin response, body temperature, EMG tracings, blood pressure, heart rate, and stomach acidity. Biofeedback is commonly used for the reduction of headache pain.

Hypnosis

Hypnosis is a state of deep relaxation and altered consciousness during which attention can be focused and suggestions received. The patient's willingness to be hypnotized is of primary importance to its success. The patient must trust the practitioner. During hypnosis, it has been shown that patients have a decreased awareness of their peripheral surroundings. Because they can focus their thoughts so completely, they can, in a sense, block, substitute, change, or forget the pain.

The overall goal of hypnosis is to provide the patient with experiences that develop their sense of mastery over their pain experiences. While some research seems to support a positive effect of hypnosis in some patients, it is not clear if that effect is a placebo response. Because hypnosis can "unlock" repressed memories, some of which could be very disturbing to the patient, the use of hypnosis should be initiated by a psychiatrist/psychologist.

Music Therapy

Two types of music can be used to decrease pain. Soothing, nonmetered music without lyrics, such as "New Age" music, helps a person to achieve a more profound state of relaxation.

Music that has a definite beat and, perhaps, lyrics can be a wonderful distraction to pain.

For this therapy to work as well as possible, one should use earphones, be in a quiet and undisturbed place, allow at least 15 minutes for the process, and use a basic relaxation exercise just before listening to the music.

To use music as a distraction, mellow music can be used to facilitate imagery exercises, or more upbeat music can be used alone. A patient can increase the volume of music if the pain worsens and lower it as it improves. The patient should be encouraged to sing along with the music, or conduct, hum, dance, keep beat, play along, etc.

Music therapy can be beneficial in intensive care unit patients, chronic pain patients, and postoperative patients.

COGNITIVE TECHNIQUES

Pain would not be experienced at all if we did not have cognitive awareness of its existence. When cognitive awareness occurs, our brain assigns a meaning to the experience. The meaning assigned to pain can depend on many factors, such as one's past history with pain, observed reactions to other people's pain, and cultural variables relating to the meaning of pain. Some of the cognitive behavior therapies are generally beneficial, including sensory and procedural information and social and spiritual support. Other therapies are more effective in those patients who have been identified as having involuntary thoughts about their pain experiences, which only exacerbate that experience. An example of a therapy used to counteract negative, involuntary thoughts is cognitive restructuring. The use of more than one of these cognitive techniques at a time has been shown to be of greater value than using just one, particularly in the headache and chronic pain patient populations.

Cognitive Restructuring

This technique focuses on teaching patients to monitor and identify their own negative interpretations of their pain experiences. Once identified, they evaluate the reality of those thoughts and then replace them with new interpretations. These new interpretations are intended to be more accurate and therefore adaptive. Cognitive restructuring is thought to influence the pain experience by decreasing distress, decreasing negative emotional and behavioral responses, and increasing adaptive behaviors and thoughts.

Preparatory Information

Preparatory information includes a detailed description of the steps of the procedure the patient will undergo as well as a specific description of the sensations the patient will likely experience during the procedure. The mechanisms by which procedural information is thought to help in the reduction of pain include reduction of anxiety and fear of the unknown and a change in the cognitive interpretation of events. The kind of information that best helps a patient varies depending on his or her overall state of anxiety. A patient with a high level of anxiety seems to do best with sensory information, and with lower anxiety, procedural information.

Social and Spiritual Support

The social context in which a person responds to pain has elements of uncertainty, perceived loss of control, social isolation, observed pain behaviors, and culture. Within the construct of culture are the elements of customs, beliefs, and values. Social and spiritual support may reduce pain by altering the patient's cognitive appraisal of his or her life to be more positive and hopeful; developing interpersonal bonds that allow the patient to share his or her feelings, thus reducing anxiety; and increasing compliance with a treatment regimen.

Conclusions

Pain is a subjective and multifactorial experience. Psychologic factors cannot be easily separated from anatomic and physiologic factors. The issue is not whether patients benefit from a placebo response or "real" physiologic bodily changes, it is that they **feel better**—an essential result of pain management.

Selected Readings

Acute Pain Management Panel. Acute Pain Management: Operative or Medical Procedures and Trauma. In: *Clinical Practice Guideline.* Rockville, MD: Agency for Health Care Policy and Research, Public Health Service, U.S. Department of Health and Human Services, Feb. 1992. AHCPR Pub. No. 92-0032. Pp. 21–26, 96, 106–107, 126–127.

Bonica J. *The Management of Pain* (2nd ed.). Philadelphia: Lea & Febiger, 1990. Pp. 28–132, 1711–1756, 1805–1821, 1862–1877.

Deyo RA, et al. A controlled trial of transcutaneous electrical nerve stimulation (TENS) and exercise for chronic low back pain. *N Engl J Med* 322:1627–1634, 1990.

Doody S, Smith C, and Webb J. Nonpharmacologic interventions for pain management. *Crit Care Nurs Clin North Am* 3:69–75, 1991.

Fields H. *Pain.* New York, McGraw-Hill, 1987. Chapters 5 and 11.

Garrison DW and Foreman RD. Decreased activity of spontaneous and noxiously evoked dorsal horn cells during transcutaneous electrical nerve stimulation (TENS). *Pain* 58:309–315, 1994.

Karlstrom E and Abel GG. Biofeedback for musculoskeletal pain. *JAMA* 270:2736, 1993.

McCaffery M and Beebe A. *Pain: Clinical Manual for Nursing Practice.* St. Louis: Mosby, 1989. Chaps 5–8.

Price DD and Mayer DJ. Evidence for endogenous opiate analgesic mechanisms triggered by somatosensory stimulation (including acupuncture) in humans. *Pain Forum* 4:40–43, 1995.

Smith I, Airey S, and Salmond S. Nontechnologic strategies for coping with chronic low back pain. *Orthop Nurs* 9:26–32, 1990.

Soeken K and Carson V. Responding to the spiritual needs of the chronically ill. *Nurs Clin North Am* 22:603–611, 1987.

ter Kuile MM, et al. Autogenic training and cognitive self-hypnosis for the treatment of recurrent headaches in three different subject groups. *Pain* 58:331–340, 1994.

Wall P and Melzak R. *Textbook of Pain* (3rd ed.). New York: Churchill-Livingstone, 1984.

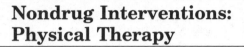

7

Nondrug Interventions: Physical Therapy

Harriet Wittink, Terry Hoskins Michel, and Melissa Wolff

> *"Life begins on the other side of despair."*
>
> J.P. SARTRE

The physical therapist identifies cardiopulmonary, musculoskeletal, and neuromuscular impairments that may cause physical/functional limitations. **Physical therapy intervenes to restore or improve function.**

Referral is appropriate when pain impairs a patient's optimal functional ability or reduces a patient's independence. Referral should include a diagnosis and precautions. Often, a request to "evaluate and treat" is sufficient.

Assessment and Treatment

An evaluation determines the patient's **ability to perform functional activities** and defines the **impairments that limit the patient's functioning**. Physical impairments are measured with procedures such as goniometry and manual muscle testing. Impairments may be the direct effect of a disease, syndrome, or lesion and relatively confined to one body system, or they may be the more generalized and indirect effects of the underlying problem. For example, in the patient with low back pain, the primary impairments of pain and inactivity cause secondary impairments such as loss of range of motion, decreased muscle strength, and decreased aerobic capacity.

The therapist determines which of the impairments related to the patient's functional limitations can be remedied by physical therapy and which require patient compensation. Treatment focuses on optimal functional restoration. Collaborative treatment with a pain center is often essential in attaining this goal through improved pain control and consistency of care.

Physical Agents

The physical agents most commonly used in physical therapy are electrical stimulation, ranging from low voltage to high voltage, ultrasound, heat, and cold. The two principal therapeutic effects of electrical energy lie in generation of heat and the stimulation of peripheral nerves and muscle.

ELECTRIC CURRENT

Electrical stimulation is most commonly used for reduction of pain, edema, and muscle spasm and stimulation of muscle contraction. There is an optimum frequency for the maximum stimulation response—typically, 0–5 Hz for sympathetic nerves, 10–150 Hz for parasympathetic nerves, and 10–50 Hz for motor nerves.

ULTRASOUND

Ultrasound is a form of mechanotherapy with both thermal and nonthermal effects, including increased blood flow, increased extensibility of collagenous tissues, and decreased pain and muscle spasm. Ultrasound may increase range of motion due to contractures of ligamentous or capsular tissues, or both types.

Exercise

Exercise has two aims: muscle strengthening and general exercise endurance. **Increased muscle strength**, or muscle hypertrophy, is achieved by high-intensity, short-duration exercise. **Endurance exercise** is performed with low-intensity, dynamic, long-duration activities. This improves neuromuscular control and coordination and prevents injury to noncontractile structures during prolonged activities. Endurance exercise is associated with increased aerobic capacity, bone, ligament, and tendon strength, and improved blood flow to joints and muscles. An increase in CNS, brain norepinephrine, and serotonin levels as well as beta-endorphin and plasma immunoglobulin levels has been demonstrated with moderate aerobic exercise (30 min, 3–5 times per wk).

Joint Mobilization

Joint mobilization techniques improve joint mobility when passive range of motion is limited by the ligamentous and capsular structures. Capsular extensibility is restored by applying carefully directed focuses across the articular surfaces. All collagenous tissues rely heavily on movement to ensure adequate nutrition and respond to the same loading forces as bone (according to Wolff's law/Davis's law). Without stretching the tissues, joint mobilization is believed to decrease pain by stimulation of types I and II mechanoreceptors. Joint mobilization is often combined with ultrasound or heat to increase tissue extensibility and render treatment more effective.

Musculoskeletal Pain

JOINT PAIN

The fibrous capsules and ligaments stabilize the articulating surfaces. Proprioceptive nerve fiber stimulation within the joint results in a compensating muscle response when strains are applied to the joint. Thus, the passive stabilization by ligaments is reinforced by the dynamic stabilization of muscle, a process integrated by the CNS.

Recent studies have shown that in the inflamed or injured joint, nociceptive afferent nerve fibers respond instead to low-threshold, non-noxious mechanical distortion of articular tissues. Arthritis appears to be associated with mechanosensitivity in afferent nerve fibers previously unresponsive to joint movement or local stimulation, and with an enhanced response of some low-threshold, non-nociceptive afferent nerve fibers. Such peripheral neural mechanisms may contribute to an individual's perception of the intensity of articular pain; to the hyperalgesia and allodynia that may occur with a traumatized or inflamed joint; and to the spontaneous pain and incident pain that is commonly seen in a damaged or inflamed joint. Thus, treatment directed toward altering peripheral mechanisms of nociception are most appropriate for inflammatory joint pain.

OSTEOARTHRITIS

Early degenerative changes may remain asymptomatic until synovitis develops with effusion, stiffness, capsular thickening, and formation of marginal osteophytes. Osteophytes may cause excessive deformity of the articular bone ends, pain due to distortion of the periosteum, and limitation of movement. Other sources of pain include bony changes at sites of ligamentous attachments and protective muscle spasms that result in joint immobilization.

During the acute phase of synovitis treatment with ice massage, joint protection techniques and gentle, active range of motion may be beneficial to reduce fibrosis and enhance transsynovial nutrient flow.

MYOFASCIAL PAIN SYNDROME

Myofascial pain syndromes include a large group of muscle disorders characterized by the presence of hypersensitive points, called **trigger points**, within one or more muscles and/or the investing connective tissue, together with a syndrome of pain, muscle spasm, tenderness, stiffness, limitation of motion, weakness, and occasionally autonomic dysfunction. A trigger point (TP) is so named because its stimulation will produce effects at another place, called the **reference zone**. The pathophysiology is not well defined but may be associated with increased calcium-ion release causing nociceptive fiber injury.

An acute episode of myofascial pain often follows overuse of unconditioned muscles, prolonged stresses on musculoskeletal structures due to poor posture during work or recreational activities, sports injuries, cervical and/or lumbar strain, or a period of intense emotional stress. There is a difference between soreness after exercise and the TP phenomenon. Muscles that are stiff and sore from exercise contain tender points, but palpation of these sites does not refer pain to other areas.

Patients with myofascial pain usually present with persistent pain, tight or aching muscles, limited range of motion, and general fatigue. The patient might not be aware of muscular involvement and may instead complain of headache, neck pain, backache, or sciatica. The pattern of referred pain from TPs and associated phenomena is relatively constant and predictable and does not follow a dermatomal pattern or nerve root distribution. TP and their referral patterns are described in detail in the classic work by Travell and Simons (1983). Diagnosis of TP is established by standard physical therapy assessment and careful palpation of the muscles involved for tender TPs and taut bands. Pressure on the tender TP will usually cause the patient to jump or cry out ("jump sign").

NECK PAIN

Total movement of the cervical spine is the composite of segmental motion of all the cervical vertebrae. The major portion of rotation occurs in the upper three cervical segments, C1–C3, and the remaining motion occurs at the lower cervical segments, C4–C7. Movement patterns on a poor postural base contribute to repetitive microtrauma of the cervical structures, including the facets, discs, ligaments, articular capsules, and muscles. These poor patterns of movement contribute to habitual overuse of isolated motion segments, while they minimize normal movement of other segments. Habitual dysfunction at isolated segments may generate bony hypertrophy, ligamentous laxity, and breakdown of disc and facet articulations. All these factors may result in pain.

Principles of exercise training include retraining the musculature to control cervical mobility and stability of the painful spinal segment. Exercise will promote the necessary strength, coordination, and endurance to maintain the cervical spine in a stable and safe position during loading, mobility, and weight-bearing activities. Exercise training optimizes the capacity of the cervicothoracic muscles to absorb loads in all directions, while it minimizes direct strain and stress on individual cervical tissues. It also reduces repetitive microtrauma to the cervical segments and limits progression of injury, allowing gradual healing.

BACK PAIN

Low back pain remains society's most costly disease. Sickness and disability due to low back pain has risen 2500% over the last 20 years. Back pain, more than any other pain, has been associated with psychologic factors including work dissatisfaction and depression. Time off from work and return to work are poorly correlated with physical findings. These two work-related factors appear to be dependent on socioeconomic and job satisfaction variables.

Assessing the etiology of back pain is challenging. There is evidence to suggest that patients who take an active role in the rehabilitation process may enhance their chances of recovery. Early exercise and return to activity appear to be the most effective treatment of the patient with back pain at this time.

There is no significant benefit from surgical treatment, transcutaneous electrical nerve stimulation (TENS), or prolonged bed rest.

Acute Back Pain

When acute back pain involves muscle spasm, heat, cold, electrical, or manual modalities may be used to decrease the spasm. Several studies have pointed out the immediate or short-term symptomatic reduction of pain of less than 1 month's duration after spinal manipulation or mobilization in patients with low back pain. **Long-term results, however, were comparable for both the experimental and control groups in most studies.**

Patients should pursue a level of activity that does not exacerbate their pain. In the spine, the health of the joints is largely dependent on repeated low-stress movements. In the same way, the intervertebral disc is largely dependent on movement for its nutrition. Treatment commonly begins with soft-tissue flexibility and joint range-of-motion exercises, followed by isometric exercises for the lower back. Flexibility training usually focuses on increasing the length of the back extensors, hamstrings, iliopsoas, rectus femoris, and gastrocnemius. After ensuring the patient executes the flexibility exercises appropriately, these are made part of their home program. The patient is then trained in active joint mobilization exercises, such as extension exercises, in the prone and standing positions. Strengthening exercises are incorporated for the lower and upper abdominal muscles, the back extensors, the multifidi, and rotatores. General aerobic exercise is an integral part of the program and includes walking, swimming, or riding a stationary bike. Steady progression is ensured by setting exercise quotas. This method of treatment teaches patients that it is safe to move while also increasing their activity level.

Sympathetically Maintained Pain

Chapter 13 provides additional information on sympathetically maintained pain.

ACUTE MANAGEMENT

The initial injury that precipitates reflex sympathetic dystrophy is usually trivial but may involve fracture, soft-tissue damage, hematoma, and nerve damage.

Early physical therapy involves desensitization techniques such as tapping, stroking, and massaging the skin of the affected area. Patients must wear gloves or socks with progressively rough inner surfaces (hair shirt analogy!). As desensitization progresses, simple functional activities are initiated, often beginning with reflexively provoked action, such as weight-bearing, catching or kicking a ball, or catching one's balance after perturbation. Functional progress is made through gait training or correction of improperly used muscles, restoration of normal muscle length and postural alignment, and work on strength and endurance to balance muscle groups around major joints.

CHRONIC MANAGEMENT

The longer sympathetically maintained pain is allowed to endure, the more dysfunctional the patient becomes, and the harder the pain and immobility are to reverse. However, much success has been found in patients who receive serial sympathetic blocks in conjunction with physical therapy and are retrained in functional activities throughout the period of receiving blocks. Thus, making use of the short-term pain relief from blocks to promote and reinforce appropriate movement patterns may provide the best chance of success long term in patients.

Chronic Pain

> *"The constant effort ... to separate the purely physiological from the purely psychological, and to label symptoms as either organic or functional has a certain futility about it. ..."*
>
> FINNESON, 1969

Treating patients with nonmalignant chronic pain is difficult. These patients often present with pain complaints that seem out of proportion to their objective findings, yet they assure their physician they are completely disabled due to their pain, often in their work life as well as in their social and recreational lives. Chronic pain patients usually present with primary as well as secondary impairments. The primary impairments result from injury and may or may not be treatable by physical therapy. The secondary impairments are the consequence of the patient's response to the initial injury with self-immobilization. Lack of exercise, poor body alignment, shortening and weakening of the joint structures, and over-guarding of the injured part of the body result in a weakened physical condition that can make normal daily activities more difficult, uncomfortable, and stressful. As a result, the patient's pain and suffering increase. These patients are commonly depressed as well, thus further spiraling into a cycle of disuse, pain, and impairment. The impairments resulting from disuse are readily addressed by an aggressive exercise program comprised of stretching; cardiovascular, strength, and endurance training; and behavioral modification tailored to the patient's individual needs.

The patient is made to progress systematically, thus learning that increased activity does not equal increased pain. The focus of exercise is on endurance training. Patients are instructed in a low-weight, high-repetition program addressing all major postural muscle groups while maintaining control of the movement. At the Massachusetts General Hospital, patients are seen 2 or 3 times per week for 1.5 hours of exercise each time. The program is tailored to their individual needs, but the components are the same:

1. Aerobic exercise: bike, treadmill, upper body exercises (UBE) at 65% to 85% predicted of maximum heart rate.
2. Stretching exercises for shortened musculature.
3. Endurance exercise for the major postural muscles, working up to three sets of 30 repetitions of each exercise.
4. Coordination/skill exercises.
5. Mobilizing exercise, if needed.

Meetings are held twice a week to discuss patients with doctors from other specialties, including behavioral medicine, neurology, and anesthesiology.

Physical therapy goals for these patients are to (1) increase functional capacity, (2) establish effective pain-coping skills, (3) decrease health care utilization, and (4) decrease dependency on medications.

Conclusions: General Principles of Physical and Occupational Therapy Interventions

The goals of rehabilitation are pain reduction, maintenance or maximization of function, prevention of complications including disability, and education of the patient and caregivers about pain and sequelae. Ultimately, the goal of rehabilitation intervention is to provide hope. Pain reduction can occur simply by decreasing the deleterious effects of gravity, pressure, tension, and muscle spasm. Protecting the affected area from exposure to cold, excessive heat, or injury; stimulating circulation to decrease the incidence and severity of trophic changes; and preventing edema and deformities will prevent some of the complications of disability. Development of fibrosis, muscle contractures, joint stiffness, and ankylosis can permanently affect the recovery of maximal function following nerve injury.

Rehabilitation can maintain or maximize function by discouraging inactivity, accelerating the restoration of function, and assisting with re-education in the absence of nerve recovery. Education of the patient and caregivers regarding the independent use of modalities for pain reduction and development of a home program to maintain or improve function is crucial in the total rehabilitation of the patient. The patient requires knowledge about the etiology of pain and injury and the expected course or recovery. There are numerous modalities available to the physical and occupational therapist that can be used in the clinic or independently by the patient. Most of these modalities were addressed earlier in the chapter and are presented here briefly.

The potential benefits of **thermal modalities** (deep and superficial modalities) may include increased blood flow, decreased pain and muscle spasm, decreased chronic inflammation, increased active movement, facilitated exercise, decreased stiffness and viscosity, and increased relaxation. When cold is used the opposite effect may occur, which is desirable in some cases of acute injury or pain. Ultrasound may relax scar tissue and increase tissue extensibility.

Nerve stimulation may decrease muscle spasm, increase relaxation, increase the ability to exercise and perform range of motion, increase blood flow and metabolism, and decrease pain. The skillful use of TENS of peripheral large-diameter afferent nerve fibers sometimes decreases pain. Difficulties with use of TENS include variability of patient response and treatment and stimulation parameters. If there is deafferentation near the painful area, use of TENS in this area may increase pain.

Massage may have positive circulatory effects. Denervated or partially innervated tissue requires gentle, monitored external pressure. **Orthotics, prosthetics, splints, and compression wraps** may yield pain reduction, injury prevention, and functional assistance. Progressive and frequently monitored joint positioning will allow for functional immobilization. The result of careful use of external appliances includes decreased formation of edema, effusion, and venous congestion.

Selected Readings

Grieve GP. *Modern Manual Therapy of the Vertebral Column.* New York: Churchill-Livingstone, 1986.

Guccione A. *Geriatric Physical Therapy.* St. Louis: Mosby, 1993.

McCaffery M and Wolff MS. Pain Relief Using Cutaneous Modalities, Positioning and Movement. In: Turk DC, Feldman CS (eds), *Noninvasive Approaches to Pain Management in the Terminally Ill.* New York: Haworth Press, 1992. Pp. 121–154.

Sullivan P and Markos P. *Clinical Procedures in Therapeutic Exercise.* Norwalk, CT: Appleton & Lange, 1987.

Timm KE. A randomized-control study of active and passive treatments for chronic low back pain following L5 laminectomy. *J Orthop Sports Phys Ther* 20:276–286, 1994.

Travell J and Simon D. Myofascial pain and dysfunction. In: *The Trigger Point Manual.* Baltimore: Williams and Wilkins, 1983.

Nondrug Interventions: Psychosocial Aspects of Pain

Tina U. Wolter and David K. Ahern

> *"Happiness is not being pained in body or troubled in mind."*
>
> THOMAS JEFFERSON

In recent years, the predominant conceptual model employed for the assessment of chronic pain has shifted from a primarily medically oriented "specificity model," in which pain is viewed as directly proportional to and reflective of the amount and degree of tissue damage, to the current perspective of pain as a "biopsychosocial" phenomenon. In this model as opposed to its predecessor, pain is viewed not as a dichotomous entity but as a combination of factors—biologic, psychologic, social, and cultural—that contribute to an individual's pain experience. For this reason, a thorough assessment of the patient's current pain status and level of functioning in all of the above-mentioned spheres is critical in formulating optimal treatment plans.

Patient Assessment

Assessment is accomplished in **two phases**: through a semi-structured clinical interview and the administration of pencil-and-paper measures. Information obtained from each phase of the assessment is then integrated to produce a picture of the individual, taking into account not only physical but also behavioral, psychosocial, and economic factors influencing the patient's current pain and functional status. Once identified, these various factors can be addressed through multicomponent treatments.

THE CLINICAL INTERVIEW

Interviewing is done in a semistructured format designed to obtain detailed information on contributing factors to the pain problem. Attention is given to relationships between individual aspects of the pain experience, and the data obtained are combined with supplementary data from the medical chart review and standardized assessment instruments to arrive at an individualized treatment plan and recommendations. Whenever possible, the interview is conducted with both the patient and spouse or significant other to obtain a more complete picture of functioning and the impact of pain on the marital and/or family unit.

Typically the interview begins by allaying the patient's fears that he or she has been referred for behavioral medicine assessment because of a physician's belief that the person is "crazy" or that the pain is "all in my head." Rather, we use this opportunity to explain that the assessment is a way for us to better understand not only the pain experience itself but also the ways in which it has affected the patient's life in general. In addition, some amount of "normalizing" of the patient's experience in terms of increased stress and disruption of routine can be helpful in reassuring the patient and establishing rapport, which are crucial not only in obtaining valid assessment information but also in establishing a positive treatment relationship.

Pain Characteristics

The actual pain complaint is addressed first. Location, intensity, duration, and fluctuations in actual pain patterns are assessed next. Subjective descriptions of pain (dull, throbbing, shooting, etc.) should be noted. The use of affective descriptors, as well, is important in obtaining a more thorough understanding of the patient's emotional response to his or her pain. Self-report pain scales are another commonly used method of assessing the individual's pain experience. The patient is asked to rate his or her pain on a scale (0 to 10, for example) for a given time period, either at that moment or for a specified period such as an hour or a day, or longer. In the initial assessment, pain ratings are usually obtained for the current level of pain, as well as the range of pain experience.

Determining overall parameters of pain leads naturally to the elaboration of influencing factors—for example, those activities associated with pain exacerbation, and conversely, those activities or factors associated with pain relief. Close attention is paid to both of these areas, because important information regarding the extent to which environmental or operant factors may affect the pain syndrome can be identified.

Consistent behavior patterns that are associated with pain exacerbations are important to note. For example, if pain is increased reliably when the patient is at work, but is relieved appreciably during work breaks or vacation, work history and job satisfaction should be investigated more thoroughly in the interview. Several presentations and variations of both pain complaints and behavior that suggest operant involvement have been identified. These include (1) pain and pain behaviors that are highly visible/audible and have a major impact on the behavior of individuals in the patient's environment, e.g., taking over the patient's chores or responsibilities, getting the patient's medication, (2) a differential tendency for aversive over pleasant activities or responsibilities to increase pain, (3) the immediate and invariable relief of pain from medication, rest, or attention, (4) constant and unvarying pain experience without periods of reduced intensity, (5) pain that is increased by any sort of activity, (6) immediate cessation of activity in response to pain, and (7) pain that reportedly interferes with daily activities but does not interfere with sleep.

Coping Behavior

Elicitation of the patient's attempts to cope with his or her pain, both successful and unsuccessful, is easily incorporated into the interview when obtaining information about pain patterns. This approach provides useful information about the patient's primary coping strategy, skill level, and ability, as well as a general sense of the patient's degree of reliance on external versus internal means of assistance (e.g., primary reliance on medications or surgical interventions, participation in physical therapy or support groups).

Pain Behavior

Paying attention to the patient's verbal and nonverbal behavior is also very informative. Besides the use of pain descriptors, patients often attempt to communicate the extent of their suffering through grimacing, groaning or moaning, and frequent postural shifts during the course of the interview. These behaviors are considered to be reflective of the patient's pain experience; consequently, they are conceptualized as pain behaviors. Frequently, patients will call attention to their suffering by pointing out their behavior or excusing themselves for it in the presence of the clinician. In other patients, these behaviors have become automatic aspects of their self-presentation and are not acknowledged. Some patients evidence the grimacing, guarding, or verbalizations noted above, but do so to a much lesser degree. Still other individuals evidence very little or no pain behavior. In these patients, particularly, it is important to note any discrepancies between their verbalized reports of pain/distress and their appearance. Pointing out such discrepancies to the patient can yield useful information about the patient's current coping status, since some patients will acknowledge that they have pain but choose not to show it, whereas other individuals sometimes become rather defensive at the perceived questioning of their self-report. Obviously, appropriate clinical judgment regarding the timing and extent of questioning along these lines is in order on the clinician's part.

Health Care Utilization

Thorough assessment of pain-relevant medical history can help establish whether health care over- or underutilization is a concern. This part of the interview can also reveal a great deal about the patient's general interaction with the health care system and identify general attitudes, beliefs, and expectations about care. Past dissatisfactions with particular health care providers or treatment approaches, for example, may point to a patient's unwillingness to take personal responsibility for his or her own health care. Conversely, unquestioning compliance with multiple invasive procedures which yield no significant improvement can indicate a lack of sophistication or assertiveness on the patient's part. Further, the pattern of health care utilization can point to lack of coordination among various health care providers. Duplication of services, contradictory interventions, and repetition of interventions in the absence of new or changed physical findings are all manifestations of a lack of coordinated care. This last item, in fact, can contribute to worsening of the patient's health status through increased risk of iatrogenic complications related to specific treatments.

History of Medication Use

Current use of medication, including dose and schedule, is basic information that needs to be collected not only for pain medications but for all medications currently used by the patient. Both prescription and nonprescription drugs should be recorded, as should use of illicit or "street" drugs, if applicable. Parameters of use, including average daily intake, as well as minimum and maximum daily intake, especially of prn medication, is also important to assess. Factors contributing to increased or decreased medication usage should be explored, since they can sometimes reveal behavioral patterns or operant factors involved in the pain problem. Similarly, the patient's pattern of medication intake should be explored. For example, does the patient take pain medication on a time-contingent basis, or does he or she wait until pain is at its highest level to take it? Does the patient take increased doses of medication in anticipation of painful activity? Do prescriptions usually last for the duration of the prescription period, or does the patient exhibit a pattern of "running out" before the next scheduled refill? Answers to these questions are important in formulating the most appropriate treatment plan.

Vocational and Financial Impact

Current job status—that is, whether the patient is still working—current job duties, number of days missed from work due to pain, physicians' visits, and other related variables are assessed to determine the impact of pain on the patient's current functioning. Is the injury job related? Comparison of current versus previous job performance (absenteeism, change in job duties, etc.) can provide useful clues about the extent of pain-related vocational disruption. In addition to premorbid job functioning in such objective terms, it is also useful to examine premorbid job satisfaction, including the patient's relationship with his or her employer and coworkers: this has been widely determined to be an important predictor of return-to-work status in a number of chronic pain populations, including chronic low back pain sufferers.

Again, during this part of the assessment the clinician should determine the extent of impact of pain on current functioning and assess whether any operant factors are influencing pain report or behavior. For example, are family members more supportive of the patient remaining at home (to be a homemaker, for example) than of having the patient work outside the home? Does the level of financial compensation associated with current disability status raise overall net income for the household? Patients who believe they might benefit from Workers' Compensation or judicial court awards for injury-related disability or suffering may be less inclined to resume normal functioning than patients who are severely financially burdened as a result of pain-related unemployment or reductions in wages. Additionally, patients whose premorbid job functioning or job satisfaction was low might regard current unemployment status more favorably than workers with high job satisfaction.

Finally, it is important to assess patient's views and expectations (as well as prior attempts, if any) regarding their return to work in terms of the conditions necessary to successfully return to work. Often, patients feel that they must be pain free to resume employment. In the absence of re-education or cognitive restructuring, in which the patient is able to accept some level of discomfort or increased sensations, prognosis for successful re-entry into the workforce is poor.

Functional Disability

Assessment of functional disability consists of the determination of the activities limited or precluded by the patient's pain. Usually, this is best achieved by having the individual first note general areas of limitation. Typically, patients will begin by stressing those areas of greatest importance to them. The interview can proceed from here in a variety of ways designed to cover remaining major aspects of functioning, including work, recreation, social interaction, household chores, and family relationships.

A useful technique in helping formulate a picture of the patient's current functional level is to ask him or her to describe a typical day in as much detail as possible. For example, times of awakening, dressing, eating breakfast (including type and amount of meal, who prepares it, kitchen cleanup), and reading the paper might be noted as standard daily routines. The amount of time required to complete each activity is also important to ascertain, because for some patients, the general routine might take 45 minutes, whereas for others, it could take 2 hours. When patients with pain lose a sense of structure to their day and find that there are many hours to fill, it is not uncommon to find that much of the day is spent lying down or resting. For these patients, treatment might focus on increasing the range and scope of daily activities to increase physical endurance as well as combat depressive syndromes resulting from inactivity and loss of reinforcing activities or social interaction. Alternatively, some individuals have full, if not hectic, schedules with little or no rest periods. Still others exhibit a pattern of prolonged periods of inactivity and "recovery" from sporadic bursts of high activity. Again, the focus of treatment will be different for each of these individuals, based on their stated level and pattern of activity.

Some conditioning factors may contribute to the development or maintenance of functional impairment or disability:

1. The patient differentially experiences a restriction of unpleasant over pleasant activities.
2. The patient experiences a restriction of activities that occurred infrequently versus often prior to the pain problem.
3. The patient experiences high cross-situational variability in one or more of his or her limitations (i.e., keeps up house and garden, car maintenance, but cannot ambulate sufficiently at work).
4. The patient shows a tendency to overextend periodically, with subsequent long periods of inability and "recovery."
5. The patient experiences a pattern suggestive of avoidance learning, whereby the patient accepts activity limitation as permanent or unchanging and makes no attempt to try the activity again.
6. The patient experiences a generalization of avoidance learning, whereby the patient is restricted in one area of functioning and extends inactivity in this area to other similar behaviors.
7. The patient experiences social environmental reinforcement of his or her disability through society's increased positive attention to impaired function, assumption of the individual's former responsibilities, or punishment or discouragement of the patient's attempts to overcome limitations.
8. The patient experiences an increase in pleasant or positive activities as replacements or substitutes for restricted activities.

Marital and Family Relationships

Assessment should document the extent of marital and/or family disruption, examine the current level of discord, determine whether pain behavior and disability are being reinforced by the marital or family unit, and evaluate whether the patient's current pain problems are serving as a means of communication in the marriage. Because prior research has shown that the marital relationship usually has a stronger influence on the pain problem than wider family relationships, greater attention is given (see below) to marital issues. In general, though, questioning and exploration of the above four assessment areas should address the larger (and possibly extended) family unit as well.

Marital satisfaction prior to pain onset and since that time needs to be assessed. One spouse's pain often causes an increased strain on the relationship, usually reported in terms of the patient being more "snappy" or irritable. Other areas of conflict and potential discord are financial, or they may relate to specific interaction pattern changes between the partners. These areas are usually seen as negative, but occasionally a couple will report that it is good they are able to be together more now, or that since going to see so many physicians together, they have found more time to talk than they used to. These answers, as well as the interactional style used during the interview, can provide the interviewer with many useful clues about marital functioning and its likely impact on the pain problem, in terms of increased stress level or anxiety contributing to the pain experience. Alternatively, overly protective or solicitous behavior on the part of the spouse toward the patient might indicate reinforcement (often unintentional) of the patient's "sick" behavior.

Emotional Distress and Psychologic Disturbance

An adverse impact on the pain patient's mood over time is likely to occur. The impact can be mild or severe, depending on a combination of factors including pain level and severity and the patient's psychologic status, both premorbidly and currently. Assessment, therefore, should include an attempt to thoroughly understand the psychologic adjustment or symptomatology in order to better understand the pain problem and suggest treatment areas. For more detail, refer to Chapters 23 and 24.

Depression can manifest as the result of a loss of ability to engage in pleasant or reinforcing activity; persistent exposure to averse stimulation (pain); a loss of rewarding, or inability to maintain social relationships; and the decreased ability to engage in activity that is productive and satisfying to the individual. As mentioned above, changes in role relationships (primary caregiver to care receiver) and attendant financial consequences can contribute to lowered self-esteem and self-deprecation. A constant battle with legal or compensatory agencies also adds to attendant stresses and, in the face of unsuccessful outcome, contributes to depression. Treatment approaches with depressed individuals must take into account the factors contributing to their depression. With some individuals, learned helplessness may prevent the individual from being able to engage productively in any kind of treatment out of the belief or fear that this attempt, too, may fail.

Other psychological factors that may contribute to or complicate the overall pain problem are coping deficits, neuropsychologic deficits, cognitive deficits, social skill problems, and major psychiatric illness. All of these should be assessed in the interview, because they must be addressed in treatment. Personality factors presenting impediments to rehabilitation (hysteria, hypochondriasis) also need to be assessed. For example, patients often present with a very persistent pain focus to the exclusion of other life events or concerns, which may represent hysterical personality features or somatization.

Concluding the Interview

The clinical interview ends with patient feedback, as well as the formulation of the initial treatment plan. For some patients, behavioral medicine intervention is not recommended, as with those patients who are very resistant to an approach that does not offer specific medical treatment or surgical intervention. Treatment is also best postponed in cases of clear-cut thought disorder, until the patient's psychopathology is under the control of medication. Usually, patients who are not appropriate for treatment will already have expressed their unwillingness for further behavioral medicine intervention. Here, the clinician's focus is on reiterating the importance of accepting a rehabilitative rather than a curative model of pain management, and pointing out that it is possible to increase or improve the patient's functioning even in the face of continuing pain. For those patients who are not yet ready to enter into rehabilitative treatment, the initial clinical encounter can serve as an educational experience and can lay a foundation for future interaction.

For patients who are ready for treatment, the interview can end with a review of important clinical features and considerations relevant to the patient (e.g., current level of inactivity, mood state, family factors), along with a brief description of the proposed treatment plan and specific interventions that might be used. For example, the clinician might say, "I see that the pain has caused you a great deal of distress. I would propose to . . . ."

PAPER-AND-PENCIL MEASURES

The use of written instruments in the evaluation of chronic pain is crucial. An instrument can provide detailed self-report information about an individual's specific condition, as well as a quick overview of the patient's problem and reliability/variability checks on verbal interview data, and in many cases the patient's responses can be compared to existing norms to assess where the individual lies in relation to other persons with the same or similar problems. Often, prior research will indicate the likelihood of success or the appropriateness of a given treatment protocol or approach. Similarly, standardized instruments are critical in research study design, allowing specificity in both subject selection and description. The instruments commonly used in the Behavioral Medicine Unit, Department of Psychiatry, Massachusetts General Hospital, are described below.

Sickness Impact Profile (SIP)

SIP is one of the most widely used measures of health status in pain clinics. It consists of 136 items, in checklist format, which assess the impact of health problems in 12 areas of functioning: ambulation, mobility, body care and movement, social interaction, communication, alertness, emotional behavior, sleep, diet, work, home management, and recreation. It is scored to form three composite scales: physical, psychosocial, and total, which includes physical, psychosocial, work, and recreational pastimes information. Its reliability and validity as a measure of dysfunction in pain patients has been well established (Follick, Smith, and Ahern, 1985).

Pain and Impairment Relationship Scale (PAIRS)

Because attitudes, beliefs, and expectations have been shown to determine response to pain rehabilitation, it is important to assess patients' beliefs regarding their pain. Often, as a result of lengthy and unsuccessful (or unsatisfactory) treatment, patients can develop beliefs and expectations that can complicate further treatment efforts. One such belief is that they are unable to live normal, productive lives as long as they experience pain. They can become caught up in searching for a pain "cure" to the exclusion of all else, and when no magic cure is found, these patients remain impaired, placing themselves at risk for further disruptions to their lives.

PAIRS was developed to assess the extent to which chronic pain patients believe they cannot function normally because of their pain. The scale is a 15-item measure designed to assess the degree to which patients perceive their functional status as related to their pain level. Each statement measures a given thought, attitude, or opinion about pain. Patients endorse each item along a 7-point Likert-type scale (strongly disagree to strongly agree). Responses are summed to obtain an overall score. High scores indicate a person's greater tendency to equate pain with impairment and to restrict functioning when pain is present. Research using PAIRS has demonstrated adequate internal consistency and significant correlations with other measures of the cognitive component of chronic pain syndrome. In addition, it has been demonstrated in a chronic low back pain population that PAIRS scores were significantly correlated to measures of physical impairment, but not to physicians' ratings of disease severity, nor to measures of favorable self-report response bias.

Minnesota Multiphasic Personality Inventory (MMPI)

The MMPI is an empirically based, 566-item, self-report measure that yields a profile of personality attributes and psychopathology. It has been used extensively in both clinical and research settings with chronic pain populations. In one such study, it was found that the MMPI successfully predicted response to surgical and conservative pain treatments; MMPI scale elevations reflecting psychopathology were associated with poor outcome.

Interventions

Intervention is based on the patient's willingness to undergo pain rehabilitation, where the focus of treatment is to help the patient attain maximal function despite residual pain experience.

The overall goals of treatment are as follows:

1. Reduction of pain behavior and degree to which patients focus on their pain
2. Increased activity level and functional capacity
3. Reduction of the distress and attendant emotional suffering experienced by patients
4. Rearrangement of contingencies to pain behavior by family and significant others

5. Reduction of excessive health care utilization

MODIFICATION OF VERBAL BEHAVIOR AND PAIN BEHAVIOR

One primary treatment goal is to decrease pain behavior and related dysfunctional behaviors while increasing functional activities and "well" behaviors. Often, specific pain behaviors targeted for elimination or reduction are enumerated in a treatment contract filled out and signed by both the patient and the therapist during the second session. More adaptive behaviors the patient should assimilate are, likewise, specified in the treatment contract.

Typically, a reduction in pain behaviors is achieved through use of learning theory techniques. For example, pain behavior is ignored by the therapist and members of the treatment team. Moans, pain complaints, grimacing, and guarding are not responded to, nor does the treatment staff engage in talk about pain-related behavior or activity, except as medically indicated (e.g., new symptomatology suggestive of objective changes in health status such as neural involvement). Instead, staff reinforce the patient for gains made in the exercise program, time spent walking, or time out of bed, for example. Emphasis is on gains in function, with increased independence.

INCREASED ACTIVITY LEVEL

The patient is reinforced for improving functional activity goals, which can include decreasing "down" time as well as increasing repetitions of exercises and engaging in other functional activities such as walking, or increasing social interactions. This is accomplished through a variety of techniques.

Self-Monitoring and Behavior Charting

Patients are encouraged to keep records of their activities on a daily basis. Items such as relaxation sessions (complete with before-and-after ratings) of both pain and tension as well as physical therapy exercises are recorded. Time spent walking or engaging in social activities is also noted. Again, patterns of behavior should be noted, with expected increases in functional and positive activities with a concomitant decrease in dysfunctional behaviors (inordinate bed-rest, social isolation, etc.). Patients quickly learn to track their own activity patterns and progress once they have become accustomed to self-monitoring. The patient's logs and notations are used in treatment sessions to pinpoint problem areas and problem-solve, or, more positively, to reinforce the patient's gains and initiatives. During later treatment phases, activity logs can be used as a goal-setting aid, with progressive increases in those behaviors leading to goal attainment.

Goal-Setting

Initially, goal-setting serves as a means of preparing the patient for behavior changes and as an educational tool. The patient learns the basic principles of taking an activity and breaking it into manageable and achievable behaviors. For example, "going out to dinner" involves building sufficient sitting tolerance to handle a multicourse meal. As skills are acquired, behaviors are shaped to resemble the goal (meeting a friend for coffee). Finally, after goals are met, new ones that build on accomplishments take their place. Not all goals involve purely physical activities; increasing contact with friends or former colleagues, seeking a job, and socializing all serve to increase patient functioning.

Pacing

The ability to regulate not only the type of activity in which one engages but also the appropriate time for doing so is part of pacing. Patients learn to engage in certain behaviors for set periods of time to prevent excessive behavior (e.g., sitting in front of the computer for 25 minutes, then taking a 2- to 5-minute break before returning). Breaking a large task into smaller components is another method of pacing (e.g., preparing a meal in phases rather than waiting until dinnertime).

Health Care Utilization

Treatment also encourages a reduction in the number of pain-related office and emergency room visits, surgeries, and pharmacists contacted related to pain impairment or function. This is achieved through coordination and communication among all members of the treatment team, so that the patient receives a consistent message and treatment approach from all relevant care providers.

Medication

Chronic pain patients frequently use a variety of pain-relieving medications. Overuse and inappropriate use have been widely documented in the literature. Treatment focuses on appropriate reduction of medication. Again, medication reduction is usually accomplished within the framework of increased strength, endurance, and physical capacity training, as well as with relaxation, stress management, and pacing skills utilization. After the initial assessment period (see above), the patient's schedule for taking pain-related medications is shifted, if necessary, from an activity- or pain-contingent basis to a time-contingent basis. This lays the groundwork for breaking the learned association between occurrence of pain and automatic use of medication. Concurrently, the prescribing physician decreases the dosage (strength or amount prescribed per allotted time period) or the patient is encouraged to decrease the dosage within preset limits established in consultation with either the physician or behavioral medicine psychologist, or both. The goal of this aspect of treatment is to achieve the greatest and most reasonable reduction in the patient's medical regimen, especially in opiate or narcotic use. Understandably, some patients will require some degree of ongoing analgesic use, but others are able to eliminate medication use entirely or can switch to less habit-forming medications.

SOMATIC THERAPIES

Dealing with Relapse

Simply because patients have learned new techniques of managing their pain, and have hopefully become fairly adept at implementing the various techniques and skills, this does not guarantee they will never again be overwhelmed by pain and its accompanying despair, catastrophic thoughts, and feelings of hopelessness. Therapists can, however, lessen the impact of these temporary setbacks in a number of ways that can make "relapse" a useful learning experience, rather than one of failure.

Predicting Relapse

Usually, the first time patients try a significantly new behavior or routine (including lengthening the time between treatment sessions), they can expect pain flare-ups due to overextension brought on by lapses in pacing and other techniques, the increased stress of adjusting to new situations, and other unexpected factors. By predicting some of these difficulties, as well as allowing for a temporary increase in pain, therapists can prepare the patient for the inevitable stress incurred by temporary pain management difficulties. Additionally, one creates a win–win situation, in that, should the patient experience difficulties, they will come as less of a surprise to him or her and serve to reinforce the notion that the therapist does have an understanding of the situation. Alternatively, should the patient not experience difficulties, he or she can derive satisfaction (by receiving reinforcement both in the treatment session and on a personal basis) from having mastered the situation without the anticipated difficulties.

Positive Self-Statements Designed to Combat Failure

A summary of cognitive interventions that patients should be taught to help them deal with the negative experience of pain management setbacks is given below:

1. Treat "slips" (whether in relaxation practice or activity-based pain management) as mistakes rather than failures. This allows for graceful resumption of "the program."
2. Realize that feelings of guilt, self-blame, and anger are common among patients who experience pain exacerbation. The focus should be on emphasizing overall strengths and positive direction rather than magnifying mistakes.
3. Use setbacks to problem-solve for the future. What triggered the episode? What can the patient do differently next time, based on what he or she has learned from the situation? Sometimes, events that are not entirely in the patient's control happen. It is important to recognize that in reality, these things might happen, and to form contingency plans for dealing with such events as well as those

which are more completely under the patient's control. Often, acknowledgment by the therapist that a given aspect of a situation was, in fact, probably out of the patient's control is enough to reduce the patient's stress and enable him or her to focus on use of his or her coping repertoire.

4. Devise a plan and ways in which setback does not dictate new negative behavioral patterns. The patient should resume usual activities, continue relaxation techniques, use pacing, and focus on activities. Review cognitive strategies and suggest variations, if appropriate. The more the patient can contribute to this phase, the more control he or she will likely feel and be able to implement in future difficult situations.

Selected Readings

Ahern DK, Adams AE, and Follick MJ. Emotional distress and marital disturbance in spouses of chronic low back pain patients. *Clin J Pain* 1:69–74, 1985.

Flor H, Fydrich T, and Turk DC. Efficacy of multidisciplinary pain treatment centers: A meta-analytic review. *Pain* 49:221–230, 1992.

Follick MJ, Ahern DK, and Aberger EW. Development of an audiovisual taxonomy of pain behavior: Reliability and discriminant validity. *Health Psychol* 17:445-449, 1986.

Follick MJ, Smith TW, and Ahern DK. The sickness impact profile: A global measure of disability in chronic low back pain. *Pain* 21:67–76, 1985.

Fordyce WE. *Behavioral Methods for Chronic Pain and Illness.* St Louis: Mosby, 1976.

Holzman AD, Turk DC, and Kerns RD. The Cognitive-behavioral Approach in Treating Chronic Pain. In: Holzman AD and Turk DC (eds.). *Pain Management: A Handbook of Psychological Treatment Approaches.* Elmsford, NY: Pergamon Press, 1986.

Pither CE, and Nicholas MK. Psychological approaches in chronic pain management. *Br Med Bull* 47:743–761, 1991.

Rachlin H. Pain and behavior. *Behav Brain Sci* 8:43–53, 1985.

Roberts AH, Sternbach RA, and Polich J. Behavioral management of chronic pain and excess disability: Long term follow-up of an outpatient program. *Clin J Pain* 9:41–48, 1993.

Schwartz DP, DeGood DE, and Shutty MS. Direct assessment of beliefs and attitudes of chronic pain patients. *Arch Phys Med Rehabil* 66:806–809, 1985.

Turk DC. Customizing treatment for chronic patients: Who, what, and why. *Clin J Pain* 6:255–270, 1990.

Diagnostic and Therapeutic Procedures in Pain Management

Donald P. Todd and Shaffin A. Mohamed

> *"Take care not to get off soundings."*
>
> JAMES C. WHITE

This chapter reflects the majority of the diagnostic and therapeutic procedures for pain management performed at the Massachusetts General Hospital (MGH) Pain Center, since its foundation in 1948 by Donald P. Todd, MD. Several other procedures performed at other pain management centers are not described here. Some of these procedures have been abandoned by MGH, owing to their lack of utility in practice or to an unacceptable rate of complications intrinsically related to the procedure. Still other procedures are not mentioned here since they have not been implemented at MGH, and because they may not have proved to be effective in either the literature or practice.

Since we are called upon to perform diagnostic and therapeutic blocks, one of us (D.P.T.) devised some of these methods over a period of several years. This involved studying anatomy texts, surgical and radiologic, as well as consulting neurosurgeons, general and orthopedic surgeons, and radiologists. After a long period of trial and error, these techniques became effective, reliable, and reasonably free of untoward effects. For more than 20 years they have been taught to the staff and fellows at MGH. Hence, many of the techniques described are advanced techniques suitable for physicians beyond residency training.

Some of the procedures found here are variants of the "standard" techniques described in the literature. This is a result of our attempts to increase the precision, ease of performance, and safety of these procedures.

Aids to Techniques

DIAGNOSTIC VERSUS THERAPEUTIC PROCEDURES

Before starting a procedure, the clinician needs to determine whether to perform a diagnostic or therapeutic procedure in order to prepare the patient accordingly.

Diagnostic blocks should reveal two issues: (1) Does the pain have an important element of maintenance by sympathetic nerves as opposed to somatosensory nerves? (2) What particular nerve carries the pain or neuromuscular function in question? For example, which of several lumbar nerves adjacent to several bulging lumbar discs is responsible for the pain? Or, which intercostal nerve or nerves carry pain in a chest wall cancer? Upon finding the answers to these questions, the correct nerves can be ablated by alcohol.

Some clinicians believe that blocking a nerve first with placebo and then with anesthetic indicates whether a patient's pain is "real" or psychologic. However, by conventional wisdom, this test merely indicates whether the patient is a placebo responder on that occasion.

Therefore, in preparing the patient, the clinician needs to be sure that the patient has sustained pain before the procedure and that the pain can be reproduced or augmented by some activity or tactile stimuli. The same activity or stimuli must be repeated after the block. Finally, by objective testing, the clinician must demonstrate that the block was, in fact, accomplished.

In performing a block for sympathetic pain, the clinician must choose a site where the anesthetic is unlikely to affect somatic nerves that would interfere with interpretation (e.g., stellate block and paravertebral lumbar sympathetic block sites). In somatic pain, a paresthesic site must be found and very small, concentrated amounts of anesthetic used there to try to localize the block to the specific nerve. This degree of accuracy requires the use of a fluoroscopic image intensifier ("C-arm").

Therapeutic blocks, on the other hand, do not require this level of preparation or accuracy.

MARKING THE SITE

When using the C-arm fluoroscopy, it is very useful to first rest the point of a Kelly clamp over the target site on the patient, as seen on x ray, and then to position it over the insertion site. Although the insertion point is usually found by measurement or palpation, it is helpful to see whether this site would make it difficult to reach the target in a particular patient due to the angle required or because a rib might be in the way (as in lumbar sympathetic or celiac plexus block). These locations can then be marked on the skin by firmly pressing the hub of a 15-gauge needle onto the skin for 30 to 60 seconds. This mark will not disappear during preparation.

NERVE BLOCKING SOLUTIONS

For sympathetic nerves, mixing equal parts of 1% lidocaine with 1:200,000 epinephrine and 0.5% bupivacaine results in a final concentration of 0.5% lidocaine, 0.25% bupivacaine, and 1:400,000 epinephrine. This solution is adequate to block sympathetic nerves, does not create toxic levels in high volumes, and has enough epinephrine to provide early warning of intravascular injection. The onset of lidocaine is rapid, and bupivacaine provides prolonged effect. It should also be noted that in some patients with reflex sympathetic dystrophy (RSD) (the emotionally labile, especially), epinephrine may cause a panic attack, so it is best avoided.

For paravertebral or any mixed nerve block, a mixture of 1.5% lidocaine with 1:200,000 epinephrine and 0.2% tetracaine injected into a paresthesic site will provide a solid block, in a total volume of 2 ml (in 0.25-ml increments to avoid nerve damage). Again lidocaine provides rapid onset, and tetracaine prolongs the block long enough (approximately 1 hr) to allow the patient to make diagnostic observations. The solution is easily made by mixing 20 mg of crystalline (niphanoid) tetracaine for spinal anesthesia with 10 ml of 1.5% lidocaine.

A 0.75% bupivacaine solution could be substituted for tetracaine, but it will excessively dilute both the lidocaine and bupivacaine when the solutions are mixed. Using 2% lidocaine seems to cause too much spread.

Specific Blocks

SYMPATHETIC NERVE BLOCKS

Sympathetic nerve blocks are done in an attempt to isolate the relevant sympathetic nerves from the somatic nerves. Apart from the thoracic paravertebral and interpleural approaches, these techniques are useful for regional, pure sympathetic nervous system blockade.

Neck extension causes the cervical spine to be more superficial and thus easier to reach and draws the esophagus behind the trachea so it is less easily pierced by the left-sided approach.

Preblock Management

Patients are requested to consume only a light meal at least 4 hours prior to the procedure. Baseline vital signs are obtained, and an 18- or 20-gauge intravenous catheter with a heplock is placed. Premedication is avoided so baseline pain is not altered, patient cooperation is retained, and neurovascular responses to the block are not altered. The patient is positioned appropriately and blood pressure, ECG, pulse oximeter, and skin temperature monitors are engaged. Baseline verbal analog scores and range-of-motion estimates are obtained. Where indicated, a baseline skin psychogalvanic response may be obtained.

Block Procedures

Cervicothoracic, or Stellate, Ganglion Nerve Block

The following technique is specifically for use with C-arm fluoroscopy. "Standard" or nonfluoroscopic techniques are widely used elsewhere. The C-arm image intensifier is required to increase the success rate for upper-extremity sympathetic blocks from a range of 27% to 70% to approximately 90%.

INDICATIONS

1. Diagnosis and therapy of sympathetically maintained pain
2. Sympathetically mediated pain due to malignancy or other causes
3. Peripheral vasospastic disease, e.g., Raynaud's phenomenon
4. Acute herpes zoster
5. Acute posttraumatic or postoperative vascular insufficiency of the face, neck, or upper extremities

TECHNIQUE

1. Position the patient supine with the neck extended and a pillow under the shoulders.
2. Palpate the space between carotid pulsation and the lateral trachea, as low as possible in the neck.
3. Make a skin wheal over the medial edge of carotid pulsation at this level, usually at C6 or C7 over the transverse process, by C-arm fluoroscopy.
4. Direct a 2½ in. 22-gauge spinal needle caudad and medialward toward the junction of the lateral portion of segments C7 and T1—the level of the stellate ganglion (Fig. 9-1A,B).
5. When bone is encountered, check your position (it should feel like the hard, flat top of a table), withdraw 1 mm, and inject 10 ml of a 0.25% bupivacaine–0.5% lidocaine solution. Epinephrine is not used because some RSD patients are hypersensitive to it and may get panicky.
6. The 10 ml will conveniently spread (as dye would show) from C1 to T4.
7. Because there is no anatomic guide to the depth of the appropriate fascial plane (Fig. 9-2), a certain percentage of blocks (about 10%) will be missed.
8. Because of the medial placement (3–5 mm, medial to stellate ganglion) complications of vertebral artery injection, brachial plexus block and pneumothorax are not produced. Recurrent nerve block is not unusual, especially if the needle passes close to trachea.
9. A typical Horner's syndrome (ptosis, miosis, enophthalmos, often with anhydrosis and nasal congestion) is often produced, but tests of upper-extremity sympathetic nerve block need to be made, since the appearance of Horner's syndrome does not ensure an adequate block of the upper extremity.
10. If only the cervical portion of the sympathetic nerves needs to be blocked, then the procedure is more easily done at C6 or C5, but C-arm fluoroscopy should be used for accuracy.

POTENTIAL COMPLICATIONS

1. Transient nerve paralysis of the recurrent laryngeal nerve (hoarseness) or phrenic nerve (shortness of breath)
2. Pneumothorax
3. Hematoma

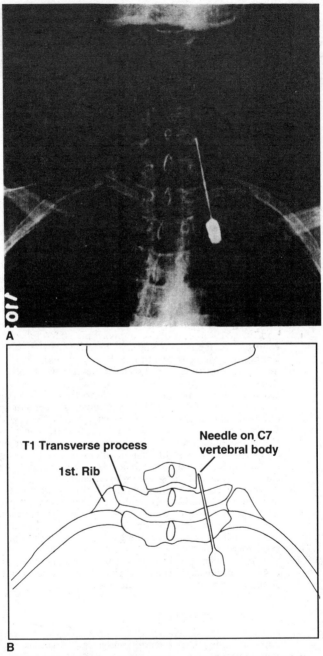

T1 Transverse process

1st. Rib

Needle on C7 vertebral body

Fig. 9-1. (A,B) Stellate ganglion block—anterior approach and diagrammatic representation.

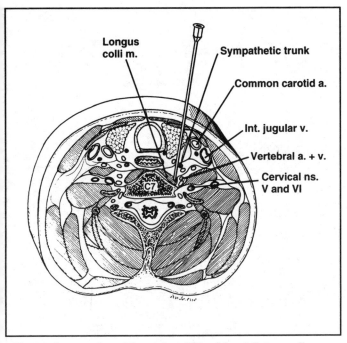

Fig. 9-2. Cross section of the neck at C7 level for stellate ganglion block.

4. Subarachnoid or epidural anesthesia by injection into the dural sleeve of the cervical root
5. Seizures, as a result of intravascular injection of local anesthetic

Stellate Catheter Block

If a prolonged block (3–7 days) is desired, the catheter may be left in place, using the method outlined below. This is an inpatient procedure, with about 7 days of block therapy indicated. It is a method that may be effective when single blocks do not produce a prolonged effect. The anterior catheter approach has been largely replaced by the interpleural catheter method due to ease of maintenance (see below). However, in patients with respiratory disease, the anterior approach is safer.

TECHNIQUE

1. Position: as for a single block.
2. Use a 16-gauge, 5½ in. Angiocath (Becton Dickinson Vascular Access, Sandy, Utah). Catheter-over-needle tends to cause less back-tracking of solution than catheter-through-needle. The extra length allows the injection port to be taped to the upper chest, so subsequent injections are less likely to displace the catheter (Fig. 9-3).

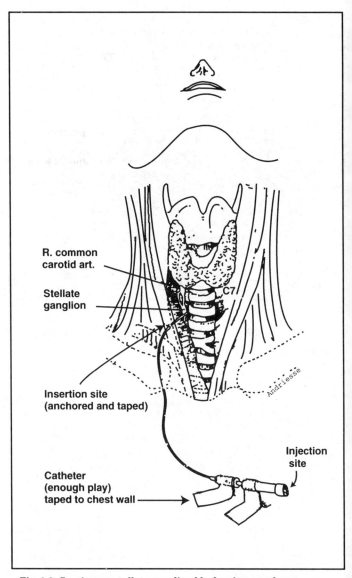

Fig. 9-3. Continuous stellate ganglion block using a catheter.

3. The entire catheter track, down to the bone, is anesthetized with a 2½ in., 22-gauge needle. If one aspirates on withdrawal and finds no blood, transvessel placement of the catheter is less likely.
4. Catheter-over-needle is then placed under C-arm fluoroscopic control, and the needle is withdrawn while holding the catheter against bone.
5. After a drop of Neosporin ointment at the entry point, the catheter can be held in the vertical position by radially placed Steri-Strips or by Tegaderm. Steri-Strips are small reinforced adhesive tapes. Tegaderm is an adhesive translucent polymer dressing (Tegaderm, 3M Medical-Surgical Division, St. Paul, MN).
6. The pillow is removed from under the shoulders, the head is returned to the neutral position, and the injection port is taped loosely to the upper chest to allow some head movement. The patient is cautioned to keep head movements to a minimum to avoid catheter displacement.
7. Inject the catheter with 10 ml of 0.25% bupivacaine.

POSTBLOCK MANAGEMENT

1. The catheter is injected with 10 ml of 0.25% bupivacaine q4h, preferably after meals.
2. If the patient's voice is hoarse, avoid oral fluids and solids.
3. Physical therapy, if indicated, should take place two or three times a day.
4. Patients must not be sent home with the catheter in place.

POTENTIAL COMPLICATIONS

1. Migration of catheter into a vessel
2. Aspiration
3. Pneumothorax
4. Hematoma
5. Intravascular injection

Thoracic Paravertebral Sympathetic Block

Sympathetic fibers from T1–T4 spinal roots can also be blocked paravertebrally by placing two needles caudad to ribs 1 and 3. However, the hazard of pneumothorax precludes practical use of this block.

Interpleural Approach

Local anesthetic deposited in the interpleural space (between visceral and parietal pleura) diffuses to the thoracic sympathetic fibers, which is a useful approach for long-term sympathetic block of at least the T1–T4 spinal levels. This catheter stays in place better than the stellate catheter, but runs an increased risk of pneumothorax, a potentially dire complication in patients with respiratory disease.

INDICATIONS

1. Continuous, unilateral sympathetic blockage (see Cervicothoracic, or Stellate, Ganglion Nerve Block above)
2. Acute, unilateral, postoperative pain relief for abdominal procedures

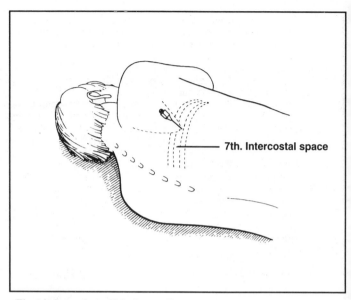

Fig. 9-4. Interpleural block—surface anatomy.

3. Thoracic acute herpes zoster or postherpetic neuralgia (not prolonged relief of the latter)
4. Pancreatic pain due to either chronic pancreatitis or pancreatic malignancy
5. Thoracic, chest wall, or esophageal pain due to either benign or malignant disease

Contraindications

1. Local infection
2. Bleeding diatheses
3. Pulmonary infections
4. Pulmonary fibrosis
5. Pleural adhesions
6. Symptomatic emphysema or bullous emphysema
7. Hemothorax
8. Pleural effusion

Technique

1. The patient's position should be lateral decubitus, with the upper shoulder rolled 45° forward (Fig. 9-4). A convenient interspace, caudad to the tip of the scapula, is chosen, and the track is well anesthetized down to the upper border of the lower rib.
2. A Tuohy needle, with hanging drop in place, is very slowly and carefully advanced to the upper border of the rib (to avoid the intercostal nerve and vessels).
3. It is then advanced above the rib, until the drop sucks in (Fig. 9-5). A second person immediately inserts the cath-

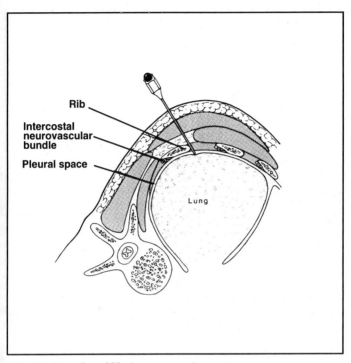

Fig. 9-5. Interpleural block—cross section anatomy.

eter through the needle and advances it an additional 15 cm or so.

4. A standard epidural catheter, preferably with a round end and side ports, such as a Portex (Concord/Portex, Keene, NH), is used because it is considered to be less traumatic.
5. The needle opening should have been directed cephalo-medial to encourage the catheter to go toward the posterior upper thorax.
6. After the catheter is in place, as much air as possible should be aspirated, while the patient takes a few breaths to move the pleura about.
7. A small test dose of lidocaine is given, and the catheter is taped in place. (Tegaderm makes a good, visible dressing; a small amount of triple antibiotic ointment at the catheter site may help to reduce infection.) A chest radiograph is obtained prior to use.
8. Sympathetic blocking doses of local anesthetic are given with the patient in the lateral decubitus position, affected side up, 10° of Trendelenberg, with the shoulder rotated **backward** 45°. This encourages the solution to flow into the costovertebral gutter and to reach sympathetic nerves beneath parietal pleura.
9. Every 4 hours 20–30 ml of 0.25% bupivacaine (no epinephrine) is given, and usually suffices to maintain a sympathetic block.

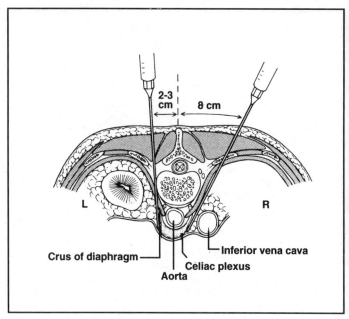

Fig. 9-6. Celiac plexus block — cross section at L1 level.

POTENTIAL COMPLICATIONS

1. Pneumothorax, including tension pneumothorax
2. Laceration of intercostal neurovascular bundle
3. Empyema and superficial infections
4. Formation of a bronchopleural fistula (rare).

Celiac Plexus Nerve Block

Since the celiac plexus is a network surrounding the celiac artery and the adjacent anterior aorta, the objective is to deposit solution anterior to the aorta. A variety of approaches are used.

1. Posterior, bilateral symmetrical approach, often without x ray.
2. Posterior approach with transfixion of the aorta.
3. Anterior approach using a CT scan and placing the needle on anterior aorta.
4. Bilateral posterior, asymmetrical approach with C-arm fluoroscopic guidance, as described below. With this technique, the right-sided needle is passed between the inferior vena cava and the aorta toward its anterior surface, and the left-sided needle is passed tangential to the aorta (Fig. 9-6). (Note: Neurolytic substances should never be injected in the vicinity of the spine without C-arm fluoroscopic and preliminary dye guidance.)

INDICATIONS

1. Pancreatic cancer pain
2. Pain of chronic relapsing pancreatitis, where the combination of local anesthetic and steroid is sometimes helpful

3. Diagnosis and therapy of sympathetically mediated abdominal, retroperitoneal, or flank pain

TECHNIQUE. The patient should be prone with a pillow under the epigastrium.

Right Side

1. Mark the skin, as in lumbar sympathetic block (see below), but at the L1 level.
2. A 20-gauge, 15-cm styletted needle is passed to the upper lateral portion of the body of L1, deviated laterally, and carried about 2.5 cm anterior to anterior surface of the L1 body.
3. Aspirate carefully as you proceed.

Left Side

1. A 20-gauge, 12-cm styletted needle is inserted vertical to the back, 2–3 cm lateral to the spinous process of L1, and just lateral to the upper lateral margin of the L1 body, using C-arm fluoroscopic visualization.
2. The needle is carried down to the lateral edge of the L1 vertebra.
3. The needle is deviated lateral, bevel toward the vertebra, and passed just beyond the lateral edge of the vertebra.
4. With the C-arm fluoroscopic image in the cross-table position, the right-sided needle is advanced 2.5 cm anterior to the anterior border of L1.
5. The left-sided needle is carefully advanced until a pulsating resistance is reached (the aorta), or until it is 2 cm anterior to L1.
6. After a 2-ml test dose, 20–25 ml of 0.5% lidocaine or 0.25% bupivacaine (or a mixture of both) is injected on each side.

Neurolytic Block

1. Prior to performing a neurolytic block, a diagnostic block should be done the day before to demonstrate pain relief. If this is done just prior to the alcohol block, the placebo effect and duration of relief cannot be evaluated.
2. Ten milliliters of 1% lidocaine is injected on either side.
3. This is followed by 5 ml of water-soluble dye (Isovue, Bristol Meyers Squibb, Princeton, NJ) 50% diluted with saline). Ideally a sausage-like pattern around the aorta is produced, but layering either anterior or posterior to the aorta is satisfactory. If dye streaks diagonally toward the diaphragm, it is in the crus of the diaphragm, and alcohol injection would be ineffective. If dye follows posteriorly toward the intervertebral foramen, the needle needs to be repositioned to avoid alcohol contacting the somatic nerves.
4. After a 20-minute wait to allow dispersal of lidocaine and dye, which can be verified with C-arm fluoroscopy, 25 ml of 50% alcohol (absolute alcohol diluted with saline) is injected on each side.
5. Usually the 10 ml of lidocaine will protect against irritative pain from the alcohol, but the patient may experience a brief aching in the epigastrium or back.

POTENTIAL COMPLICATIONS

1. Intravascular injection
2. Great-vessel perforation and retroperitoneal hematoma
3. Puncture of a viscus
4. Injection into kidneys, pancreas, peritoneal cavity, or liver
5. Epidural, subarachnoid, or lumbar plexus injection, possibly with neurolytic agents (not seen if performed under fluoroscopy)
6. Acute abdominal and chest discomfort, lasting approximately 30 minutes
7. Orthostatic hypotension, as a result of profound sympathetic neural blockade, lasting 48 hours or longer, following a neurolytic injection
8. Thrombosis or pressure occlusion of the spinal branch of the aorta, with resultant paraplegia (extremely rare)

Lumbar Sympathetic Nerve Block

Since the principal spinal segmental sympathetic supply to the lower extremities comes from L1–L3, it seems logical to place a needle at L2, and rely on volume and diffusion of local anesthetics to cover the whole outflow.

INDICATIONS

1. Diagnosis and therapy of sympathetically maintained pain syndromes of the lower extremities
2. Evaluation of potential benefit of neurolytic blockade or sympathectomy
3. Acute peripheral vascular insufficiency
4. Acute herpes zoster of the lower extremities
5. Some peripheral neuropathic pain syndromes of the lower extremities, with a sympathetically mediated component

TECHNIQUE

1. Accurate placement of the needle requires C-arm image intensifier guidance.
2. The patient should be prone with a pillow beneath the epigastrium.
3. Identify the lateral cephalad border of the body of the L2 vertebra (cephalad to transverse process, to avoid spinal nerve) by x ray.
4. Mark the skin projection.
5. Using x-ray visualization, mark 8 cm lateral to the spinous process of L2, slightly cephalad to the first mark.
6. Check to see that the mark is inferior or medial to the twelfth rib; if not, move medially.
7. Infiltrate lidocaine down to the body of the vertebra.
8. A 20-gauge, 12.5-cm (5 in.) needle is then carried down to the first target (lateral-cephalad portion of the body of L2).
9. Withdraw, redirect laterally with the needle bevel medial, and advance so the needle slides easily by the lateral surface of vertebra (Fig. 9-7).
10. Change to the cross-table C-arm fluoroscopic view. Advance the needle 1–2 mm anterior to the anterior surface of L2 (Fig. 9-8A,B).

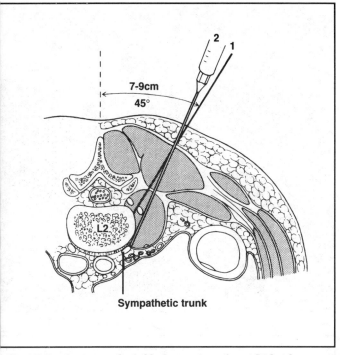

Fig. 9-7. Lumbar sympathetic block—cross section at L2 level.

11. Inject 20–30 ml of 0.5% lidocaine and 0.25% bupivacaine.

POSTBLOCK MANAGEMENT. Within minutes, flushing and warming of the foot should occur, and skin temperature should rise from 22°C to 34°C (see below). Sometimes, if the patient is very apprehensive and hyperreactive, the skin temperature will not rise for 20 to 30 minutes, presumably because circulating epinephrine maintains vasoconstriction. Once the patient relaxes in the recovery room, the foot usually warms up.

POTENTIAL COMPLICATIONS

1. As for celiac plexus block, above
2. Ureteral or renal perforation
3. Lumbar somatic nerve block and possible genitofemoral nerve block
4. Hypoalgesia in the L1/L2 distribution of the thigh

Hypogastric Plexus Nerve Block

This block may be useful in certain pelvic pain syndromes. Techniques have been suggested that resemble lumbar sympathetic blocks, but at L5. We have not had enough experience to discuss this block; it is mentioned for the sake of completeness.

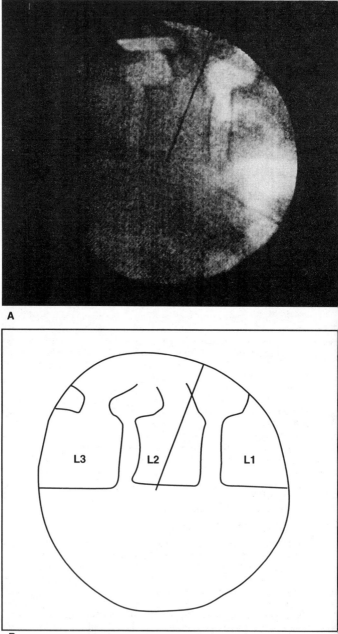

A

B

Fig. 9-8. (A, B) Lumbar sympathetic block—lateral radiograph and diagrammatic representation.

Confirmation of Sympathetic Blocks

This is an essential element in sympathetic blocks, especially for diagnostic ones. Because there are no sensory measures of block efficacy, other means are needed.

Skin Temperature

Skin temperature is simple to measure with a thermocouple, best placed on the pads of the fingers or toe tips, to record maximum temperature swings. This applies, of course, only to blocks involving the upper or lower extremities. No clear-cut means of assessing completeness of sympathetic block of the trunk has been devised. Temperature tests are best performed in a cool room (68°F–70°F) after the patient has fasted for at least two hours, with the arms and legs exposed to air. This allows a baseline skin temperature close to room temperature. The contralateral temperature should be continually compared. A complete sympathetic block should cause a rise in temperature from 72°F (22°C) to 93°F (34°C) in a patient with normal peripheral circulation. With vascular insufficiency (unusual in RSD), skin temperature does not fall as low or rise as high. Other signs of sympathetic block should appear, such as flushing and dry skin.

Psychogalvanic or Galvanic Skin Response

A more clear-cut end point is provided by the psychogalvanic or galvanic skin response (Cousins and Bromage, 1988). It is easily performed by a standard, existing ECG, used as a galvanometer: Any two opposing leads (RA–LA, or lead I, is simple) are placed on the palm and dorsum of the hand or sole and the dorsum of the foot, depending on the extremity involved. Other leads are attached at random for stability of recording (preferably not in ECG configuration to avoid ECG tracing). To "discharge" the sympathetic nerves, a single deep breath, a sudden unexpected noise, or painful stimuli are used. This produces, with intact sympathetic nerves, a biphasic response seconds later (Fig. 9-9), returning to baseline in about 5 seconds. If the sympathetic nerves are completely blocked there is no response (flat line). The response may not be present in very old people or in diabetics with peripheral neuropathy. The electrophysiologic mechanism is not understood.

Postblock Management

The patient is observed for 1 hour in the postanesthesia care unit to evaluate for potential complications that do not appear immediately. The patient is then discharged with an escort. A patient having received a stellate ganglion nerve block is tested with small amounts of fluid to detect possible aspiration prior to feeding. If hoarseness is present, oral intake should be avoided. Other potential complications should be anticipated prior to discharge. A patient who has received a lumbar sympathetic block requires only 1 hour of observation, as described above. For neurolytic blocks, extended observation (24–48 hr) is required.

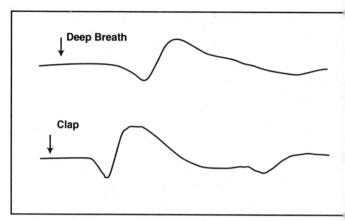

Fig. 9-9. Psychogalvanic reflex galvanometer (ECG) tracing.

A patient with an interpleural catheter usually stays at the hospital. Injections of 0.25% bupivacaine, 5–15 ml q4–6 h can be given to maintain a sympathetic block of the unilateral upper extremity. Blood pressure and vital signs should be evaluated regularly. A chest radiograph should be checked for clinically significant pneumothorax prior to using the catheter.

Regular monitoring of vital signs following a celiac plexus block, for up to 4 hours with a local anesthetic block, and 24 hours or longer with a neurolytic block, may be necessary. Evaluation for the other potential complications is also necessary.

Evaluation of Blocks

In sympathetically maintained pain, there should be immediate, complete relief, lasting hours to weeks. Partial relief is thought to indicate a "sympathetic element" in the pain. Yet in some patients with a clinical diagnosis of sympathetically maintained pain there is no relief. In practice, the results of sympathetic blocks indicate whether blocking procedures would be useful in therapy.

Block Treatment Protocol

In treating RSD with sympathetic blocks, our practice is to give one block per week for 3 weeks. If, in conjunction with physical therapy, the blocks allow the disease to improve they are continued. If the duration of relief from the block is not useful, and the disease fails to improve, then a 1-week continuous block on an inpatient basis is indicated. If improvement is sustained after the week in the hospital, but symptoms recur, a second or even third attempt at hospitalized continuous catheter treatment is tried. If all of this fails a surgical sympathectomy may be recommended. Our neurosurgeons and general surgeons believe that surgical sympathectomy is followed by fewer complications than neurolytic blocks with alcohol. If only a 4- to 6-week sympathetic ablation is desired, then aqueous phenol (7%) may be used.

Spinal cord stimulation is also a more recent alternative; however, we have not been performing this procedure and therefore cannot comment further on it.

CENTRAL NERVE BLOCKS

Lumbar Epidural Block

This section pertains to the catheter approaches in pain management. Because the intrathecal space is not used extensively in chronic pain management, this subject is not discussed. Hence, this section focuses on epidural catheters for the thoracic or lumbar regions. We do not employ cervical epidural catheters.

The epidural block is usually a central one, of both the somatic and sympathetic nerves. However, a predominantly sympathetic block, continuous or intermittent, can be achieved using more dilute local anesthetic solutions (e.g., 0.10–0.25% bupivacaine), when indicated. Somatic blockade is easily achieved by increasing the local anesthetic concentration (e.g., 0.25–0.50% bupivacaine), when necessary. For prolonged use, tunneled epidural catheters are placed.

Indications

1. Pain syndromes due to peripheral vascular insufficiency, including ischemic vasospastic pain
2. Prolonged sympathetic blockade for treatment of sympathetically maintained pain, unilateral or bilateral
3. Management of acute herpes zoster, and sometimes for postherpetic neuralgia
4. Treatment of acute thoracic or lumbar strain, with radiculopathy
5. Treatment of regional pain syndromes due to malignancy
6. Diagnostic or therapeutic (temporary or neurolytic) blocks

Preblock Management

Patients are requested to consume only a light meal at least 4 hours before the procedure. Baseline vital signs are obtained, and an 18- or 20-gauge intravenous catheter with a heplock is placed. Premedication is avoided so patient cooperation is retained and neurovascular responses to the block are not altered. The patient is positioned appropriately and blood pressure, ECG, and pulse oximeter monitors are started.

Block Procedures

MIDLINE APPROACH

1. The patient takes the lateral position, with maximal flexion of the back and with the knees to the abdomen.

2. Obese patients should sit bent forward, with the knees to the abdomen or the legs resting on a stool. This helps to identify the midline, and may widen the posterior interspinous space.

3. The spinal cord terminates at L1 or L2 in the adult; therefore, the spinous process, intervertebral space, and midline are carefully palpated below this level. An appropriate interspace is located.

4. The overlying skin is prepared with antiseptic solution (such as alcohol or povidone-iodine), and a sterile, fenestrated cloth draped over the site.

5. A skin wheal is made with a ½-in., 25-gauge needle, using 1% lidocaine, and deeper infiltration is performed with a 1½ in., 22-gauge needle.

6. A 17- or 18-gauge Tuohy needle is directed perpendicular or slightly cephalad in the interspinous space with the bevel pointing cephalad and advanced to the ligamentum flavum.

7. The stylet is removed and a glass syringe containing 3–4 ml of air is attached to the Tuohy needle. The needle is advanced, while rapidly oscillating the plunger on the syringe, until there is a loss of resistance and some of the air escapes. This maneuver can be performed using sterile saline in the syringe, but with continuous pressure on the plunger until there is a loss of resistance. We do not recommend the hanging drop method, because we have noted a higher incidence of dural punctures.

8. Medication or saline can be injected into the Tuohy needle to distend the epidural space, and the epidural catheter is advanced through the needle at least 5 cm into the epidural space.

9. The Tuohy needle is removed while maintaining the catheter in position, and the distance between the catheter mark and the skin is measured to assure that the catheter has not been moved during removal of the needle.

10. The catheter is then secured to the skin with a transparent dressing and tested for intravascular or intrathecal placement with 3 ml of 2% lidocaine with epinephrine. Aspiration is also performed for blood or cerebrospinal fluid.

11. To decrease displacement of the catheter tip, it is wise to bring the excess catheter around the flank to the epigastrium, rather than up the back and over the shoulder, as is done in operative cases. This is because flexing the spine inevitably pulls the nonstretching catheter back from the epidural space.

12. The catheter is then ready for use, either with bolus or continuous infusions.

PARAMEDIAN APPROACH

1. A skin wheal is made 1 cm lateral and 2 cm caudad to the interspinous space to be entered.

2. A 17- or 18-gauge Tuohy needle is aimed from the lateral skin wheal to the top of the target interspace, i.e., the needle is aimed medially and slightly cephalad.

3. The needle is advanced to the ligamentum flavum, and an air- or saline-filled syringe is attached.
4. After obtaining a loss of resistance, the catheter is threaded in, the Tuohy needle is removed, and the catheter is tested and secured, as above.

TUNNELED EPIDURAL CATHETER

1. Place the epidural catheter as instructed above.
2. Anesthetize a subcutaneous tract horizontally across one side of the back.
3. Tunnel a long 14-gauge intravenous catheter through the tract, starting farthest away from the epidural placement site and emerging in the same skin nick as the epidural catheter. (Note: Do not puncture the epidural catheter with the intravenous needle.)
4. Remove the needle from the intravenous catheter and thread the epidural catheter through the intravenous catheter.
5. Remove the intravenous catheter and secure the epidural catheter at the lateral skin exit wound with transparent dressing.
6. The epidural catheter is tested (as above) and used for intermittent boluses or continuous infusion.

Potential Complications

1. Dural puncture, possible postdural puncture headache
2. Subarachnoid injection with high spinal anesthesia and hypotension
3. Intravascular injection, e.g., into epidural veins, with possible seizures
4. Broken epidural catheter
5. Potential neural damage
6. Epidural hematoma
7. Epidural abscess
8. Vasovagal syncope
9. Arachnoiditis

Postblock Management

If the catheter is to be used for continuous block, the patient is admitted to the hospital for 7 to 10 days. Vital signs are monitored every hour for the first 4 hours, every 2 hours for the next 4 hours, and then every shift. The patient is admitted for the purpose of intensive physical therapy, following pain relief.

Pain relief is usually achieved using a continuous infusion of 0.1% bupivacaine, up to 10 ml/hr, sometimes with the addition of 3 or 10 μg/ml fentanyl. Diet and other activities are based on patient preference.

If the catheter is to be used for pain relief (e.g., cancer pain), the 0.1% bupivacaine solution is tried. If relief is not achieved, 0.25% bupivacaine, with or without fentanyl, can be used as necessary. Vital signs are monitored as described above. Activity and diet are as tolerated by the patient. The catheter should be removed in 7 to 10 days. If prolonged infusions are required, the catheter is tunneled subcutaneously at the time of placement.

Thoracic Epidural Block

This procedure is performed in the same way as for the lumbar epidural catheter. Indications may vary for the location of the catheter, but the technique varies only in that additional care is required in approaching the epidural space, because the distances are less than those for a lumbar approach. In addition, the needle must be aimed in a more cephalad direction to traverse the thoracic interspinous space. Management and complications are essentially identical to those of the lumbar epidural catheter.

Caudal Epidural Block

Although caudal injections are performed under fluoroscopic guidance, we rarely place caudal epidural catheters for pain management in adults.

PARAVERTEBRAL NERVE BLOCKS (SELECTED NERVE ROOT BLOCKS)

Standard textbook procedures for paravertebral nerve blocks were designed to produce anesthesia for surgery and not for diagnostic or therapeutic purposes. Standard procedures emphasize safety (i.e., less likely to enter the subarachnoid space) and blanketing the area with large volumes. This does not allow isolation of a single nerve root for diagnosis, nor the likelihood of entering the epidural nerve root space for therapy.

We briefly discuss the concept of injecting into paresthesias. Local anesthetic injections into nerves damage them through disruption. This is due to the volume and force of the injection. The needle itself does not produce clinically detectable damage, unless the nerve is repeatedly speared. Hence, if one injects small amounts (0.25–0.50 ml) very slowly (only moderately painful to the patient), no discernible clinical damage is done, and the block is assured. This has been my experience in over 40 years of injecting into paresthesias of many types of peripheral nerves (D.P.T.).

Preblock Management

If the purpose of the block is diagnostic, it is essential that the patient experience pain before the block, which may be produced or exacerbated by some motion or activity. It is difficult to make observations about the simple statement: "I have pain." Analgesic or sedative medications should be avoided before the block, if at all possible. If not, then medication effect alone should be tested before the block, to be sure that the pain is still present. Short-acting anxiolytics are preferred over analgesics.

Patients are also asked to eat lightly up to 4 hours before the block. An intravenous catheter may not be used, but vital signs are monitored.

Indications

1. Determination of the nerve root(s) involved in a pain syndrome. The surgeon is then able to proceed with more confidence in removing a disc or decompressing the root that carries the pain.
2. Therapeutic steroid injection at a scarred or compressed root, for pain not relieved by midline epidural steroid. This is particularly useful in lumbar radicular pain.

Block Procedures

Cervical Paravertebral Nerve Block

Recall that cervical nerves leave the spine **above** their respective vertebra. Furthermore, the C1 root has no sensory function. The C2 root emerges laterally between the C1 and C2 vertebrae, passes over the articular process of C1, and emerges between the posterior arches of C1 and C2. It is distributed mainly to the greater occipital nerve.

TECHNIQUE FOR C2 NERVE ROOT BLOCK. The C2 root is best blocked as it passes over the posterior surface of the superior articular process of C2. Generally, it is simpler to block the occipital nerve, if that fulfills the need. With C-arm fluoroscopic guidance, and with the patient prone, the needle is directed vertically down to the articular process, where paresthesia may be obtained.

TECHNIQUE FOR C3–C6 NERVE ROOT BLOCKS

1. Position the patient with no pillow support and with the head in the neutral position or rotated away from the side to be blocked. The patient's anatomy is more symmetrical in the neutral position, but it is more difficult to palpate and to guide the needle. With the head rotated (it may be necessary to elevate the shoulder on padding) it is easier to look into the intervertebral foramen and to palpate and guide the needle, but the anatomy of the neck becomes spiral (Fig. 9-10).
2. Using C-arm fluoroscopy, a skin mark is made over the posterior border of the intervertebral foramen image and slightly cephalad to it. The cervical plexus can be avoided by approaching the cervical nerve in its foramen from a posterior position, since the cervical plexus lies lateral and anterior to the transverse processes.
3. A 2½ in., 22-gauge spinal needle is advanced so it encounters the superior surface of the groove in the transverse process that supports the nerve. The needle is then deviated toward the intervertebral opening until paresthesia is obtained (Fig. 9-11).
4. The C-arm fluoroscope is then rotated to the anteroposterior position to observe the medial progress of the needle. The needle point should not go beyond the cephalad-directed lip on the lateral border of the body of the vertebra, which marks the lateral extent of the epidural space. The needle point should also be at least halfway into the mass of the transverse process image to avoid spread to anesthetic to other roots (Fig. 9-12).

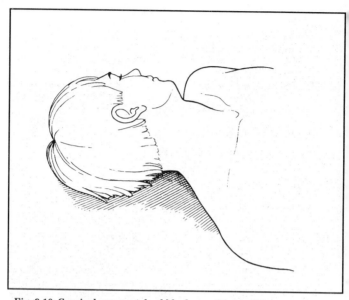

Fig. 9-10. Cervical paravertebral block—patient position.

5. A single nerve root can be anesthetized with 1–2 ml of a mixture of equal parts of 1.5% lidocaine and 0.2% tetracaine, with 1:400,000 epinephrine, or with 0.5% bupivacaine in place of tetracaine (it is simple to mix 2 ml of 0.2% tetracaine from a spinal ampule with 2 ml of 1.5% lidocaine with 1:200,000 epinephrine in a syringe). Inject 0.25–0.50 ml at a time.

Technique for C7 nerve root block. The C7 lies on the anterior surface of the flattened transverse process of C7. •

1. Position the patient supine.
2. Insert the needle lateral and superior to the transverse process and advance to touch it.
3. Then move the needle about on the process until paresthesia is achieved.
4. Perform the injection as above.

Technique for C8 nerve root block. The C8 root emerges between the C7 and T1 vertebrae and is blocked in the same manner as for the thoracic nerves (see below).

Thoracic Paravertebral Nerve Block

Most clinicians have found that single paravertebral thoracic nerve blocks are difficult to perform without producing a pneumothorax. This accounts for the variety of techniques suggested.

1. Direct the needle from the rib above the nerve, medial and caudad for 1 cm into the intercostal space, and reach the nerve through diffusion of a large volume (3–5 ml) of local anesthetic. This is recommended for surgical procedures.

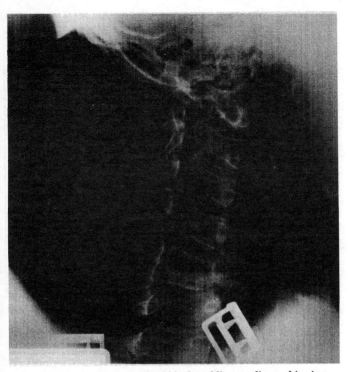

Fig. 9-11. Cervical paravertebral block—oblique radiographic view.

2. Start much closer to the midline and "walk off" the lateral part of the lamina in a caudad direction, using similarly large volumes.
3. Insert the needle 5 cm lateral to the midline until it contacts the rib below the nerve and redirect the needle just cephalad to the rib on an acute angle (about 30°–45° with skin surface) toward the intervertebral foramen. In this manner a single nerve root can be anesthetized for diagnostic purposes. This technique is described below.

Owing to the considerable hazard of pneumothorax with all these approaches, one should consider the necessity of using the paravertebral approach, as opposed to the standard intercostal block. Furthermore, unless it is essential to block the posterior primary division of the nerve root, intercostal nerve blocks serve just as well and seldom produce a pneumothorax. A nearby skeleton is of great assistance in interpreting bony landmarks encountered by the needle.

TECHNIQUE

1. Position the patient laterally with a pillow under the chest and rotate the patient forward about 45° to make the ribs as superficial as possible.

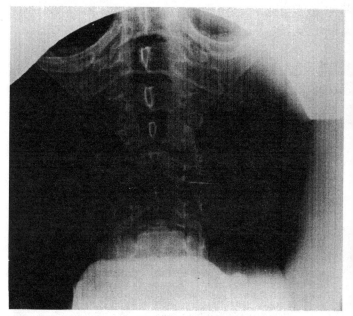

Fig. 9-12. Cervical paravertebral block—anteroposterior radiographic view.

2. Using fluoroscopy (a necessity for accuracy), locate the appropriate rib and intervertebral foramen.
3. Anesthetize the skin entry site with 1% lidocaine using a short 25-gauge needle.
4. Insert a 2½-in., 22-gauge needle 5 cm (5–7 cm in heavy-set people) lateral to the midline until it encounters the rib.
5. With the intervertebral foramen in view on the lateral x ray, advance the needle above the rib and toward the foramen until paresthesia is achieved. It is reassuring to encounter the lateral portion of a vertebra, before entering the foramen, to indicate proper depth.
6. Rotate the C-arm fluoroscope into the anteroposterior position to check that the needle is lateral to the epidural (or spinal canal) space.
7. Inject 1–2 ml on 0.25-ml increments until anesthesia is achieved.

Lumbar Paravertebral Nerve Block

There are two principal techniques: direct the needle either caudad from the transverse process above the nerve or cephalad from the process below the nerve. As with thoracic blocks, greater accuracy and an increased possibility of spreading solution along or into the perineural epidural sheath are achieved using the latter approach; however, subarachnoid injection is also a more frequent hazard.

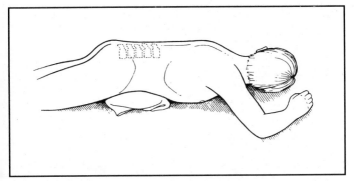

Fig. 9-13. Lumbar paravertebral block—patient position. (Used also for lumbar sympathetic and lumbar epidural injections.)

TECHNIQUE FOR L1–L4 NERVE ROOT BLOCKS. In the lumbar region, as opposed to the thoracic region, if one heads for the intervertebral foramen from the transverse process below the nerve, it is very easy to enter the spinal epidural space or intrathecal canal, so the diagnostic value of a single nerve root block is lost. In addition, the lumbar spine offers considerably more space in which to maneuver, so paresthesia is readily achieved when the needle encounters a nerve as it emerges just caudad to the pedicle of the vertebra. This is approached from the transverse process cephalad to the nerve.

1. Position the patient prone with a pillow under the belly using C-arm fluoroscopy (Fig. 9-13).
2. Visualize the caudad border of the desired vertebral pedicle and mark this target skin projection.
3. Insert the needle 5 cm lateral to the midline (4–7 cm, depending on body mass) to encounter the caudad border of the transverse process above the target nerve.
4. Then advance the needle from the transverse process, caudad and medial, toward the pedicle of the vertebra, which projects as an oval shadow on an anteroposterior view of the spine, until paresthesia is obtained. A lateral C-arm fluoroscopic view will confirm position of the needle at the intervertebal foramen (Fig. 9-14).
5. Inject into the paresthesic site 1–2 ml of solution in 0.25-ml increments. For therapeutic purposes, 50 mg of triamcinolone (Aristocort or Kenalog) is adequate.

TECHNIQUE FOR L5 NERVE ROOT BLOCK. Owing to the close proximity of the L5 transverse process to the sacrum, it is often difficult to maneuver the needle in this narrow space from an insertion point 5 cm lateral to the midline in order to achieve paresthesia. One is usually more successful in choosing a more lateral insertion point, so the needle passes either caudad or anterior to a posteriorly inclined transverse process.

1. Position the patient prone with a pillow under the lower belly.
2. The skin entry site is well anesthetized.

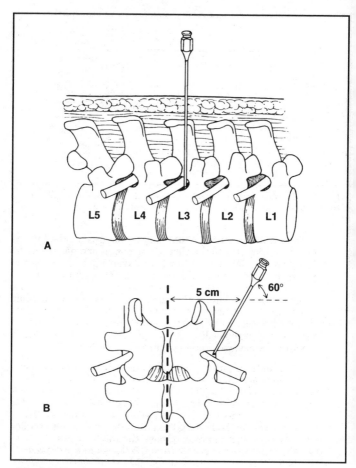

Fig. 9-14. Lumbar paravertebral block—lateral (A) and anteroposterior (B) views.

3. A 3½-in., 22-gauge spinal needle is inserted 8 cm lateral to the midline, just above the iliac crest, by C-arm fluoroscopy.
4. It is advanced medial and somewhat caudad to strike the L5 transverse process.
5. The needle is then redirected slightly caudad and anteriorly to encounter the posterior surface of the lateral body of L5, just caudad to the pedicle, and about 2 cm deeper.
6. The point is maneuvered as for other lumbar nerves to achieve paresthesia.
7. The position is checked using a lateral C-arm fluoroscopic view, and the same injection is made.

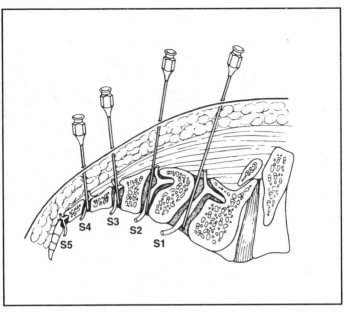

Fig. 9-15. Sacral nerve blocks—parasagittal section.

Sacral Paravertebral Nerve Block

For diagnostic, individual sacral nerve root blocks, it is necessary to find a place where each root is anatomically separated from adjacent roots. This is at the anterior sacral foramen, where the anterior primary division emerges from the sacral epidural space, and courses into the posterior pelvis to join the lumbosacral plexus (Fig. 9-15). To concentrate steroid near the affected sacral root (but not exclusively to one root), sacral epidural injections can be made, once the needle is through the posterior foramen. At S1, the epidural space is about 2 cm deep; at S2, 1½ cm; at S3, 1 cm; and at S4, ½ cm.

TECHNIQUE FOR S1 NERVE ROOT BLOCK. Scan the sacral area briefly with the C-arm fluoroscope at different angles (remember, sacrum takes off posteriorly from the lumbar spine at about 45°) to see if the posterior foramen can be made to lay over the anterior foramen. Usually only the anterior foramen is seen. Bowel shadows (gas or feces) may partially obscure landmarks, but attempts to clean out the bowel using enemas or cathartics only tend to make matters worse.

1. Position the patient prone with a pillow under the lower belly using C-arm fluoroscopy for visualization.
2. With a rubber marker on a 3½ in., 22-gauge spinal needle, insert the needle at the level of the L5 vertebra (C-arm in straight anteroposterior direction) level, just lateral to the image of the anterior S1 foramen.
3. The needle is advanced at 45° caudally to strike the posterior surface of the sacrum.

4. The rubber marker on the needle is set 1 cm from the skin.
5. The needle point is then moved about until it falls through the posterior foramen (Fig. 9-16A,B).
6. The posterior foramen is usually found somewhat cephalad and lateral to the superomedial border of the elliptical image of the anterior foramen.
7. For epidural injections, the needle point is advanced 1 cm through the posterior foramen, as measured by the rubber marker (described above).
8. To block the S1 root, the needle is advanced another centimeter until paresthesia is achieved at the anterior foramen (Fig. 9-17A,B).
9. If no paresthesia is achieved after two to three thrusts of the needle, it must be withdrawn and inserted through a new skin wheal, either 1 cm medial or lateral to the initial wheal. One of these three positions usually achieves paresthesia.
10. Intraneurally, 1–2 ml of solution is injected 0.25 ml at a time.

TECHNIQUE FOR S2–S4 NERVE ROOT BLOCKS. Remember that the sacrum is curved and that needles will appear in a radial array, starting from the S1 root.

1. Position the patient prone with a pillow under the lower belly using C-arm fluoroscopy for visualization.
2. Skin wheals are made slightly lateral and vertical to the image of the anterior foramen.
3. As described above, anterior foramina and paresthesia will be found approximately 1.5 cm, 1.0 cm, and 0.5 cm through the posterior foramina of S2, S3, and S4, respectively.

TECHNIQUE FOR S5 NERVE ROOT BLOCK. In most people, there is no S5 posterior or anterior foramen. This is not an accurate block, nor is accuracy often required. The S5 root can be anesthetized (without paresthesia) by passing a needle just inferior and lateral to the tip of the sacrum (Fig. 9-18).

Postblock Management

Patients are observed for potential, late-appearing complications for 1 hour. If motor and sensory functions are intact, the patient is discharged with an escort.

SOMATIC (PERIPHERAL) NERVE BLOCKS

These procedures are frequently performed with local anesthetics for diagnostic and therapeutic reasons. Some are then repeated with neurolytic agents or surgical ablation. Cryotherapy is also performed at some centers; however, we do not currently use this modality.

Preblock Management

No special preparation is necessary. Pain should be present at the time of the block for diagnostic purposes.

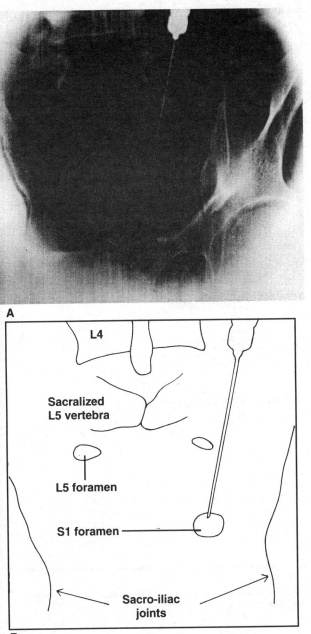

Fig. 9-16. (A,B) First sacral (S1) nerve block—anteroposterior radiographic view and diagrammatic representation.

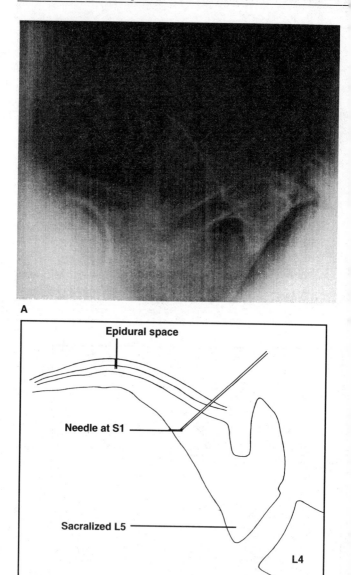

A

B

Fig. 9-17. (A,B) First sacral (S1) nerve block—lateral radiographic view and diagrammatic representation.

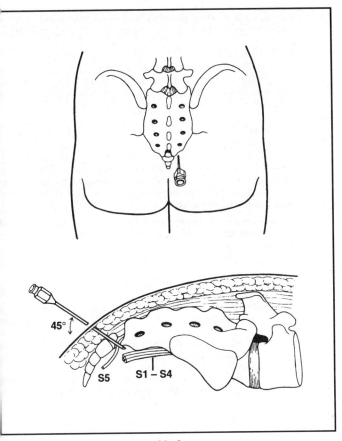

Fig. 9-18. Fifth sacral (S5) nerve block.

Trigger Point Injections

These blocks are performed for a vague and broad entity called **myofascial pain syndrome**. Patients present with localized, palpable, swollen muscle bundles, which reproduce the pain when pressure is applied, called **trigger points**. Trigger points can be detected by light palpation with the flats of the fingers. When "swelling" is detected, pressure will elicit the referred pain. If the referred pain is not reproduced, this is not a trigger point, but merely a muscle in spasm.

The pain is temporarily relieved by injection of a local anesthetic into the trigger point. However, prolonged relief is obtained through local anesthetics and steroid injections, sometimes in conjunction with adjunctive therapies. These therapies include physical therapy, particularly stretching, massage, and heat. Stretching can be painful, so a vapocoolant, such as ethyl chloride, and local anesthetic injectio should precede stretching, i.e., "spray-and-stretch" techniqu

Technique

1. Inject 3–5 ml of 0.25% bupivacaine, with 10 mg of tr amcinolone, into and around the trigger point using a 2! gauge, 1½-in. needle, and aspirating before injecting.
2. Repeat as needed, and wherever required.

Peripheral Nerve Blocks

Occipital Nerve Block

Occipital neuralgia can result from stretching or entrapmen of the occipital nerve. The nerve is sometimes trapped in th fascia overlying the posterior surface of C2, or in occipita ligamentous attachments.

INDICATIONS. Occipital neuralgia either as tension head aches or following injury, e.g., auto accidents with whiplash falls, or work injuries.

TECHNIQUE

1. Position the patient sitting on a stool with the elbows lean ing on a table and with the forehead in the hands.
2. Palpate the posterior occipital protuberance and mov 1.5–2.0 cm laterally and feel for occipital artery pulsatio and groove (Fig. 9-19).
3. Inject 5 ml of 0.5% bupivacaine, with 30 mg of triamcin olone, down to the bone and fan out. Occipital nerve an algesia should occur very rapidly.
4. Inject some of the solution more caudally for occipital mus cle attachment pain and spasm, which often respond t steroid injections.

Intercostal Nerve Block

INDICATIONS

1. Rib fractures—acute, traumatic, and pathologic
2. Chest-wall metastases or tumor
3. Postthoracotomy pain or pain due to percutaneous drain age tubes
4. Diagnostic or therapeutic blocks for abdominal pain ver sus abdominal wall pain.

TECHNIQUE

1. Position the patient in the semilateral position, with the sites to be injected made prominent by placing a pillow under opposite thorax.
2. The injection site should be at the posterior axillary line to 5–7 cm lateral to the vertebral spinous processes. (One cannot get posterior division without injecting via the par avertebral approach: hazard of pneumothorax.)
3. Make a skin wheal (and injection in a thin person) with a 25-gauge, ½-in. subcutaneous needle. Enter vertical to skin, "walk" the needle just below the rib and forward 2 mm. Inject 3 ml of 0.5% bupivacaine with epinephrine at

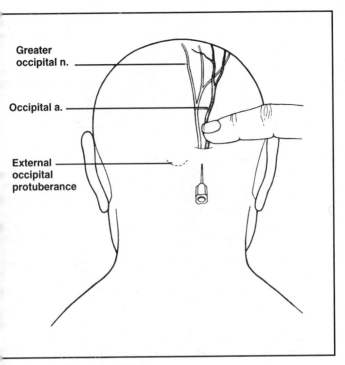

Fig. 9-19. Occipital nerve block.

each rib (Fig. 9-20). (Note: anesthetic is absorbed as rapidly as if given intravenously.)

4. Neurolytic intercostal block: First block the nerve proximally with 0.5% bupivacaine, and then inject 2–3 ml of 100% ethyl alcohol lateral to the anesthetized site (alcohol is initially very painful).

POTENTIAL COMPLICATIONS

1. Pneumothorax (low incidence)
2. Intravascular injection
3. Seizures
4. Alcoholic neuritis

Lateral Femoral Cutaneous Nerve Block

This condition is believed to be associated with obesity or pregnancy or the wearing of a tight belt. It is thought to be due to entrapment of the lateral femoral cutaneous nerve as it passes through the inguinal ligament. Neurolytic blocks are not recommended; however, surgical dissection may be considered.

INDICATIONS. Meralgia paresthetica: burning pain, numbness, and tingling in the anterolateral aspect of the thigh.

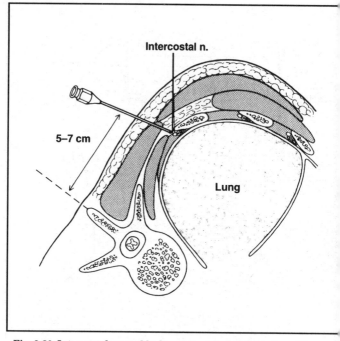

Fig. 9-20. Intercostal nerve block — patient in semilateral position.

TECHNIQUE

1. Position the patient supine.
2. Palpate the anterior superior iliac spine and insert a 1½-in., 25- or 22-gauge needle 2–3 cm medial to it (Fig 9-21).
3. Proceed through the fascia (feel a "pop") and inject 10 m of 0.5% bupivacaine with 30 mg of triamcinolone, fanwise from the medial surface of the iliac spine medial to be neath the insertion point.

EVALUATION OF BLOCK. Analgesia of upper two thirds o anterolateral thigh should be produced.

Ilioinguinal Nerve Block

INDICATIONS

1. Postherniorraphy pain, which is usually due to trauma to the genitofemoral nerve in the floor of the inguinal canal
2. Diagnostic block, prior to surgical dissection or neurolytic block (hazardous).
3. Testicular pain, with or without a history of trauma or surgery.

TECHNIQUE

1. Position the patient supine.

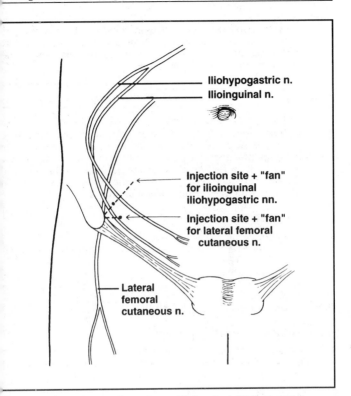

Fig. 9-21. Lateral femoral cutaneous, ilioinguinal, iliohypogastric nerve blocks.

2. Produce a skin wheal with local anesthetic, 2 cm medial to the anterior superior iliac spine.
3. Infiltrate all layers of muscle toward the umbilicus with a 1½ in., 22-gauge needle and 20 ml of 0.5% bupivacaine, for a distance of 10 cm (Fig. 9-21).

EVALUATION OF BLOCK. Variable distribution of analgesia is noted in the medial thigh and groin, which should relieve the groin pain if the ilioinguinal nerve is involved.

Genitofemoral Nerve Block

INDICATIONS

Groin or testicular pain, unrelieved by ilioinguinal block (although we have found testicular pain is often helped with lumbar sympathetic block).

TECHNIQUE

1. Position the patient supine.
2. Inject 5 ml of 0.5% bupivacaine around the spermatic cord at the base of the scrotum.

EVALUATION OF BLOCK. If pain relief occurs, but the pai
returns, the only option is a rhizotomy of L1 and L2. A lum
bar sympathetic block should be considered, as it sometime
provides relief of testicular pain.

Epidural Steroid Injections

In theory, the salutory effect of steroid is to reduce inflam
mation, swelling, and scar that arise as a consequence c
nerve pressure and extruded disc (at least such an effect o:
inflammation and scar is seen elsewhere in the body, such a
tendinitis). Pathologically, it has been observed that the bul:
of a scar is reduced by diminishing the hyaline portion of sca:
while leaving the fibrinous skeleton intact.

INDICATIONS

1. Acute herniated or bulging disc
2. Herniated nucleus pulposus, with nerve root irritation o:
   compression
3. Spinal stenosis
4. Spondylolisthesis
5. Scoliosis
6. Chronic degenerative disc disease

PREBLOCK MANAGEMENT

Patients are requested to consume only light meals up to ∢
hours before the procedure. An intravenous catheter is sel
dom placed, but vital signs may be monitored.

EQUIPMENT

Glass table, C-arm fluoroscopy, basic needle set ("Prep Set")
22-gauge, 2½-in. or 3½-in. spinal needle, short bevel (length
depends on patient's body build) 1% lidocaine with epineph
rine 1:200,000, triamcinolone as either: Aristocort (in poly
ethylene glycol), which may irritate; Kenalog (in methyl
cellulose), which is less irritating and allergenic; o:
methylprednisolone as Depo-Medrol (in polyethylene glyco
with or without 0.9% benzyl alcohol).

BLOCK PROCEDURES

Technique

Position the patient prone with the feet over the end of the
table and a bunched-up pillow under the abdomen (between
iliac crests and costal margin) to reverse lumbar lordosis and
for patient comfort. Provide a small support under head, if requested. The arms should be relaxed over the sides of the table

Lumbar Approach

1. Locate appropriate interspinal process with C-arm fluoroscope using the tip of a Kelly clamp as a marker. Mark
   the spot on the skin with the hub of No. 15 IV needle.
2. Prepare the skin with 70% alcohol and drape widely.

3. Infiltrate intra- and subcutaneous 1% lidocaine slowly and in small amount. Deep interspinous infiltration is achieved to full depth with a 22-gauge, 1½-in. needle.
4. Set rubber depth marker on 2½-in. (or 3½-in.) spinal needle at previous depth of epidural space, or at estimated depth if first injection.
5. Insert the spinal needle in the plane of the C-arm fluoroscope image (usually a little cephalad) down to the ligament.
6. Attach a well-lubricated 10-ml glass syringe to needle with about 4 cc of air in it. Holding the syringe (not needle) with one hand and pressing firmly with the finger or thumb of the other hand on plunger, maintain positive pressure constantly while rapidly oscillating the plunger. Advance the needle slowly and steadily (not intermittently) until sudden loss of resistance is achieved (allow only minimum air to escape).
7. If depth of loss-of-resistance seems inappropriate, withdraw the needle 3 mm and repeat.
8. Inject 2 ml of 1% lidocaine to test if the needle is in the subarachnoid space: allow 5 minutes to develop anesthesia. *Exception:* In spinal stenosis, test with only 1 ml, as prolonged and extensive anesthesia can occur with 2 ml.
9. Take permanent x ray, if required.
10. If demonstration of epidural placement is desired, inject 3 ml more of 1% lidocaine. This will usually produce some spotty anesthesia in the back or legs.
11. Inject 75 mg Aristocort (or equivalent), diluted with saline if desired.
12. Replace the stylet in the needle (to avoid tracking steroid through skin), push the marker down to skin surface for later measurement, and withdraw the needle.
13. With gauze, press on the needle hole, slide skin back and forth to stop bleeding, and close the tract.
14. Apply Band-Aid, to be removed upon reaching home.
15. Slowly sit the patient up and do not leave unattended until safely in a wheelchair (legs may be weak and buckle).

ALTERNATIVE APPROACHES

Paramedian

1. A skin wheal is usually made 1 cm lateral and 1 cm caudad from the interspinous puncture.
2. Remember, there will be no interspinous ligament to provide resistance to air in the syringe. Only when the ligamentum flavum is reached will there be resistance.
3. Proceed as in the midline approach.

Caudal

1. This approach is useful if the patient has had multiple laminectomies, with much scarring, and an alteration of the normal anatomy.
2. A total volume of 25–30 ml is needed to fill the caudal canal and reach the L5–S1 junction.

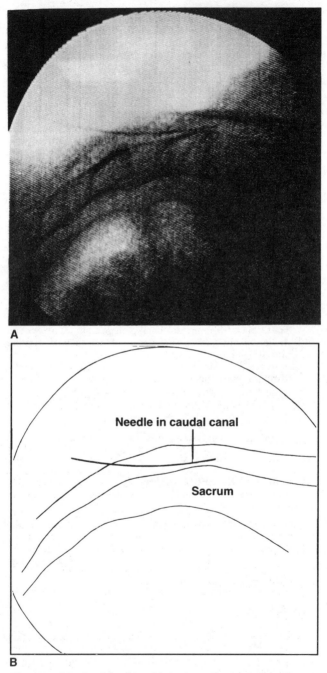

A

B

Fig. 9-22. (A,B) Caudal epidural injection—lateral radiographic view and diagrammatic representation.

3. The standard sacral hiatus approach is used. A lateral fluoroscopic view will ensure needle placement in the sacral canal (Fig. 9-22A,B).

Through Posterior S1 Foramen

1. This is useful if the epidural space is not otherwise available, and especially when symptoms are confined to the S1 or S2 levels.
2. Approximately 15 ml total volume is needed to reach the L5–S1 junction, the usual site of pathology.
3. See S1 paravertebral block for details of technique.

Paravertebral

1. This approach is useful if symptoms are mainly radicular and previous midline injections have not helped.
2. The dose is usually reduced to 50 mg Aristocort; dilution is not needed.
3. The technique is discussed under paravertebral blocks.

Potential Complications

1. Dural puncture, with intrathecal blockade
2. Postdural-puncture headaches
3. Epidural hematoma
4. Epidural abcess; cutaneous infections; meningitis
5. Intrathecal steroid blocks are not recommended, owing to potential complications such as anterior spinal artery syndrome, arachnoiditis, meningitis, urinary retention, cauda equina syndrome, as well as a lack of effect.

Postblock Management

The patient is observed for potential, late-appearing complications for 1 hour. If motor and sensory functions are intact, the patient is then discharged, with an escort.

Block Treatment Protocol

Our custom is to give three epidural injections at 2- to 4-week intervals, as needed, to ascertain response. A reprieve is given for 3 to 6 months to avoid possible ligamentous atrophy from steroid injections. Injections may then be repeated as required.

Facet Joint Injections

Pathophysiology of facet arthritis (zygapophyseal joint):

1. Disc degeneration, leading to joint malalignment and arthritis (Fig. 9-23).
2. Part of the generalized process of degenerative joint disease.

INDICATIONS

1. Diagnosis: local anesthetic injection into a joint or joints to determine if the joint is the source of back pain. This is done to aid the orthopedic surgeon in making a decision on spinal fusion.

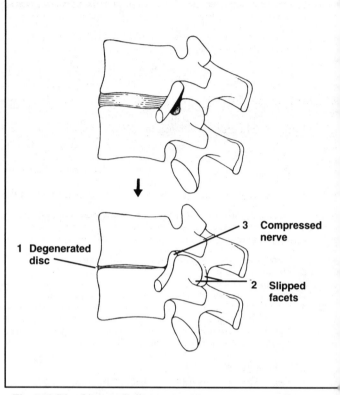

Fig. 9-23. Disc degeneration consequences.

2. Some people think it is worthwhile injecting steroid into the joints. My opinion is that it provides relief for only up to 2 weeks (D.P.T.).
3. As a predictive tool, prior to denervating the joint with alcohol, or radiofrequency ablation of the joint nerve of Luschka. (The jury is still out on this procedure.)

PREBLOCK MANAGEMENT

Patients should only eat light meals up to 4 hours before the procedure. Vital signs may be monitored, but an intravenous catheter is usually not used, except for cervical facet blocks. Sterile preparation and draping are performed prior to all procedures.

BLOCK PROCEDURES

Lumbar Facet Block

Prior to commencing with the block, the pain should be evaluated by back bending. Extension characteristically produces facet pain.

Technique

1. The patient should be in the modified Sims' position: 10°, 10°, 20°, 30°, 45° of rotation, block side up for L1–2, L2–3, L3–4, L4–5, and S5–S1 joint injections, respectively.
2. Rotate the C-arm fluoroscope to get the best view into the joint: the "scotty dog" image is characteristic—the vertically oriented joint image is behind his ear.
3. Usually an entry point 2 cm lateral to the midline leads to entry into the joint. However, entering directly over the joint image or even lateral to it may be required, depending on arthritic overgrowth of the joint.
4. A 22-gauge, 3½-in. spinal needle is carried with minimal local anesthetic to the edge of the joint. The needle is then "walked" in 1-mm steps medial or lateral, cephalad or caudad, until it drops into the joint. A characteristic curve is seen at the distal needle, showing it is following the joint, usually medially.
5. An intact joint will accept up to 1 ml of fluid (0.5% bupivacaine) to anesthetize the joint. If the joint capsule is disrupted, it will, of course, have infinite capacity. One should be careful not to inject more than 1 ml, preferably in 0.5-ml increments, or it will spread to other innervating branches and cause a false-positive response.
6. If relief is obtained, relief should not outlast the duration of the anesthetic (1–2 hr), or one would suspect a nonspecific response.

Cervical Facet Block

The indications are the same as for lumbar facet blocks, although they are especially useful after abnormally moving facet joints have been identified by previous continuous fluoroscopy. Whiplash injuries tend to disrupt facet motion.

Technique

1. An intravenous catheter is placed, vital signs are monitored, and fluoroscopy is employed.
2. Position the patient prone with a pillow under the chest, the neck somewhat flexed, and the forehead resting on an intravenous fluid bag for comfort.
3. With the C-arm fluoroscopic image in the anteroposterior direction, make the entry point directly over the transverse process mass, usually 1.5–2.0 cm lateral to the midline, and about three vertebrae caudad to the desired level (see angle of joints).
4. With minimal local anesthetic, a 22-gauge, 3½-in. spinal needle is advanced at about 30° with the skin until bone is encountered, at the desired level.
5. The joint space is then visualized by placing the C-arm fluoroscope in the lateral position, and the needle is "walked" 1 mm at a time until it drops into the joint. The final position of needle tip is halfway through the joint (Fig. 9-24A,B).
6. The lateral–medial position of the needle needs to be checked again with the C-arm fluoroscope in the posteroanterior view. The needle point should be in the middle of transverse process mass (Fig. 9-25A,B). (Slipping too far medially would produce epidural or spinal anesthesia!)

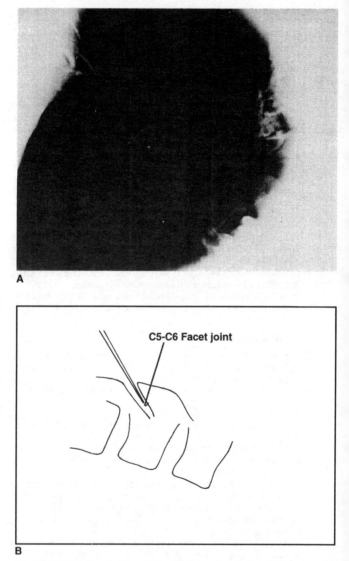

A

C5-C6 Facet joint

B

Fig. 9-24. (A,B) Cervical facet block—lateral radiographic view and diagrammatic representation.

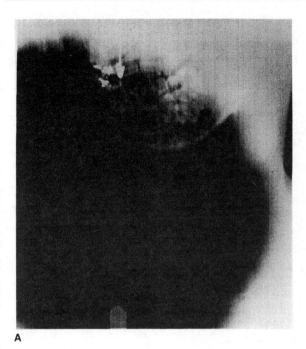

A

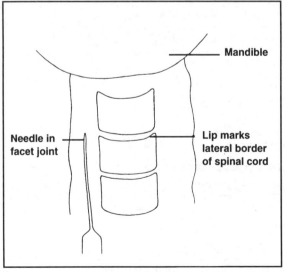

B

Fig. 9-25. (A,B) Cervical facet block—anteroposterior radiographic view and diagrammatic representation.

7. Again, 1 ml of 0.5% bupivacaine in 0.5-ml increments is sufficient to anesthetize the joint.
8. If the joint is the source of pain, painful motion of the neck before the block should be immediately painless following the block.

Sacroiliac Joint Block

Although not a facet joint, the technique is so similar to the facet techniques that it is included here. The temptation to inject this joint is great since tenderness over the S1 joint is a very common finding in lumbar disc disease. In fact, this was the reason back pain used to be treated by sacroiliac fusion, before Mixter and Barr, in the early 1930s, demonstrated that the herniated disc is a cause of sciatica. The sacroiliac joint is rarely the cause of back pain, except possibly in Marie-Strumpel arthritis and pelvic disruption.

Indications

Diagnosis or therapy of low back or sacral pain, with or without steroid.

Technique

1. As the joint region is so easily palpable, its injection would seem simple. Actually it is not, and C-arm fluoroscopic guidance is needed.
2. The patient should be in the modified Sims' position, and the pelvis is rotated until the joint appears clearly under fluoroscopy.
3. The insertion point usually needs to be almost in the midline (depending on the amount of subcutaneous tissue) and is anesthetized prior to proceeding with the block.
4. A 22-gauge, 3½-in. spinal needle is carried deeply into the joint. The needle tip will show its usual deviation, as it does in the lumbar facet, under C-arm fluoroscopic visualization (Fig. 9-26A,B).
5. To anesthetize this joint 2–3 ml of 0.5% bupivacaine should be adequate. Steroid is an option.

POTENTIAL COMPLICATIONS

1. Infection
2. Penetration of the pelvic viscus if the needle traverses the joint (remote).

POSTBLOCK MANAGEMENT

Patients are observed for potential, late-appearing complications for 1 hour. If motor and sensory functions are intact, the patient is discharged, with an escort.

Additional Diagnostic and Therapeutic Techniques

INTRAVENOUS LIDOCAINE INJECTION

Indications

Neuropathic pain syndromes, particularly with continuous or lancinating dysesthesias, e.g., diabetic neuropathy, phantom

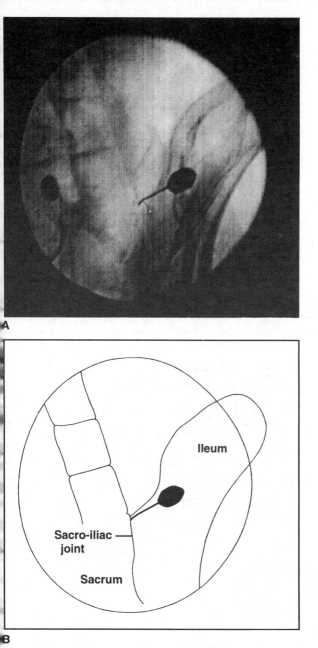

A

B

Fig. 9-26. (A,B) Sacroiliac joint injection—anteroposterior radiographic view and diagrammatic representation.

limb, neuralgia, and myofascial pain syndromes. The proce‐
dure is performed to evaluate the utility of oral local anes‐
thetics for pain relief.

Preblock Management

1. The patient is asked to eat lightly prior to the procedure
   and to fast for 4 hours immediately preceding the pro‐
   cedure.
2. A baseline ECG and liver function tests (LFTs) are ob‐
   tained. Conduction abnormalities are a contraindication to
   this procedure. Abnormally elevated LFTs are a contra‐
   indication to Mexiletine.

Procedure

1. Vital signs are monitored frequently.
2. The patient is supine on a bed, and an 18- or 20-gauge
   intravenous catheter is placed in an upper extremity.
3. A preblock verbal analog scale (VAS) pain rating is ob‐
   tained (0–10). Pain must exist at that time to evaluate
   the efficacy of the block.
4. Over 10 to 15 minutes 1–2 mg/kg lidocaine without epi‐
   nephrine is injected. We usually inject 100 mg for the av‐
   erage adult. Tinnitus, perioral numbness, metallic oral
   taste, and dizziness are often experienced; injection speed
   should be reduced at this time and restarted with reso‐
   lution of symptoms.

Evaluation of Procedure

1. VAS scores are obtained before, during, and after the
   block.
2. A 50% or greater reduction in pain would indicate a trial
   with oral Mexiletine.
3. Specificity of response can be tested by injecting 10 ml of
   normal saline prior to intravenous lidocaine, and by ob‐
   taining VAS scores. The responses are self-explanatory.

Potential Complications

1. Cardiac arrhythmias
2. Syncope
3. Hypotension
4. Ataxia
5. Tremors
6. Dizziness
7. Nervousness
8. Skin rash
9. Visual changes
10. Seizures
11. Anaphylaxis

Postblock Management

The patient is observed for 30 minutes, in the sitting position
and then allowed to ambulate. If stable, the intravenous cath‐
eter is removed and the patient is discharged. When starting

Mexiletine it is advisable to start on 150 mg at bedtime for 3 days, then tid. This seems to allow more patients to accept the drug, without having to stop as a result of side effects.

INTRAVENOUS PHENTOLAMINE INFUSION

Indications

1. Diagnosis, and sometimes therapy, of sympathetically maintained pain.
2. Diagnosis or therapy of sympathetically maintained pain, when sympathetic blocks are contraindicated, e.g., with anticoagulated patients, infection of needle entry site.

Preblock Management

1. Patients are requested to eat lightly up to 4 hours before the procedure.
2. The patient is evaluated for cardiac disease or other conditions that may be affected by hypotension.

Procedure

This is performed at our institution, essentially according to the protocol described by Raja and colleagues.

1. With the patient supine, ECG, blood pressure, and oxygen saturation monitors are placed.
2. An 18- or 20-gauge intravenous catheter is placed.
3. Baseline pain levels are elicited (VAS scores).
4. A bolus of 500-ml lactated Ringer's solution is administered via continuous infusion. This helps counteract hypotension and can act as a placebo test.
5. Stimulus-independent pain evaluations (VAS scores) and stimulus-evoked pain evaluations (VAS, mechanical test, cold test, etc.) are performed.
6. Propranolol, 2 mg intravenously, is administered to counteract reflex tachycardia.
7. Phentolamine, 35–70 mg intravenously in 250 ml normal saline, is infused over 20 minutes, without the patient's direct knowledge of initiation of the infusion.

Evaluation of Procedure

Pain testing and vital signs are evaluated for another half hour, prior to discharge. The data are used to indicate the presence of sympathetically maintained pain, particularly if the pain is relieved. If the pain is not relieved, we have not found this to definitively exclude the diagnosis, and either corroborative blocks or sympathetically independent pain may be considered.

Potential Complications

1. Hypotension, mild to profound, possibly leading to hypoperfusion states.
2. Dizziness, lightheadedness
3. Reflex tachycardia

4. Orthostatic hypotension
5. Syncope

Postblock Management

Patients are observed for 30 minutes after the block, and somatosensory and pain evaluations are conducted. Patients are then allowed to sit up, and stand up, as tolerated. If they are stable, they are discharged; if not, they are observed for as long as necessary, prior to discharge with an escort.

INTRAVENOUS REGIONAL SYMPATHETIC BLOCKS (BIER BLOCK)

These blocks are done in an attempt to create a sympathetic block at the level of the extremity (peripheral). Several medications can be used, including guanethidine, bretylium, labetalol, prazosin, clonidine, and reserpine. Intravenous guanethidine and reserpine are not readily available in the United States. We currently use the mixed alpha- and beta-antagonist, labetalol, for its alpha-antagonist and antisympathetic effects.

Indications

1. Therapeutic sympathetic blockade of an upper or lower extremity.
2. Diagnostic blocks when patients refuse needle blocks or are on anticoagulants, or when needle blocks are contraindicated or unsuccessful.

Preblock Management

1. Patients are requested to eat lightly up to 4 hours before the procedure.
2. Baseline vital signs (ECG, blood pressure, oxygen saturation) are obtained.

Procedure

1. The patient is supine.
2. A 20- or 22-gauge intravenous catheter is placed in a nonaffected extremity for intravenous access and prehydration.
4. The affected extremity is exsanguinated by elevating it and tightly rolling an Esmarch bandage distally to proximally.
5. A pneumatic cuff is applied proximally at a pressure of 250 mm Hg for 20 minutes.
6. Inject into an upper extremity 20–30 mg of labetalol plus 100 mg of lidocaine added to a 20-ml solution with normal saline.
7. Inject into the affected lower extremity 30–40 mg of labetalol plus 200 mg of lidocaine added to a 35-ml solution with normal saline.
8. The cuff is either deflated slowly or deflated and reinflated over 5 to 10 minutes, while monitoring vital signs closely.

Evaluation of the Procedure

1. Baseline and postprocedural pain evaluations are performed, including VAS score.
2. A time course of the pain relief is noted, as relief can range from hours to months.

Potential Complications

1. Hypotension, mild to profound, particularly when deflating the pneumatic cuff, or with a leaking cuff
2. Dizziness
3. Ischemia or neuropathy in the affected limb, usually transient
4. Orthostatic hypotension
5. Syncope

Postblock Management

The patient's vital signs are monitored for 1 hour following deflation of the cuff, and, if stable, the patient is discharged with an escort.

Selected Readings

Benzon HT. Epidural steroid injections for low back pain and lumbosacral radiculopathy. *Pain* 24:227–295, 1986.

Bonica JJ. *The Management of Pain* (vols 1 and II; 2nd ed). Philadelphia: Lea & Febiger, 1990.

Cousins MJ and Bromage PR. *Neural Blockade* (2nd ed). Philadelphia: JB Lippincott, 1988.

Dellemijn PLI, et al. The interpretation of pain relief and sensory changes following sympathetic blockade. *Brain* 117:1475–1487, 1994.

Eisenberg E, Carr DB, and Chalmers TC. Neurolytic celiac plexus block for treatment of cancer pain: A meta analysis. *Reg Anesth Pain Management* 80:290–295, 1995.

Haddox JD. Lumbar and cervical epidural steroid therapy. *Anesthesiol Clin N Amer* 10:179–203, 1992.

Mercadante S. Celiac plexus block versus analgesics in pancreatic cancer. *Pain* 52:187–192, 1993.

Moore DC. *Regional Block* (4th ed). Springfield, IL: Charles C. Thomas, 1965.

Raj PP. *Practical Management of Pain* (2nd ed). St. Louis: Mosby–Year Book, 1992.

Raja SN, et al. Systemic alpha-adrenergic blockade with phentolamine: A diagnostic test for sympathetically maintained pain. *Anesthesiology* 74:691–698, 1991.

Rowlingson JC. Epidural steroids: Do they have a place in pain management. *Am Pain Soc J* 1:20–27, 1994.

Rowlingson JC and Hamill RJ. Treatment of low back pain. *Int Anesthesiol Clin* 29:57–68, 1991.

Treede RD, et al. The plasticity of cutaneous hyperalgesia during sympathetic ganglion blockade in patients with neuropathic pain. *Brain* 115:607–621, 1992.

Wall PD and Melzack R. *Textbook of Pain* (3rd ed). New York: Churchill-Livingstone, 1994.

An Approach to Neurosurgical Interventions for Persistent Pain

David M. Frim and G. Rees Cosgrove

> *"Pain is the psychic adjunct to an imperative protective reflex."*
> CHARLES SHERRINGTON

A multidisciplinary approach to patients with chronic pain is the best way to individualize treatment plans and optimize clinical results. Neurosurgical participation in the management plan is variable. In general, neurosurgical consultation is sought only after the patient's pain has been proved refractory to all appropriate medical therapy. In some institutions, neurosurgery is considered during the initial evaluation of the chronic pain patient.

Timing of Neurosurgical Interventions

All patients should undergo a reasonable trial of conservative therapy before neurosurgical intervention is discussed. Specifically, oral analgesics, parenteral agents, and usually short-term anesthetic interventions (e.g., local blocks, temporary infusion catheters) should be tried as treatments. Enhancing the chronic pain patient's quality of life is paramount, and when it is clear that the overall goals of pain management are not being met by less invasive treatment, surgical approaches should be considered. In particular, early neurosurgical intervention can optimize function and greatly improve pain control during the final months of life in terminal cancer patients. Surgical treatment for the most debilitated patient reduces its functional benefit and increases surgical risk. Unfortunately, there are no rules for when neurosurgical alternatives are appropriate, and individual clinical situations must be carefully assessed.

Augmentative Versus Ablative Procedures

Neurosurgical approaches to chronic pain can be loosely grouped into two broad categories: **augmentative**, where a device or substance is "added," such as a pump system designed to infuse opiates or electrodes for electrical stimulation, and **ablative**, where nervous input is severed, such as the many spinal cord lesions for treating chronic pain of malignant origin. Augmentative techniques have the advantage of being reversible and can be discontinued if they prove ineffective with no loss of function. Many procedures, however, suffer from technical problems inherent in managing infusion pumps and chronic stimulator systems. Research on the development of biologic delivery systems may, one day, simplify this aspect of neuroaugmentation. Ablative approaches to chronic pain carry with them the finality of neural tissue destruction as well as the inevitable loss of function that accompanies destruction of nervous tissue. In addition, chronic pain frequently recurs months to years after an initial successful ablative procedure. In pain of malignant origin, where the patient's life span is limited, this concern is less problematic than in pain associated with benign causes.

Scope of Neurosurgical Manipulations

Functional neurosurgical interventions for pain are directed at various levels of the nervous system, including the peripheral nerves, spinal cord, and brain. When selecting a surgical intervention, it is important to balance the **potential benefit to the patient versus the risk of *expected* loss of function,** *likely* **loss of function, and** *possible* **loss of function.** The technical requirements of the procedure and postoperative management issues as well as the general condition of the patient must also be considered. Many pain complaints can be addressed by some neurosurgical intervention—the important issue is, at what cost?

Variability of Approach

There is no uniformity of approach in evaluating the pain patient for neurosurgical intervention. Although algorithms exist for choosing specific procedures designed to relieve certain complaints, each patient merits careful evaluation before a surgical procedure is even suggested. This way, inappropriate expectations on the part of the patient can be prevented and the greatest flexibility in designing a course of therapy best suited to the patient is possible. Indeed, a given neurosurgical procedure used to treat identical complaints in different patients can produce vastly different results. For these reasons we caution against a rigid approach to neurosurgical intervention.

Appropriate Selection and Evaluation of the Neurosurgical Pain Patient

MEDICAL WORKUP AND TREATMENT

Prior to considering any procedure for control, it is extremely important to exclude an underlying treatable medical condition. Unrecognized causative pathology or correctable structural lesions must be excluded before any functional neurosurgical procedure is undertaken.

All candidates for neurosurgery require the usual preoperative evaluations for anesthetic management and surgery. Patients at high risk for surgery (e.g., those with end-stage malignancy) may be eager for intervention but may be unable to survive surgery. Medical optimization of preoperative status may require manipulations not in accord with a patient's wishes or with the approach of the care team. This situation can be avoided through the neurosurgeon's early involvement with the patient who is difficult to manage on an oral or parenteral analgesic regimen.

MALIGNANT VERSUS BENIGN PAIN

The common differentiation of pain into that of malignant or benign origin is useful. In general, ablative approaches are more suitable to pain of malignant origin, where quality of life may be paramount to functional outcome. Ablative surgery for pain of benign origin, albeit some specific conditions such as trigeminal neuralgia, is a "tricky business," where other conditions—notably, disability status, concurrent litigation, and psychosocial status—are far more important.

A second, more practical consideration in the differentiation between benign and malignant pain is that patients who have benign pain and a normal life expectancy must be managed for decades after their surgical procedure. For example, the maintenance requirements for both the technical and emotional support of every patient can be significant after implantation of chronic stimulators in the spinal canal or drug infusion systems.

MULTIDISCIPLINARY TEAM APPROACH

The comprehensive pain service, with its neurologic, anesthesiologic, psychiatric nursing, and social service components, remains the best resource for ensuring optimal patient care. Neurosurgeons who elect to treat chronic pain patients without this support network may find that care is compromised. Similarly, the treatment of chronic pain is significantly hampered without the surgical team's input. Early involvement of the surgical team in patients who are poor responders to conservative measures, careful evaluation of each patient's needs and status, and deliberate review of all nonsurgical and surgical options will likely produce the best results.

Specific Neurosurgical Interventions Encountered by the Pain Service: Description and Results

ABLATIVE PROCEDURES

Peripheral Ablative Procedures

There is very little published information on peripheral neurotomy outside the cranial nerves, except in the case of pain related to spinal facet innervation. Peripheral lesions in the extremities can eventually result in a deafferentation pain syndrome. The procedure of choice for appendicular mononeuralgias is currently chronic stimulation, as described below. Results of facet denervation are variable, and although good results for chronic back pain have been reported, these have not been reproducible.

Surgical intervention for craniofacial pain syndromes has met with much greater success. Trigeminal neuralgia can be treated with peripheral neurectomy with excellent results. Unfortunately, as in all peripheral lesions, nerve regeneration will usually recur, as will the pain syndrome. For these reasons, peripheral neurolytic procedures are generally not performed for chronic pain.

The craniofacial pain caused by trigeminal and glossopharyngeal neuralgia can be treated by percutaneous peripheral nerve or ganglionic ablation in the intracranial space. This is generally done by radiofrequency lesions (RFLs) or by injection of a sclerosing agent such as glycerol. The results of these ablations are variable, but in the case of RFLs for trigeminal neuralgia, initial pain relief followed by several years of comfort can be expected in 70% to 80% of patients. Open craniotomy for microvascular decompression or cranial nerve section is also an option for younger patients with craniofacial pain or for those who have failed percutaneous rhizotomy. The results of these interventions are similar, but operative risk is higher for open surgical procedures.

Spinal Cord Ablative Procedures

The rationale for ablative lesions in and around the spinal cord is based on the anatomy of nociceptive pathways, from the periphery to the spinal cord and its central connections. The approach to spinal cord lesioning can be divided into lesions of the ganglia and dorsal root entry zones, lesions of the fibers crossing the spinothalamic tracts, and lesions of the ascending tracts (Fig. 10-1).

The **dorsal ganglia** can be surgically excised (**ganglionectomy**) in an open or percutaneous procedure, providing relief of pain in a roughly dermatomal distribution. This procedure must be performed at multiple levels but provides pain relief with concurrent loss of sensory input. Attempts have been made, with variable success, to limit the ablation to nociceptive input only. For defined pain of the thoracic or upper lumbar roots, this procedure can be of great benefit.

Dorsal rhizotomy was one of the first operations used for pain control, and although generally effective, it is also accompanied by complete sensory loss in the appropriate dermatomal distribution. Extensive dorsal root sectioning in an extremity leads to a useless limb and is not recommended. Partial or incomplete posterior rhizotomies have therefore been employed for certain chronic pain states and painful spasticity, and have been especially useful in occipital neuralgia.

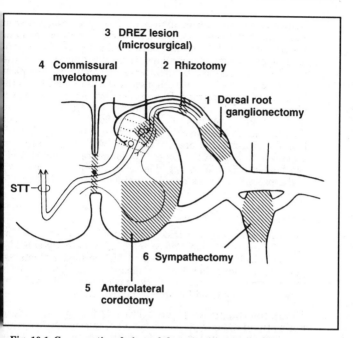

Fig. 10-1. Cross-sectional view of the spinal cord showing approximate sites of common spinal cord ablative interventions — midline myelotomy, cordotomy, sympathectomy, dorsal root entry zone (DREZ) ablation, dorsal root ganglionectomy, and peripheral rhizotomy. (STT = spinothalamic tract.)

Pain of deafferentation related to root avulsion or phantom limb pain has been successfully treated with an open operation to cause lesion of the **dorsal root entry zone (DREZ)**. Small thermocoagulation lesions are made in the posterior spinal cord in the DREZ at multiple levels, presumably interrupting nociceptive pathways in Lissauer's tract or destroying neurons in the substantia gelatinosa. Significant pain relief lasting several years has been achieved in a variety of chronic pain states, including postherpetic neuralgia and phantom limb pain. Early results are generally good, but recurrence of pain is common.

Spinothalamic tract input from a specific dermatome crosses in the midline over several levels before ascending into the anterolateral aspect of the spinal cord. Localized bilateral pain, such as that seen with sacral tumors, can be addressed by **midline (commissural) myelotomy**. Good bilateral pain relief can be achieved, though the potential for functional loss is great. The likelihood of postoperative neurologic deficit restricts this approach to pain of malignant origin in patients who have functional disturbances (e.g., bladder dysfunction) preoperatively.

The procedure of **interruption of the ascending lateral spinothalamic tract** with either a percutaneous or open **anterolateral cordotomy** has been used successfully for pain of malignant origin. As in all ablations of the spinal cord, the risk for functional loss is high. Lower-extremity pain is most easily approached by open thoracic cordotomy and bilateral lesions can be performed. Bilateral cordotomy increases risk of neurologic deficits. Cordotomy at the cervical levels above diaphragmatic input on one side and below it on the other (i.e., C3 and C6) can avoid postoperative respiratory difficulties. For reasons that are unclear, pain will often return 1 to 2 years postoperatively. Repeat cordotomy at a higher level can be performed, although this is an infrequent occurrence if the procedure is restricted to patients with a limited life span.

Central Ablative Procedures

Accurate lesioning of nociceptive pathways in the mesencephalon, diencephalon, and cortex has been greatly aided by the technical advances in CT- and MRI-guided stereotaxis. Long-term results, however, are disappointing, and for these reasons, the use of central ablations is controversial and generally only considered for pain of malignant origin.

The general approach to deep brain lesioning, as in deep brain stimulation, is placement of a stimulating or lesioning electrode into a stereotactically identified site. The area is then stimulated as the electrode position is adjusted to achieve the desired effect. At this point a lesion is created, or in the case of stimulation, the electrode is secured in place.

Lesioning the spinothalamic and secondary trigeminal tract in the midbrain (**mesencephalotomy**) can provide relief of head and neck pain that is unilateral. More rostral lesions in the medial thalamus (**thalamotomy**) can also provide unilateral or, in some cases, bilateral pain relief. A procedure for destroying the cingulate gyrus and bundle in the frontal lobe (**cingulotomy**) has also been used in cases of diffuse chronic pain associated with depression. These approaches should be reserved for the experienced, functional neurosurgeon.

For reasons that are unclear, pain from hormonally responsive tumors that produce bony pain (carcinoma of the prostate and breast) is sometimes very amenable to **pituitary ablation**, either stereotactically or via a transsphenoidal approach. The sudden and complete relief of bony pain evident on emergence from anesthesia in many of these cases is well worth the expected postoperative endocrine deficits.

AUGMENTATIVE PROCEDURES

Implantable Stimulator Systems

Peripheral Nerve

Pain arising from a mononeuropathy may be treated by chronic stimulation, particularly when the pain is due to nerve injury. Cancer pain has also been treated in this way, but with less success. The long-term implantation of a stimulating electrode requires a significant investment of time and effort to manage the technical aspects of the device. Newer hardware designed for this purpose has simplified these techniques.

Spinal Cord and Deep Brain

Spinal cord stimulation is frequently used for treating chronic pain, particularly of nonmalignant origin, because of its reversibility. It remains popular despite the high cost and maintenance of the systems. Spinal cord stimulators can be inserted percutaneously or during open procedures. The scientific basis for pain relief is unclear, though—as in peripheral nerve stimulation—the principle remains to cause paresthesia over the painful areas, which somehow moderates pain perception. Unfortunately, no specific entities have emerged as "best responders" to spinal cord stimulation. Common entities that have responded to this type of therapy include failed back syndrome, lower-extremity pain of vascular origin, and other neurogenic pain syndromes. Published reports predict an approximately 50% long-term success rate for all patients treated with spinal cord stimulation.

Deep brain stimulation (DBS) is confined to pain centers where there is significant interest in the procedure and a commitment to the management of patients with implanted stimulators. The two targets are the periaqueductal gray matter areas in the brain stem and nuclei ventralis posteromedialis and ventralis posterolateralis thalami. Reports of DBS used for a variety of chronic pain states suggest that initial success is often followed by decremental effectiveness over time. Relief can be expected in 50% to 80% of patients initially, but the long-term results seem to indicate that not many more than half of DBS patients derive significant benefit. The most appropriate use of this methodology appears to be in addressing chronic pain refractory to all other approaches in patients with a long life expectancy.

Implantable Infusion Systems

The infusion of spinal epidural opiates or local anesthetic solutions is now an accepted and frequently used procedure for extremity and occasionally truncal pain. The role of the neurosurgeon in the management of spinal infusion technique is to offer the long-term surgical implantation of subcutaneously tunneled catheters leading to a reservoir, or the placement of catheters that exit the anterior abdominal wall that can be injected externally. In general, surgically implanted catheters have a longer life and lower complication rate.

Opiate infusion into the spinal intradural space or through the intraventricular route will involve a neurosurgeon for catheter placement and avoidance of complications. It would appear that these intradural routes provide superior analgesia to epidural routes; however, there is an increased incidence of postoperative deficits and infectious complications and a risk of overdose. A spinal intradural or frontal intraventricular catheter can be adapted to any of several commercially available infusion systems. For short-term pain relief requiring relatively minor surgery, the intradural routes are likely underutilized.

Miscellaneous Neurosurgical Interventions

TRIGEMINAL AND GLOSSOPHARYNGEAL NEURALGIA

The neurosurgical approach to trigeminal and glossopharyngeal neuralgia includes percutaneous rhizotomy, open partial cranial rhizotomy, and microvascular decompression. These options are mentioned in a separate section because of their major use and effectiveness. For any patient who has a trigeminal pain syndrome that is not controlled well by medication, the likelihood of satisfactory pain relief without medication is nearly 90% with any of these approaches. Recurrent trigeminal neuralgia can also be treated with repeat rhizotomy with good relief. Complication rates are extremely low for all these procedures, but the specific procedure recommended must be tailored to each patient's needs and risks.

LOW BACK PAIN

Low back pain is a problem commonly encountered by the neurologist and the neurosurgeon. In particular, the failed back syndrome is a frequent management problem for the pain service. Most of these patients can be managed with an aggressive medical regimen, but a detailed evaluation of patients with a failed back should be considered, as with any other pain syndrome. In carefully selected patients with continued underlying spinal structural pathology, reasonable success has been achieved with reoperation for recurrent disc disease or root compression. In addition, spinal cord stimulation or epidural opiate infusion can be of value in these patients.

SYMPATHECTOMY

Sympathectomy for autonomic and visceral pain is now almost exclusively performed by the anesthesiologist via percutaneous methods. For specific cases of reflex sympathetic dystrophy (RSD), surgical sympathectomy may be necessary due to difficulty in achieving adequate technical results via a percutaneous approach. The advantage of open sympathectomy is the excellent anatomic definition of the lesion. However, sympathectomy performed in an open fashion will still suffer from pain recurrence, like percutaneous approaches. Selective peripheral nerve stimulation has also been used for RSD confined to a single nerve distribution or extremity.

Summary and Conclusions

NEUROSURGICAL PARTICIPATION IN THE TREATMENT PLAN OF THE PAIN PATIENT

Although the surgical treatment of chronic pain should always follow a reasonably exhaustive trial of more conservative approaches, there is a role for surgical intervention in many chronic pain patients. The neurosurgeon's participation in the overall treatment plan of the chronic pain patient will provide an opportunity for this intervention early in the patient's course, before worsening of the disease or frustration with lack of progress renders neurosurgical intervention impossible. A judicious approach by the referring pain specialist, as well as frank discussions with the patient, family, and care providers, is likely to yield the best results for a patient who has not responded to medical management. Unfortunately, multiple factors and individual variability still render the surgical outcome for each patient somewhat unpredictable.

NEUROSURGICAL OUTCOME IN THE MULTIDISCIPLINARY PAIN SERVICE

As with all chronic pain patients, the entire multidisciplinary pain service should take responsibility in the preoperative and postoperative care. No one specific neurosurgical intervention will totally relieve persistent pain; it should only be considered as one therapeutic tool in the overall treatment plan. The management of chronic pain can, at times, be greatly improved by timely, selective neurosurgical interventions to provide an excellent quality of life in the face of intercurrent disease.

Selected Readings

Gybels JM and Sweet WH. Neurosurgical Treatment of Persistent Pain. In: PL Gildenberg (ed), *Pain and Headache* (vol 11) Basel: Karger, 1989.

Schmidek HH and Sweet WH. *Operative Neurosurgical Techniques: Indications, Methods, and Results* (3rd ed). Philadelphia: Saunders, 1995.

Tasker RR. Neurosurgical and Neuroaugmentative Intervention. In: RB Patt (ed), *Cancer Pain*. Philadelphia: JB Lippincott, 1993.

Tasker RR. The recurrence of pain after neurosurgical procedures. *Qual Life Res* 3: S43–S49, 1994.

Wall PD and Melzack R. *Textbook of Pain*. Edinburgh: Churchill-Livingstone, 1989.

Chronic Pain Rehabilitation

Suzanne LaCross and Sharona Soumekh

> *"Like an alarm bell stuck in the 'on' position . . . such is chronic benign pain."*
>
> BRUCE SMOLLER AND
> BRIAN SCHULMAN

Chronic pain is defined as pain that is persistent, is attributed to a physical cause, and lasts beyond the normal healing period. Often patients with chronic pain have had extensive medical evaluation and have undergone numerous medical, anesthetic, and surgical approaches without marked improvement. Chronic pain is a multidimensional problem that often leads to significant life disruption for patients and their families. Many chronic pain patients feel isolated in their suffering. These patients are often frustrated with their physician, and physicians may also feel helpless in that they have little more to offer these patients. Such patients are experiencing what has commonly been referred to as "chronic pain syndrome," and they may be appropriate candidates for a multidisciplinary or interdisciplinary pain management program.

Multidisciplinary and Interdisciplinary Approaches to Pain Management

The multidisciplinary approach to treating chronic pain patients was developed by John Bonica in 1961, and became the model both nationally and internationally. This method was described as a collaborative effort on the part of several disciplines to treat the patient suffering from chronic pain. More recently, the focus has been on an interdisciplinary approach, which involves more ongoing communication, integration, and coordination of treatment goals by team members.

The interdisciplinary team can consist of several medical disciplines, a psychosocial team, rehabilitation specialists, and a case manager to coordinate assessment, treatment goals, and discharge plans for the patient. It is important to note here that not all patients with chronic pain necessarily need a comprehensive pain management program. Patients commonly referred to such a program either on an inpatient or outpatient basis, are experiencing disability in many facets of their lives, e.g., physically, emotionally, vocationally, interpersonally. In other words, these individuals can no longer separate their lives and themselves from their pain experience. In addition, patients who are appropriate for a comprehensive pain rehabilitation program are those who are motivated to break this maladaptive cycle and alter their life-style, rather than those who focus on complete pain relief. Not every patient who can benefit from such a program needs every service offered by each discipline available. The individual differences and needs of each patient must always be accounted for. Neglecting to do so would be a disservice to the patient and would wrongly promote "pain patient homogeneity." As care givers we must consider the option of integrating conventional medical treatment as part of interdisciplinary chronic pain rehabilitation when appropriate. For example, the use of narcotic analgesics in a number of patients with chronic pain may be warranted. In other instances a patient may benefit from regional blocks as an adjunct to participation in a chronic pain rehabilitation program.

Chronic Pain Syndrome

Once again, it is important to emphasize that not all patients with chronic pain suffer from the syndrome, which is typically identified by a series of maladaptive behavior patterns with emotional sequelae, resulting in life disruption. Such patterns on the part of the patient are typically referred to as "pain behavior" or "illness behavior" and may include the following: doctor shopping; demands for additional diagnostic testing; seeking out surgical interventions; utilizing large doses of narcotics, alcohol (ETOH), or recreational drugs to alleviate pain; isolation from family and friends and alienation from others by constantly focusing on the pain; ineffective communication skills; disruption in sleep patterns; and, in most cases, a general overuse of the health care system. In addition to these overt behavior patterns, concomitant emotional experiences may include depression, anxiety, feelings of helplessness and hopelessness, frustration, poor self-esteem, fears about the future, feelings of suicide, and, in some cases, actual suicidal gestures. These mixed feelings and behaviors are a threat to the individual's existence and have been aptly referred to as "pain-go-round." When this pattern is identified, the goal becomes clear: The chronic pain patient must break these patterns and replace them with a more adaptive life-style.

CHRONIC PAIN PREDICTORS

Although the individual experiencing chronic pain syndrome is usually identified long after he or she is trapped in this cycle, it may be beneficial to consider specific variables as possible predictors. For instance, the premorbid psychologic state or preexisting personality profile may help determine whether an individual is at risk for developing this pattern. Individuals who may have a history of depression, anxiety disorder, or perhaps untreated posttraumatic stress disorder (PTSD) may be more vulnerable to serious life disruption following the onset of chronic pain. In addition, individuals with

diagnosable personality disorders, such as those that are his
trionic or borderline, may not only be more likely to demon
strate the chronic pain cycle, but may also have a poor treat
ment prognosis in a self-management pain rehabilitatio
program (Lebovits, 1991). In addition, these patients may b
disruptive to a program where the milieu is an importan
part of treatment.

A less complex but nonetheless important variable to conside
is a person's life-long coping skills. An individual who ha
learned and practiced adaptive coping skills may use thes
same skills to deal with a chronic pain problem, and therefor
may never fall into this disabling pattern. An individual wit
a polysubstance history, however, may resort back to ETO.
or recreational drugs or may even abuse prescribed narcoti
to deal with pain, and therefore may be more at risk. Othe
variables that should not be ignored include familial system
sociodemographic variables, and ethnocultural difference
Although these are crucial determinants for understandin
pain perception and expression, not enough effort has bee
made toward understanding how these variables affect th
chronic pain experience.

Many patients develop maladaptive patterns because the
are unable to accept that their pain is chronic in natur
Some are entangled in a web of anger toward whomever the
believe is to blame; the health care system itself or anyor
around them who is not suffering. These individuals are u
able to move forward to better their lives despite their pai
rather, they search for someone responsible who shou
therefore pay for their suffering. On the other hand, son
patients believe that they alone are responsible for their pr
dicament and grow to believe that pain and suffering are e
tirely their fault. They tend to catastrophize all situatio
and feel enormous guilt about their pain, their perceived la
of usefulness, and the effect this has on those around the
The fact remains, however, that some patients have be
failed by the system and given contradictory messages
their health care providers. For instance, a patient taki
prescribed narcotics may later be referred to as an "addic
Another more common example is the patient whose treati
doctors imply that the pain is "all in their head." In eith
case this contributes to the patient's self-doubt and serves
destroy the therapeutic alliance between the patient and h
or her care giver. As a result, the patient may feel that he
she has nowhere else to turn.

To summarize, individuals who have fallen into the chro
pain syndrome are more likely to benefit from a multi- rath
than unidimensional treatment approach. The philosophy
these programs is one of self-management, which takes in
account individual differences as well as general similariti
of this patient population. Providing this flexible and co
prehensive approach and integration of services requires th
the patient assumes a greater responsibility for the day-
day management of his or her life.

Patient Evaluation

Now that we have determined what portion of the chronic pain population to consider for a multi- or interdisciplinary pain rehabilitation program, careful assessment is crucial. During the evaluation we identify patients who demonstrate behavior and feelings indicative of the chronic pain cycle and who may be finally moving toward accepting the chronicity of their painful condition. These patients may have exhausted all medical forms of treatment and may now be approaching readiness for a self-management protocol.

To determine a patient's appropriateness for a chronic pain rehabilitation program, a multifactorial assessment should be used. When referred, the patient is first seen by a physician, although the physiologic etiology of the pain has usually been clearly determined long ago. During the second step of the evaluation the patient is customarily seen by a psychologist or psychiatrist to assess a wide range of psychosocial issues. During this in-depth interview a comprehensive history is obtained and the patient is closely observed. In addition, verbal and written self-report measures as well as more objective assessment tools may be administered at the evaluator's discretion.

ASSESSMENT TOOLS

Self-report inventories and rating scales are commonly used to obtain information about the patient's pain perception and experience. The McGill Pain Questionnaire (MPQ) provides the evaluator with descriptive measures of a patient's pain perception and experience that are then rated and quantified. This questionnaire can help determine patterns that may contribute to the chronic pain cycle.

Other popular assessment tools include the Coping Strategies Questionnaire (CSQ) and the Beck Depression Inventory (BDI). Since cognitive pain coping activity appears to correlate to the chronic pain syndrome, it would be advantageous to assess for this prior to considering a patient for admittance to a pain rehabilitation program. The BDI is a widely used tool that is administered to chronic pain patients due to the contribution of depression to the maladaptive cycle of pain and disability.

Other self-report inventories useful in assessing chronic pain patterns are the Pain Disability Index (PDI) and the Illness Behavior Questionnaire (IBQ). The PDI is helpful in assessing pain behaviors in patients as well as their perceived level of disability. The IBQ also assesses psychosocial distress in patients and identifies the existence of poor coping skills.

Yet another widely used measure for assessing chronic pain patients is the Sickness Impact Profile (SIP). This questionnaire measures the level of dysfunction for a sample of chronic pain patients. The Multidimensional Pain Inventory

(MPI) is effective in categorizing patients into one of these levels—dysfunctional, interpersonally distressed, and minimizer/adaptive coper. The MPI can help identify psychosocial distress and therefore determine the patient's appropriateness for a chronic pain rehabilitation program.

In addition to an interview with the patient and a brief battery of self-report measures, an evaluator may find it appropriate to administer a Minnesota Multiphasic Personality Inventory (MMPI). This inventory may be helpful when physical etiology is questionable, when the level of physical disability far exceeds the medical diagnosis, or when there is a question of psychopathology that may be contributing to the illness or interfering with the patient's ability to benefit from a self-management program. Other important variables to consider during the assessment phase include family response to the patient with chronic pain, the existence of secondary gains to the patient, and malingering. More recently clinicians have been focusing on PTSD in the form of early childhood sexual and physical abuse and its correlation with the development of chronic pain syndrome.

LEVEL OF MOTIVATION

In addition to the aforementioned tools and techniques used to assess a patient's appropriateness for a chronic pain rehabilitation program, and what many clinicians consider the most important criterion for acceptance, is level of motivation. Since this type of treatment focuses on self-management techniques, it is mandatory for a patient to be ready and willing to redefine his or her life with the existence of pain. The variable of motivation may be more difficult to assess by the novice evaluator. Take the following example: During an evaluation, when asked for goals, a patient may exclaim, "I just want to get my life back!" The determination to be made at this point is whether the patient is ready to work toward disrupting the maladaptive cycle and replace it with positive life-style changes, or whether the patient needs complete pain relief before attempting to resume any normal life pattern. If the former is the goal, one must inquire about the steps the patient is willing to take to reach these goals and assess his or her willingness to work in such a program.

Treatment

THE INTERDISCIPLINARY APPROACH

Owing to the nature of the chronic pain syndrome, successful intervention usually requires the coordinated efforts of an interdisciplinary treatment team. In fact, the model of team collaboration and intervention has become the treatment of choice for this patient population. The majority of these interdisciplinary inpatient and outpatient programs provide a merging of various services. They are, however, philosophically similar in approach, with the general emphasis on the psychosocial components and an overall cognitive–behavioral theme.

The Commission on Accreditation of Rehabilitation Facilities (CARF) recommends that an interdisciplinary treatment team consist of a **core** staff of one or more physicians, a psychologist or psychiatrist, and a physical therapist. Although staffing may differ among treatment facilities, the common thread appears to be the working methodology of the treatment team, with the patient being the pivotal member of that team. Once accepted into an interdisciplinary pain management program, the team and patient coordinate efforts toward general pain rehabilitation, with an emphasis on a comprehensive discharge and follow-up plan to help prevent relapse.

Other disciplines often included in an interdisciplinary treatment team are occupational therapists, social workers, stress-management counselors, vocational rehabilitation counselors, exercise physiologists, nurses, and a case manager. Regardless of the composition of a particular treatment team, the general goals for rehabilitation of the chronic pain patient are as follows:

Learning to cope more adaptively with chronic pain (through assertive communication, relaxation methods, etc).

Reducing the misuse or dependence on narcotics.

Learning alternative methods and modalities to reduce pain (ice massage, heat, meditation, etc).

Improving overall functioning both physically and psychologically (through proper body mechanics, relaxation, decreased depression and anxiety, etc).

Focusing on goals of reconditioning rather than complete elimination of pain.

Decreasing muscle tension and altering the stress response to prevent exacerbation of pain (through biofeedback, diaphragmatic breathing, decreased muscle guarding, etc).

Decreasing isolation and enhancing socialization and communication with family and friends (through work with social services).

Altering pain perception and belief systems by decreasing negative outlook and catastrophizing (through cognitive restructuring, affirmations, etc).

Reducing the use of health care system.

Returning to work as soon as possible.

A model interdisciplinary pain management program includes meeting the aforementioned objectives through time-limited individual and group treatment. Individual treatment by physical and occupational therapy helps the patient set and reach realistic goals specific to the needs of the individual. Exercise programs designed to strengthen and recondition will vary from patient to patient, as will functional goals set by the patient and his or her occupational therapist. The patient may learn to employ a modality such as ice massage just prior to a therapeutic outing. In addition, a patient may learn and practice diaphragmatic breathing techniques

Table 11-1. Spaulding pain rehabilitation program

	Monday	Tuesday	Wednesday	Thursday	Friday	Saturday	Sunday
7:20 AM	Breakfast	Breakfast	Breakfast	Breakfast	Breakfast	Breakfast	Breakfast
8:15 AM	Stretch 8:15–9:00	Stretch 8:15–9:00	Stretch 8:15–9:00	Stretch 8:15–9:00	Functional Activity and Exercise Group 8:15–9:00	Occupational Therapy Movement 8:15–9:00	
9:00 AM	Medication	Medication	Medication	Medication	Medication	Medication	Medication
9:00 AM	Dr.'s rounds 9:00–11:15	Dr.'s rounds 9:00–11:15	Dr.'s rounds 9:00–11:15	Dr.'s rounds 9:00–11:15	Dr.'s rounds 9:00–11:15	Dr.'s rounds 9:30–11:30	Therapeutic LOA
10:00 AM	Focus A 10:15–11:15		Focus A 10:15–11:15		Focus A 10:15–11:15		
10:45 AM						Tai Chi/ Movement Group 10:45–12:15	
11:15 AM	Focus B 11:15–12:15	Stress Mgt. 11:15–12:15	Focus B 11:15–12:15	Stress Mgt. 11:15–12:15	Focus B 11:15–12:15		
12:00 PM							
12:15 PM	Lunch	Lunch	Lunch	Lunch	Lunch	Lunch	
12:30 PM	Medication	Medication	Medication	Medication	Medication	Medication	

Time						
1:00 PM						Discharge group 1:00–2:00
1:30 PM						
2:00 PM	Ed. Group 2:00–3:00	Ed. Group 2:00–3:00	Ed. Group 2:00–3:00	Ed. Group 2:00–3:00	Leave of Absence Group 2:00–3:00	Ed. Group 2:00–3:00
2:30 PM						
3:00 PM				Community Meeting		Pain Control Modalities Group 3:00–4:00
4:00 PM		Team II Family focus		Team I Family focus	Meditation 4:00–5:00	
5:00 PM	Medication	Medication	Medication	Medication	Medication	Medication
5:05 PM	Dinner	Dinner	Dinner	Dinner	Dinner	Dinner
6:30 PM		Psychoeducational/ Substance Abuse Group 6:00–7:00	Meditation 6:30–7:30	Family Group Education 6:30–8:00		
6:45 PM			Spaulding Pain Support Group			

Table 11-1 (continued)

	Monday	Tuesday	Wednesday	Thursday	Friday	Saturday	Sunday
7:00 PM	Vocational Counseling and Leisure Activity Group 7:00–8:30					Fun night	
7:15 PM							
8:00 PM							
9:00 PM	Medication	Medication	Medication	Medication	Medication	Medication	Medication

LOA = leave of absence.
Source: Spaulding Rehabilitation Hospital, Pain Rehabilitation, Boston, MA.

taught by the stress-management counselor during activities throughout the day. It is important that the therapists be aware of goals set for the patient with each member of his or her treatment team so they can reinforce the goals of pain management by ensuring consistency and continuity of care.

Individual treatment is also provided by the psychosocial team. Psychiatrists are responsible for the management of psychotropic medications and provide consultation to the team for the more psychiatrically compromised patients. Psychologists work closely to help patients alleviate depression and focus on restructuring thought patterns. Social workers treat a patient's family members, since the cycle affects not only the patient but also those around him or her. Vocational counselors work on individual plans to return to work. This is an important goal and often one that is resisted by patients.

GROUP MEETINGS

Group meetings are an integral part of any pain management program. Along with maintaining cost-effectiveness, groups serve to reinforce the importance of the milieu by providing patients with the opportunity to receive feedback, gather support, and learn from others in chronic pain. Groups may be didactic and educational in nature. Examples of such groups found in pain management programs include social skills and assertiveness, stress management and meditation, family education, skills training (problem solving), substance abuse, and educational groups of posturing, body mechanics, and nutrition. Other groups facilitated by a psychosocial member of the team may be more psychotherapeutic in nature, with emphasis on sharing feelings and providing emotional support to one another. In either case, groups provide additional opportunities for learning and are important in the structure of a pain management program. An example of a group schedule is demonstrated in Table 11-1.

ALTERNATIVE THERAPIES

In addition to more traditional methods of treatment, the use of "alternative" therapies is gaining more recognition in the treatment of chronic pain. The use of acupuncture has recently been sited in the literature as an effective treatment of choice. In addition, methods such as Feldencris, tai chi, and yoga are being considered as viable therapies in the treatment of chronic pain.

Outcome Data

The general goal of chronic pain rehabilitation is to help individuals regain control of their lives despite the existence of chronic pain. Multidisciplinary and interdisciplinary programs are gaining recognition as an effective treatment for a majority of these patients. A study in 1973 by Fordyce and colleagues was one of the first to report positive outcomes from a multidisciplinary treatment approach with chronic pain patients. Since then, studies continue to support their conclusions.

Roberts and Reinhardt (1980) and Deardorff and associates (1991), in two separate studies, compared a group of chronic pain patients treated in a multidisciplinary pain program with a group of patients who were rejected or refused admission. The result of these studies demonstrated that treated patients did better in terms of reduction of use of medication, increase in functional activity, and return to work rate.

In another study, Flor and colleagues (1992) analyzed the efficacy of multidisciplinary treatment centers through a multianalytic review. The study included 65 centers employing a multidisciplinary treatment approach. It was concluded that this approach is superior to single-discipline treatment or no treatment approach in improving behavioral variables such as return to work and decreased use of the health care system. Even at long-term follow-up, patients who were treated in a multidisciplinary setting are functioning better than 75% of a sample that was either untreated or treated by conventional unimodal approaches. This was also demonstrated in a 3-year follow-up study in 1990 by Maruta and associates.

In other outcome studies of multidimensional treatment approaches, pain rating is not necessarily correlated to functional capacity. Two separate studies demonstrated improvements in physical activity and range of motion and a reduction in medication use with no decrease in pain rating scores.

In addition to patient outcome data, some studies support multidimensional approaches as being cost effective. Cost-effectiveness may be examined in a variety of ways and should continue to be addressed according to categories as they are identified.

Conclusion

The data from multi- and interdisciplinary approaches in chronic pain rehabilitation are promising. More recent literature focuses on cost-effectiveness and the problems with long-term adherence and relapse prevention. In addition to helping patients comply with an ongoing regimen to ensure continuation of therapeutic benefits, attempts should be made to train and educate primary care givers in the treatment of patients disabled by chronic pain.

Selected Readings

Beck AA. *Depression Inventory*. Philadelphia: Center for Cognitive Therapy, 1978.

Belgrade M. Two decades after ping-pong diplomacy: Is there a role for acupuncture in American pain medicine? *J Am Pain Soc* 3:73–83, 1994.

Bonica JJ. Multidisciplinary/Interdisciplinary Pain Programs. In: JJ Bonica (ed), *The Management of Pain* (2nd ed). Philadelphia: Lea & Febiger, 1990. Pp. 197–208.

Caudill M, et al. Decreased clinic use by chronic pain patients: Response to behavioral medicine intervention. *Clin J Pain* 7: 305–310, 1991.

Deardorff WW, Rubin HS, and Scott DW. Comprehensive multidisciplinary treatment of chronic pain: A follow-up study of treated and non-treated groups. *Pain* 45:35–43, 1991.

Ektor-Anderson J, Janzon L, and Sjolund B. Chronic pain and the sociodemographic environment: Results from the Pain Clinic at Malmo General Hospital in Sweden. *Clin J Pain* 9: 183–188, 1993.

Flor H, Fydrich T, and Turk DC. Efficacy of multidisciplinary pain treatment centers: A meta-analytic review. *Pain* 19:221–230, 1992.

Fodyce WE, et al. Operant conditioning in the treatment of chronic pain. *Arch Phys Med Rehabil* 54:399–408, 1973.

Hanson RW and Gerber KE. *Coping with Chronic Pain: A Guide to Patient Self-Management.* New York: Guilford Press, 1990.

Jensen MP, et al. Relationship of pain-specific beliefs to chronic pain adjustment. *Pain* 57:301–309, 1994.

Kabat-Zinn J. An outpatient program in behavioral medicine for chronic pain patients based on the practice by mindfulness meditation: Theoretical considerations and preliminary results. *Hosp Psychiatry* 4:33–47, 1982.

Lebovitz AH. Chronic pain: The multidisciplinary approach. *Int Anesthesiol Clin* 29:1–7, 1991.

Melzack R. The McGill Pain Questionnaire. In: R Melzack (ed), *Pain Measurement and Assessment.* New York: Raven, 1983. Pp. 41–48.

Maruta T, Swanson DW, and McHardy MJ. Three year follow-up of patients with chronic pain who were treated in a multidisciplinary pain management center. *Pain* 41:47–53, 1990.

Muse M. Stress-related, posttraumatic chronic pain syndrome: Criteria for diagnosis and preliminary report on prevalance. *Pain* 23:295–300, 1985.

Pilowsky I and Spence ND. Patterns of illness behavior in patients with intractable pain. *J Psychosom Res* 19:279–287, 1975.

Roberts AH and Reinhardt L. The behavioral management of chronic pain: Long-term follow-up with comparison groups. *Pain* 8:151–162, 1980.

Schug SA, Merry AF, and Acland RH. Treatment principles for the use of opioids in pain of nonmalignant origin. *Drugs* 42: 228–239, 1991. Review.

Skinner JB, et al. The evaluation of a cognitive behavioural treatment program in outpatients with chronic pain. *J Psychosom Res* 34:13–19, 1990.

Stieg RL, et al. Cost benefits of interdisciplinary chronic pain treatment. *Clin J Pain* 1:189–193, 1986.

Tait RC, Chibnall JT, and Krause S. The Pain Disability Index: Psychometric properties. *Pain* 40:171–182, 1990.

Turk EC and Stieg RL. Chronic pain: The necessity of interdisciplinary communication. *Clin J Pain* 3:163–167, 1987.

Turner JA and Jensen MP. Efficacy of cognitive therapy for chronic low back pain. *Pain* 52:169–177, 1993.

Williams AC, et al. Evaluation of a cognitive behavioural programme for rehabilitating patients with chronic pain. *Br J Gen Pract* 43:513–518, 1993.

Zbrozek AS. Cost-effectiveness issues to consider in designing and interpreting pain studies. *Am Pain Soc Bull* 4:5–6, 1994.

Placebo

Terry Rabinowitz

> *"Take this. It's good for you."*
> SAID BY PARENTS EVERYWHERE

The ninth verse of the 116th psalm in the Old Testament begins with the words "et-ha-lech," which means, "I shall walk." It was ultimately translated into Greek and then into Vulgate Latin as "placebo," the first-person, singular, future tense of the verb, meaning to please or to serve. Its use as a noun dates back to the twelfth century when the word was used to indicate vespers sung for the dead in the Roman Catholic Church. The term derived a negative connotation because these vespers were usually sung for a substantial fee. Chaucer used the word to mean a flatterer, sycophant, or parasite (Lasagne, 1986).

The first medical definition of placebo is found in 1785 in Motherby's *New Medical Dictionary*, where it is referred to as a "commonplace method or medicine." Later editions of the dictionary implied that placebos were inert and harmless (Lasagne, 1986). Hooper's *Medical Dictionary*, of 1811, defines it as "an epithet given to any medicine adapted more to please than benefit the patient" (Rosenzweig, Brohier, Zipfel, 1993).

For a long time the term has been associated with deception, and for centuries many therapies for medical illnesses were, in fact, placebos. Placebos were in use by the early twentieth century, but no article describing placebos was issued until 1945, when Pepper published "A Note on Placebo." (Rosenzweig, Brohier, Zipfel, 1993.)

There are various meanings of **placebo**, many of which are complex. For the purposes of this chapter, the definition proffered by Brody suffices: **"a form of medical therapy, or an intervention designed to simulate medical therapy, that at the time of use is believed not to be a specific therapy for the condition for which it is offered and that is used for its psychological effect or to eliminate observer bias in an experimental setting."**

In a **double-blind, placebo-controlled study** (DBPC) of a particular treatment, neither the subjects nor the administrators or, perhaps, the evaluators of the treatment or placebo know who is receiving what. A **single-blind study** allows the investigators to know which treatment, but the subjects are "blinded," i.e., they do not know what they are receiving. In an **open-label study**, both the investigators and the subjects know who is receiving treatment. A **crossover trial** involves switching treatments at some point in the study to determine later whether those who originally received treatment had a response that changed. One problem in drug/placebo trials has been the lack of a **nonplacebo control group**. Furthermore, placebos are not often used in clinical trials; instead, an innovative treatment is compared with a current treatment.

The Placebo Response

When a subject has a response to placebo that would not be expected based on the composition of the placebo, we call this a "placebo response" or "placebo effect." This might occur in a trial of antidepressants, where subject A was given a drug and subject B received placebo. Both subjects' depressive symptoms might improve, so subject B is said to be displaying a placebo response. However, subject B might also complain of dry mouth, anxiety, dizziness, or hallucinations—symptoms that would not be expected from an "inert" substance. Here, too, subject B is showing a placebo response.

The **placebo response** occurs in the treatment of a variety of diseases and at varying rates, but a placebo response rate of about 30% has historically been accepted as the norm. Response rates, however, show great variability across studies and are generally high (range, 24% to 74%) and occur not only with medical but also with surgical or mechanical interventions. For example, a placebo response rate of 13% was obtained in pain patients who reported a reduction of more than 50% in various kinds of pain when treated with an impressive-looking but medically inert mechanical device.

The **placebo effect** has also been demonstrated in healthy volunteers receiving placebo as a single dose or in repeated doses. In 1993, Rosenzweig and colleagues reviewed 109 nontherapeutic DBPC European trials. They found an overall incidence of unfavorable events of 19% following placebo administration. Complaints were more frequent after repeated doses and in elderly patients. The most common adverse events included headache, drowsiness, and asthenia.

Pain and Placebo

The fact that placebo treatment of a myriad of diseases and symptoms including pain results in symptomatic as well as objective improvement is widely accepted. So, for a new drug or therapy to be considered effective, it must perform better than placebo. However, the mechanisms of the placebo response remain somewhat of a mystery, although careful observations have raised interesting hypotheses about the phenomenon.

The simplest, but often overlooked, explanation for the placebo effect is that most acute and many chronic conditions resolve on their own—no intervention at all is necessary. Also, patients with chronic conditions often seek treatment for their symptoms when they are at their worst. The next change in the symptom is one of improvement. This is often observed on inpatient pain treatment units, where, after admission and before any treatment is administered, patients report symptomatic improvement.

In 1959, Henry Beecher, an early worker in the field of placebo research, reported that only 25% of men wounded in battle required morphine for pain relief, compared with 80% of civilian patients with postoperative wounds. He concluded that suffering was more widespread in the civilian group because it signified anxiety and concern about the surgery, but in the military group it represented a respite from battle and possible stateside transfer. It is obvious that this was an observation of the pain-modulating effects of endogenous opioids.

Women in labor were shown to have less pain after receiving placebo compared with no treatment (Liberman, 1964). The issue of whether the analgesic effects of the placebo response could be a learned response was studied by Laska and Sunshine (1973). Patients were given 1 of 3 doses of an analgesic on the first day but placebo the second day. Patients experienced a small decrease in analgesia, but each group responded in the same manner relative to their previous dose; i.e., patients who had received a higher opioid dose responded better to the placebo than patients who had received a lower opioid dose. *What was so interesting about this study is that it showed that previous analgesic experience predicts the efficacy of placebo.* However, this effect may "wear off," as shown in a study of placebo effects on dysmenorrhea (Fedele et al, 1989): The initial placebo regimen produced the same effect as the drug, but the effectiveness of the placebo wears off during subsequent periods of dysmenorrhea.

In a randomized DBPC trial, Levine and associates (1978) studied dental patients whose impacted teeth were extracted and who were asked to evaluate their pain using a visual analog scale (VAS) before administration of any pain treatment and after receiving naloxone (a pure opioid antagonist) or placebo as their first pain treatment. Patients given placebo first and whose pain was either reduced or unchanged were labeled "placebo responders"; "nonresponders" experienced increased pain. Naloxone given as a second drug led to no increase in pain in the nonresponders but resulted in increased pain in the responders. The investigators hypothesized that endogenous opioid peptide release was responsible for the placebo-induced analgesia in these patients; the expectation of pain relief might help to activate the release of this substance.

A later report on the same experimental population showed that in subjects who were placebo responders and who rated their postextraction pain as greater than or equal to 2.6 on the VAS (range, 0.0–10.0), placebo-induced analgesia was significantly greater than in a comparable group with VAS-rated pain of less than 2.6. From these observations the investigators concluded that placebo helps to determine both the likelihood and magnitude of the placebo response. A subsequent investigation by Levine and colleagues (1981) showed that placebo analgesia was equivalent to between 4 and 6 mg of intravenous morphine in placebo responders.

In 1984, Fields described "an endogenous central nervous system pain-modulating network, with links in the midbrain, medulla and spinal cord." This system works through the release of endogenous opioids, including enkephalins and endorphins, and may be stimulated by stress or the administration of placebo. The more intense the painful stimuli, the more likely that endorphin release will occur. Opiate-induced analgesia is produced by imitation of the action of endogenous opioids in the brain. **What was so useful about the discovery of the endogenous/descending pain-modulating pathway is that it provided a neurobiologic model for the placebo effect**.

In support of the endogenous opioid hypothesis of placebo response is the work of Lipman and associates (1990), who showed that there was a reduction of peak beta-endorphin (PBE), an endogenous opioid, in the cerebrospinal fluid of chronic pain patients but not in normal controls. They also found that PBE levels rose only in subjects who had reduced pain following administration of placebo, i.e., placebo responders. PBE, a potent central analgesic in animal studies, is a mu opioid receptor ligand.

Not all investigators entirely agree with the endogenous opioid hypothesis of placebo action. Gracely and associates (1983) administered naloxone or naloxone vehicle immediately before administration of fentanyl (an opioid) or saline placebo, or no treatment, to patients whose impacted teeth were extracted. Patients completed the McGill Pain Questionnaire (see Chap. 3) 60 and 10 minutes before the naloxone treatments. They found that pain reduction occurred in placebo recipients who were administered naloxone. There was a tendency for naloxone to increase postextraction pain in placebo recipients, but it also caused increased pain reporting in subjects who had not received placebo or fentanyl. These investigators concluded that there were at least two separate mechanisms influencing postsurgical pain in their subjects: one opioid-related and one non–opioid-related. Further support for this conclusion comes from the observation that naloxone does not block hypnosis-produced analgesia.

Grevert and Goldstein (1985) reported that naloxone is a specific blocker of the mu type opioid receptor with 10 to 15 times **less** affinity for the delta and kappa types. If naloxone failed to block a placebo response, it might be because it was administered in doses too low to sufficiently block **all** classes of opioid receptors. In an effort to further elucidate the contribution of endorphins in the placebo response, the investigators suggested that identical doses of the L-(+) and D-(−) stereoisomers of naloxone be administered. Only the D-(−) stereoisomer occupies opioid receptors. Thus, if the L-(+) stereoisomer were effective in blocking placebo analgesia, the hypothesis of endorphin-mediated placebo analgesia could be rejected.

Placebo may be more effective in highly anxious versus less anxious subjects. The effects are sometimes attributed to possible anxiety-lowering properties of placebo. It is not yet clear, however, whether anxiety reduction is a cause of or a component of the placebo response.

Conditioning of the placebo responder also influences the response. If there has been a prior association of symptom attenuation by a drug or other treatment with a particular person, procedure, or venue, a new symptom may respond to placebo if treatment is administered by that person, includes that procedure, or is given in that location.

Remember that the hypotheses above are **not** mutually exclusive. Most likely, there is more than one mechanism acting at any time to produce a placebo effect.

Who Responds to Placebo?

As with the mechanisms underlying the placebo response, the general characteristics of placebo responders are not universally agreed upon. There are conflicting reports in the literature regarding responder characteristics—one example being disagreement about subject anxiety levels. Some investigators report better responses in more anxious subjects. Others have observed better responses in less anxious participants.

What follows is a brief review of selected studies of placebo responders. The clinician is advised to consider each patient he or she treats individually, and not to expect a particular **type** of patient to show or not to show a response to placebo. This will facilitate objectivity of observations, more accurate and reliable collection of data, and provision of better patient care.

Many investigators have reported that a **subject's expectation** or belief that treatment of his or her symptoms will cause relief is a powerful predictor of the placebo response. These positive expectations are related to the subject's viewing his or her problem more positively and to the "goodness" or "badness" of the physician–patient relationship.

Jensen and Karoly (1991) examined both motivation and expectancy in the placebo response. They gave normal healthy subjects instructions designed to either increase or decrease their motivation to respond to a "sedative" placebo pill: High-expectancy subjects were given instructions that a certain personality type, B, was a more desirable type and was associated with response to the placebo administered. Type A personalities were less desirable and had no response to the placebo. Subjects were also randomly assigned to high- and low-expectancy groups based on the "dose" of the placebo they were to receive: High-expectancy subjects received high doses. These investigators observed that motivation factors were more important than expectancy factors in predicting placebo response; i.e., those subjects who were encouraged to have a stronger desire to respond to a placebo sedative tended to report greater sedation than those who were not motivated. There was limited support for expectancy factors having a role in the placebo response.

In a study of four investigations into the effects of orally administered analgesics and opioids for chronic cancer pain in a total of 288 patients, Moertel and associates (1976) reported that patients who responded to placebo also had greater responses to active drugs. Characteristics of placebo responders also included those with a professional occupation, those with a high level of education, women working outside the home, and patients who were widowed, separated, or divorced. Those resistant to placebo were patients with a low educational level, unskilled workers, housewives, married women without children, and smokers.

In a study of drug-treated and placebo-treated patients complaining of anxiety or mild depression, Rickels and Downing (1967) observed that 69.2% of high-anxiety and 65.4% of low-anxiety patients responded to real "tranquilizers," primarily chlordiazepoxide (Librium). In the placebo-treated group, 38.9% of high-anxiety patients and 78.9% of low-anxiety patients had symptomatic improvement. Placebo-treated patients with high anxiety also had the most frequent complaints of treatment side effects.

In a retrospective evaluation of predictors of placebo response in 197 depressed patients, Wilcox and colleagues (1992) examined six variables—age, gender, marital status, education, duration of illness, and severity of illness—to determine if any predicted a positive response. They found that a positive response could be predicted by married versus single status (38.2% vs. 21.9%) and by severity of illness, where less severe illness ratings predicted a better placebo response (40.8% vs. 23.4%). No significant predictions of placebo response could be made based on gender, age, education, or duration of illness. Another retrospective study of three randomized DBPC studies of 241 placebo-treated depressed patients showed that predictors of placebo response included relatively short duration of illness, a precipitating event, depression of only moderate severity, and good response to previous antidepressant treatment.

A recent report by Bystritsky and Waikar (1994) is intriguing because it showed that there may be difficulty in controlling supposed randomized DBPC trials. They observed that, based on the presence of clinical improvement and side effects, 21 of 28 patients (75%) could correctly determine whether they were receiving active drug or placebo. Thus, there may be confounding variables that are not easily controlled and that may positively or negatively influence placebo responses.

Many investigators believe that a positive placebo response is predicted by a treating physician who is interested and concerned. Moreover, a physician who believes in the potential efficacy of the treatment, whether or not it is placebo, may also be a predictor of a favorable response.

Ethical Considerations

Should placebos be used? The answer to this question is not easily reached. Consider what decision you might make if you knew from in vitro studies that a new drug was highly effective against a certain tumor or for a particular type of pain but that to get it for your patient it would first have to be subjected to DBPC trials and that some participants would surely not receive the drug and might suffer or die. Would you be willing to wait or to make the drug unavailable to some patients? This section deals with the ethical questions surrounding the use of placebos.

Although placebos have been used for centuries, their use in controlled clinical trials began only about 50 years ago when randomized DBPC trials of new therapies were made the gold standard by which the treatment under investigation was judged. If the treatment performed significantly better than placebo, it was considered a potentially usable new therapy.

During the early period of DBPC studies and certainly in the centuries before, patients were often not informed that they would be receiving placebo. This happened, in part, because the physician was considered to have a paternalistic position in the community and most of the population assumed that anyone in that position would not intentionally cause a patient harm or deceive him or her for any reason other than to help the patient.

Patients did indeed suffer for want of a treatment other than placebo, and the physician–patient relationship also became threatened. What seemed a benevolent gesture by the physician was felt by the patient, and sometimes by the community, to be a violation of the patient's autonomy. This has become more important as medical science has advanced. In times past, there were few effective treatments for most diseases. Patients got better on their own, were given ineffective treatment and died, or were given no treatment and died. The administration of placebo versus a "real treatment" was not a consideration—a "real treatment" did not exist and placebo may have actually caused an improvement in symptoms.

Contemporary medicine is different. Today there are effective treatments for many diseases that would have been deadly only decades ago. The same holds true for the management of pain and other symptoms that are not life-threatening. Should we knowingly withhold an effective treatment from some patients to determine whether a new treatment performs better than placebo?

Many investigators in the field believe that it is unethical to give placebos to uninformed subjects when alternative effective forms of therapy exist. They argue that if a patient is

informed that he or she might receive placebo instead of active drug or treatment and consents to participate in such a study, the obligation to apprise the patient has been met. Some experts suggest, however, that a better approach would be to use a treatment that has been previously shown to be effective for the condition under investigation as the "control" to which the new therapy is compared. This would allow control subjects the opportunity to receive some form of effective therapy. This type of experimental design would have its greatest utility in cases where life-threatening diseases were under investigation and recipients of placebo might die.

Not all investigators agree with these recommendations. Fields, a clinician, takes a slightly different tack and writes, "The use of placebos as a punitive measure or diagnostic test for patients suspected of malingering or exaggerating their complaints is unethical and, furthermore, that the 'information' derived is misleading." However, he suggests that as long as the patient's best interests are served, the use of placebo is justifiable.

The decision to use placebo in a particular individual must be made only after thoughtful consideration is given to the presenting clinical situation. It may be appealing to use placebo in a case where hypochondriasis or drug-seeking is suspected, but remember that normal individuals also respond to placebo. Thus, no real "incriminating evidence" may be gotten from this approach, and it may produce undue stress and suffering in the patient. Here is a situation where psychiatric consultation to help rule out nonmedical causes of the patient's complaint would be helpful.

We are left, in large part, to rely on our ethical system, our fund of medical knowledge, and the quality of our patient relationship to decide whether to use placebo. The novice clinician in pain control should certainly rely more heavily on the advice of his or her seniors when trying to make a decision. Don't work without a safety net!

Conclusions

The placebo response is real and robust. It is an individual response. Severe pains may respond to placebo, and the response may be learned and conditioned. The mechanisms by which it operates are certainly multifactorial and are not yet fully elucidated, although the descending analgesic pathway is currently our best model. There is no one specific set of characteristics that describes the placebo responder; in fact, a responder one day may be a nonresponder the next. Be vigilant when testing new drugs and therapies; a placebo effect may occur and go unnoticed, confounding the results of a costly clinical trial.

Whether placebos should be used remains a controversial topic. The decision should be guided by sound medical principles and the obligation to the patient to "first do no harm"— whether by omission or commission.

Selected Readings

Beecher HK. *Measurement of Subjective Responses. Quantitative Effects of Drugs.* New York: Oxford University Press, 1959.

Bok S. The ethics of giving placebos. *Sci Am* 231:17–23, 1974.

Brody H. *Placebos and the Philosophy of Medicine. Clinical, Conceptual, and Ethical Issues.* Chicago: University of Chicago Press, 1977.

Brody H. The lie that heals: The ethics of giving placebos. *Ann Intern Med* 97:112–118, 1982.

Brown WA, Johnson MF, and Chen M-G. Clinical features of depressed patients who do and do not improve with placebo. *Psychiatry Res* 41:203–214, 1992.

Bystritsky A and Waikar SV. Inert placebo versus active medication. Patient blindability in clinical pharmacological trials. *J Nerv Ment Dis* 182:485–487, 1994.

Fedele L, et al. Dynamics and significance of placebo response in primary dysmenorrhea. *Pain* 36:43–47, 1989.

Fields HL and Levine JD. Biology of placebo analgesia. *Am J Med* 70:745–746, 1981.

Fields HL. Pain II: New approaches to management. *Ann Neurol* 9:101–106, 1981.

Fields HL. Neurophysiology of pain and pain modulation. *Am J Med* 77:2–8, 1984.

Fields HL. *Pain.* New York: McGraw-Hill, 1987.

Gracely RH, et al. Placebo and naloxone can alter post-surgical pain by separate mechanisms. *Nature* 306:264–265, 1983.

Grevert P and Goldstein A. Placebo Analgesia, Naloxone, and the Role of Endogenous Opioids. In: L White, B Tursky, and GE Schwartz (eds), *Placebo: Theory, Research, and Mechanisms.* New York: Guilford Press, 1985. Pp. 332–350.

Jensen MP and Karoly P. Motivation and expectancy factors in symptom perception: A laboratory study of the placebo effect. *Psychosom Med* 53:144–152, 1991.

Kluge E-H. Placebos: Some ethical considerations. *Can Med Assoc J* 142:293–295, 1990.

Lasagna L. The placebo effect. *J Allergy Clin Immunol* 78:161–165, 1986.

Laska E and Sunshine A. Anticipation of analgesia: A placebo effect. *Headache* 13:1–11, 1973.

Levine JD, et al. Role of pain in placebo analgesia. *Proc Natl Acad Sci USA* 76:3528–3531, 1979.

Levine JD, Gordon NC, and Fields HL. The mechanism of placebo analgesia. *Lancet* 2:654–657, 1978.

Levine JD, et al. Analgesic responses to morphine and placebo in individuals with postoperative pain. *Pain* 10:379–389, 1981.

Liberman R. An experimental study of the placebo response under three different situations of pain. *J Psychiat Res* 2:233–246, 1964.

Lipman JL, et al. Peak β endorphin concentration in cerebrospinal fluid: Reduced in chronic pain patients and increased during the placebo response. *Psychopharmacology (Berl)* 102:112–116, 1990.

Long DM, Uematsu S, and Kouba RB. Placebo responses to medical device therapy for pain. *Stereotact Funct Neurosurg* 53:149–156, 1989.

Moertel CG, et al. Who responds to sugar pills? *Mayo Clin Proc* 51:96–100, 1976.

Rickels K and Downing RW. Drug- and placebo-treated neurotic outpatients. *Arch Gen Psychiatry* 16:369–372, 1967.

Rosenzweig P, Brohier S, and Zipfel A. The placebo effect in healthy volunteers: Influence of experimental conditions on the adverse events profile during phase I studies. *Clin Pharmacol Ther* 54:578–583, 1993.

Rothman KJ and Michels KB. The continuing unethical use of placebo controls. *N Engl J Med* 331:394–398, 1994.

Turner JA, et al. The importance of placebo effects in pain treatment and research. *JAMA* 271:1609–1614, 1994.

Wilcox CS, et al. Predictors of placebo response: A retrospective study. *Psychopharmacol Bull* 28:157–162, 1992.

Treatment of Specific Pain Syndromes

13

Neuropathic Pain

Nicolas A. Wieder and David Borsook

> *"Doctors think a lot of patients are cured who have simply quit in disgust."*
>
> DON HEROLD, 1889

Neuropathic pain—with many etiologies, proposed pathophysiologies, and clinical manifestations—is one of the most challenging and complex pain syndromes. It can disable without disfiguring and challenge the patience and tolerance of both patient and physician. Neuropathic pain is the symptom resulting from neural injury—peripheral or central, or both—to a portion of the neuronal pain transmission system. Such pain is often severe, delayed in onset following the injury, often burning or electrical in quality, and present in the absence of an ongoing primary source for the pain. The severity or chronicity of this pain is not directly related to a specific etiology.

Most neuropathic pain problems involve the peripheral nerves, at least initially. Relatively few clinical problems, by comparison, involve the CNS. Pain arising from the CNS usually involves damage to the spinothalamic tract anywhere along its course between the dorsal horn and cerebral cortex.

Biologic Basis for Neuropathic Pain

Why should a transected or an avulsed sensory nerve cause pain? What creates exaggerated painful responses to minor nociceptive stimuli or causes surgical lesions of central spinal pain pathways to fail to keep patients pain free? These and other perplexing clinical observations challenge pain practitioners. In the past few years, new animal models for neuropathic pain have been developed and have increased our understanding of the syndrome at the neurobiologic level, thus helping us to develop improved treatment strategies. These models generally describe abnormal signals of reception, modulation, or transmission.

EPHAPTIC CROSS-TALK

The ephaptic model of pain transmission has been extensively studied in animals and is described as the artificial junction of the efferent and afferent fibers. This phenomenon can exist in cases of neuroma and may be involved in the syndrome of sympathetically mediated pain. See Table 13-1.

Table 13-1. Pathogenesis of neuropathic pain

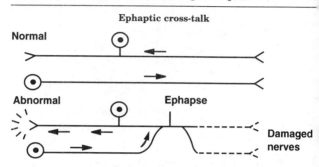

Under normal conditions, activity in a nerve remains
confined to that nerve. With nerve damage the formation
of abnormal contacts (ephapses) may result in activity in
one nerve producing electrical activation in another. This
activity is therefore not generated by normal sensory
transduction.

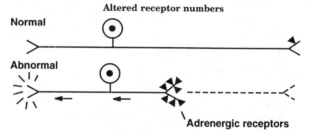

In neuroma formation, for example, increased numbers
of adrenergic receptors on the sprouting nerve terminals
are present. Increased neural activity is seen under
conditions that would not normally activate these nerves,
e.g., stress and the release of adrenaline or with
pressure over the neuroma. Microneuromas form even
after apparently minor trauma, e.g., skin incision,
postherpetic neuralgia.

ALTERED RECEPTOR NUMBER OR
ADRENERGIC RECEPTORS

Another model that has been implicated in the production of
pain and sympathetic pain states is that of altered receptor
number. After an injury, regenerating nociceptors become
sensitive to noradrenaline, which is released by the sympathetic efferent fibers. This increased sensitivity may be due to
an up-regulation of adrenergic receptors on damaged peripheral afferent fibers. Other examples include the changes in
opioid receptors in the dorsal horn in models of neuropathic

Table 13-1 (continued)

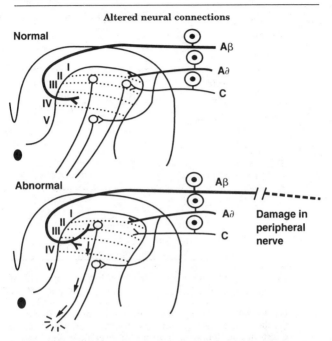

Under normal conditions of activity A-delta and C fibers make connections in the dorsal horn, predominately in laminae I and II. A-beta fibers synapse centrally in lamina IV. Thus, light touch does not activate painful sensation. Following nerve injury, however, A-beta fibers make new connections into lamina II, presumably synapsing onto spinothalamic tract neurons: Now light touch activates painful sensations. Altered connections are also known to take place in the dorsal root ganglion with increased noradrenergic synapses and may also take place within the CNS after damage to the thalamus, for example.

pain—a possible explanation for the relative refractoriness to opioids seen in chronic neuropathic pain syndromes.

ALTERED NEURAL CONNECTIVITY

The concept of neuronal plasticity helps us to understand how peripheral injury interacts with central pain transmission. In this model central pain transmission neurons are activated as a result of chronic activation of nociceptive afferent fibers, deafferentation, or alternate afferent fiber sources such as ipsilateral pathways whose primary nociceptive afferent fibers have suffered varying degrees of deafferentation.

Table 13-1 (continued)

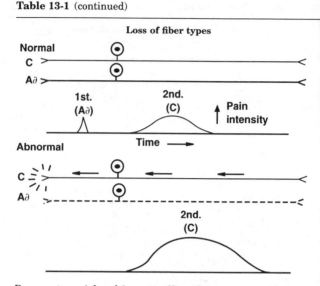

Damage to peripheral (or central?) pathways may result in a loss of specific fiber types. For example, in the Bennett model, a small ligature produces the loss of predominately large fiber types. The effect is a neuropathic pain syndrome in the rat similar to that seen in humans. Another example of this is the effect on pain following blockade of large fiber types with a blood pressure cuff. Prior to the cuff, pain is perceived as a first (A-delta-fiber transmission) and a second (C fiber) pain. After blockage of the larger fiber types, which include A-beta fibers, there is an increase in the intensity of the second pain.

Ectopic impulses

Under basal conditions, there is no activity in pain fibers. However, following nerve damage, even at a microscopic level, abnormal spontaneous activity is present in these nerves. The activity may account for constant pain and for shooting pains seen clinically.

Table 13-1 (continued)

Enlargement of receptive fields

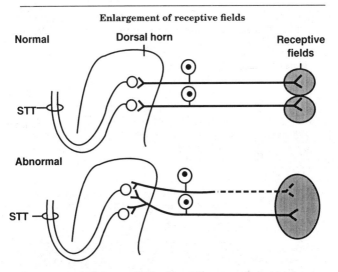

Some neuromodulators in the dorsal horn are excitatory (e.g., glutamate, calcitonin gene related peptide [CGRP], substance P [SP]) and others are inhibitory (e.g., enkephalin, galanin). With nerve damage there may be excessive release of **excitatory transmitters** producing damage to central neurons and even permanent alterations in the levels of various peptides. **Inhibitory** systems act as "protectors" and inhibit this process (e.g., galanin, enkephalin). Providing opioids prior to nerve damage may inhibit this excitatory amino acid–induced damage to neurons in the dorsal horn. In damaged conditions there may be an **enlargement of receptive fields** of spinothalamic neurons.

Recent evidence has demonstrated that following nerve injury, new connections are formed in the dorsal horn. Under basal conditions, light touching of the skin is not painful (with normal activation of A-beta fibers). After nerve damage, new connections are made by A-beta fibers (which normally synapse in lamina IV) by sending new collaterals to laminae I and II. Now, with these new connections, light touch sensations connect to second order neurons normally involved in pain transmission.

LOSS OF FIBER TYPES

The loss of fiber types has alternately been hypothesized as a mechanism of painful neuropathy.

ECTOPIC IMPULSES

Peripheral fibers that convey nociceptive information are normally inactive under basal conditions and are only activated

Table 13-1 (continued)

Coupling of sympathetic nerves and primary afferent fibers in
the dorsal root ganglion. (Adapted from EM Mclachlan, et al.
Peripheral nerve injury triggers noradrenergic sprouting within
dorsal root ganglia. *Nature* 363:543–546, 1993.)

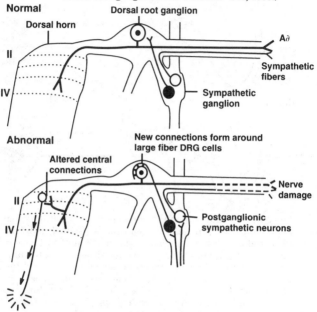

After nerve injury, noradrenergic axons sprout in the dorsal
root ganglion and form basket-like structures around large-
diameter injured neurons. Activity in sympathetic nerves
activates the large primary afferent neurons, which now send
sprouts to synapse on lamina II.

by painful stimuli. Following peripheral nerve damage, however, abnormal electrical activity is present. Such neural discharge may produce the clinical symptoms of constant pain
and superimposed shooting pains due to the continuous and
sometimes variable activity of afferent nociceptive input. Abnormal activity has also been demonstrated in patients with
central pain syndromes. For example, there are abnormal
electrical discharges in the thalamus of patients with central
(and also peripheral) pain syndromes.

SYMPATHETIC–AFFERENT COUPLING

Under normal conditions, the sympathetic nervous system
has no effect on primary afferent neurons. However, following
nerve damage, this system affects afferent neurons primarily
through noradrenergic mechanisms. Coupling between sym-

pathetic neurons and primary afferent neurons may take place peripherally at or distal to the lesion site or in the dorsal root ganglion (DRG). Coupling of these systems has been shown in the periphery following nerve injury: Stimulation of the sympathetic system activates primary afferent neurons via alpha$_1$ receptors. Furthermore, after damage to the peripheral sensory nerve, there is an increase in noradrenergic terminals surrounding neurons in the DRG. This sprouting of noradrenergic axons in the DRG takes place around the neurons of the damaged, projecting neuron. There may also be new noradrenergic sprouting on the contralateral DRG, which might be a possible explanation for a mechanism by which sympathetically maintained pain (SMP) spreads with time and why surgery for this disease (sympathectomy) has not been successful.

Clinical Presentations of Neuropathic Pain

See Table 13-2. The typical patient with neuropathic pain presents to the clinician with complaints of strange or unusual painful sensations, usually burning or tingling in quality. Often the pain is described as shooting, stabbing, or electrical. The pain usually increases in intensity toward evening as well as over time. Characteristically, the pain intensity eventually reaches a plateau.

There may be a history or findings of previous neural trauma such as thoracotomy, mastectomy, amputation, or spinal cord trauma. This trauma has, however, usually taken place many weeks before the onset of pain and the primary injury has healed.

Major **signs of neural injury** include hypersensitive skin (hyperalgesia, allodynia), a pronounced increased response and after-reaction to repetitive pain stimulation (summation), and sensory loss. Vasomotor changes, including absence of sweating, cooling of the affected area, and dystrophic changes of the skin and nails, may also occur in cases of sympathetically maintained or ischemic pain. Disuse atrophy of

Table 13-2. Clinical findings in neuropathic pain

Symptoms	Signs
Burning or electrical quality	Decreased sensation
Hypersensitivity	Allodynia
Delay in onset after precipitating injury	Hyperalgesia
	Summation
Pain in areas of decreased sensation	Associated vasomotor changes
No detectable ongoing tissue damage	
Constant pain	
Difficult to treat	

underlying muscle may also occur, especially in pain involving the knee joint.

NEUROPHYSIOLOGY OF CLINICAL FEATURES IN NEUROPATHIC PAIN

The state of painful dysesthesia, which occurs following injury to sensory neurons, may begin immediately, be delayed, or begin acutely and develop other delayed features such as those found in SMP. These features may depend on fiber type, location of nervous system involvement, or extensive deafferentation. Experimental models of deafferentation have helped us to understand some of the neurophysiologic correlates of patients' clinical symptoms (see Table 13-3).

Neuropathic Pain Syndromes: From Peripheral Nerve to Cortex

A summary of various neuropathic pain syndromes at each level of the neural axis is given in Table 13-4. Common clinical examples at each level are discussed below.

INJURY TO THE PERIPHERAL NERVES

Diabetic Neuropathy

Diabetic neuropathy is the most common peripheral neuropathy in the United States. Nervous system involvement is varied and may affect peripheral, autonomic, and cranial nerves. Three distinct types of diabetic neuropathy are described: autonomic neuropathy, symmetric distal polyneurop-

Table 13-3. Symptoms of neuropathic pain

Symptom	Characteristic
Evoked pain referred to anesthetic region (anesthesia dolorosa)	Burning Triggered from stimulation of nearby or distant areas
Nonevoked pain not referred to anesthetic region	Reduced sensibility to pinprick and cold stimuli with light touch intact
Border zone hypersensitivity	Sensitivity in areas adjacent to injury
Allodynia	Pain elicited by usually nonpainful stimuli
Hyperalgesia	Increased sensitivity to a usually painful stimulus
Variability of pain tolerance	Pain increase with emotional stress

Table 13-4. Neuropathic pain syndromes

Source	Clinical examples

Peripheral nerve	Acquired neuropathies
	  Endocrine: diabetic, distal, truncal,
	    proximal
	  Isolated: tic douloureux
	  Cancer pain
	  Infection: AIDS, Guillain-Barré
	    syndrome
	  Vasculitis
	  Toxic: clioquinol, alcohol, thallium,
	    arsenic, drugs
	Inherited neuropathies
	  Fabry's disease
	  Hereditary sensory neuropathy
	    (HSN)
	  Neurofibromatosis
	Entrapment neuropathies
	  Carpal tunnel
	  Prolapsed disk
	Herpes zoster
	Trauma: amputation, postoperative
	Sympathetically maintained pain
	Postsympathectomy pain
	Demyelination

Dorsal root ganglion	Herpes zoster
Dorsal horn	Avulsion injuries
Spinal cord tracts	Trauma Tumors Syringomyelia Cervical disk Demyelination
Midbrain/pons	Stroke Demyelination
Thalamus	Stroke Tumor Demyelination
Cortex	Stroke Seizures Demyelination

athy, and mononeuritis multiplex or mononeuropathy. The last is of more acute onset and may resolve without treatment, whereas symmetric neuropathy is of more gradual onset and more sustained.

Pathophysiology

The pathophysiology of diabetic neuropathy is that of both axonal degeneration and segmental demyelination, primarily of small nerve fibers. This pattern of an altered fiber size population with a shift toward larger nerve fiber diameter is a feature also shared by amyloid neuropathy and Fabry's disease. Other painful neuropathies differ in nerve fiber populations affected, and it is not reasonable to assume that selective loss of nerve fiber populations is solely responsible for the production of pain. Rather, the combination of axonal degeneration, spontaneous discharges from both large myelinated and small demyelinated nerve fibers, hyperglycemia, and possibly microangiopathic changes and ischemia contributes to this painful syndrome.

Treatment

Treatment consists of a comprehensive approach that relies, to a great extent, on preventive care. Hyperglycemia must be strictly controlled and is an important means a physician has of improving the substrate for the development of painful neuropathy in the patient. The possibility of other reversible causes of painful neuropathy must also be ruled out. The extent of concomitant peripheral vascular disease must be established and good foot care must be a priority.

The medical management of diabetic neuropathic pain may apply to neuropathic pain syndromes in general, with some disorders responding variably to different agents. Therefore, pharmacologic therapy of neuropathic pain is discussed next and is referred to in the content of other neuropathic syndromes.

Standard analgesics for mild somatic pain, such as acetaminophen and **nonsteroidal anti-inflammatory drugs**, are rarely effective in treating diabetic neuropathy. All of these patients are considered candidates for a trial of **tricyclic antidepressants**, unless there is a clear contraindication. Support for the use of the tertiary amines, such as amitriptyline, doxepin, and imipramine, has been extensively documented in the literature, and they are commonly the first agents of choice. This patient population, however, is at risk for autonomic dysfunction on the basis of their primary disease. Therefore, many of these patients may not tolerate the anticholinergic effects, in which case a trial of secondary amines, such as desipramine or nortriptyline, should be considered (see Chap. 5).

A general treatment principle in using tricyclic antidepressants is to start with a low dose of 10–25 mg and increase the dosage, as tolerated, every few days. This escalation, in some cases, may reach antidepressant levels for the particular agent. Care must be taken to monitor both the ECG and serum levels during significant dosage escalation.

We have begun to routinely consider the use of a **local anesthetic** as an analgesic in the management of neuropathic pain. We begin with a test dose of 100 mg of lidocaine IV infusion over 10 minutes. Other protocols use higher doses over a longer period of time, though we have found that the doses we presently use are usually sufficient for deciding on a trial of medication. Those patients who have near-complete or complete relief of pain are begun on oral mexiletine (Mexitil), a lidocaine analog, at 150 mg/day, with gradual dose escalation, as tolerated. The average effective dose in our patients is 600–900 mg. The most common side effects are nausea and gastric irritation. Serum levels of lidocaine may be useful in monitoring side effects. The ECG must be observed in all cases of dose escalation. Patients may become "tolerant" to mexiletine, and we have found taking them off it and placing them on oxycodone or codeine for a month beneficial prior to the resumption of the mexiletine.

Anticonvulsants may be helpful in cases of lancinating dysesthesias as well as for constant neuropathic pain. Clonazepam, which is both a benzodiazepine and an anticonvulsant, is usually the first agent tried in our clinic, followed by carbamazepine (Tegretol), phenytoin (Dilantin), and valproic acid (Depakene). Although the effective doses of tricyclic antidepressants for pain are usually not as high as those used for depression, the effective doses of anticonvulsants usually are in the same range as those used for patients with seizure disorders.

Capsaicin cream, at both 0.025% and 0.075%, has been used in our clinic with minimal benefit, primarily because of patients' intolerance to the burning sensation associated with topical application. We do not routinely use **neuroleptics** or **muscle relaxants** in the treatment of diabetic neuropathy. The use of **opioids** in nonmalignant pain is controversial and should probably be reserved for those physicians primarily practicing pain management. However, we have found opioids very useful in carefully selected patients (see Chap. 22).

HIV Neuropathy

HIV infection may present with and is frequently associated with peripheral nervous system involvement. HIV is a known neurotropic organism and thus has direct effects on the peripheral nerves, in addition to its well-known indirect and immune-mediated effects. There are four pathologically distinct neuropathic processes known in patients with peripheral nervous system involvement from HIV. Symmetric distal sensory motor neuropathy is the most common neuropathy; it is present in over one third of HIV patients. This is presumed to occur by direct viral invasion of the axoplasm and demyelination, with subsequent progressive axonal degeneration. Other peripheral nerve injuries are similar to those that occur in the non-HIV population, but may present treatment problems unique to patients with HIV. These include immune-mediated acute or chronic demyelinating polyneuropathy such as Guillain-Barré syndrome and chronic intermittent demyelinating polyneuropathy (CIDP); multiple mononeuropathy with vasculitic involvement; and herpes zoster, which is discussed in the section dealing with injury to the DRG.

Treatment of these disorders is similar to their treatment in the non-HIV population. It is important to point out, though, that the presence of HIV is not an absolute contraindication to steroid therapy, which may be used when appropriate Steroids may be indicated in the treatment of acute herpes zoster or CIDP. Also, although controversy exists regarding the use of opioids in nonmalignant pain, their use should be kept in perspective and a reasonable opioid regimen should be decided on by both the physician and the patient. Sometimes the nontraditional use of traditional therapy such as an epidural or intrathecal infusion of an anesthetic agent may be indicated, especially in patients with advanced symptoms of AIDS. These patients may be cachectic and unable to tolerate some of the respiratory depression and sedation produced by the medications commonly used to treat these disorders. Chapter 20 provides additional information about HIV neuropathy.

Amputation

Two distinct, nearly universal types of pain are experienced by those patients who have had a limb amputation—**stump pain** and **phantom pain**. Stump pain, which is believed to exist on the basis of persistent neural activity within a neuroma, may also be related to infection, myofascial trigger points, poorly fitted prostheses, and various other etiologies. The pain is typically both lancinating and continuous. Treatment consists of resection of the neuroma, local injection of anesthetic drugs, treatment of infection or prosthetic device, and the use of medications such as carbamazepine and other anticonvulsants that are effective in the treatment of lancinating neuropathic pain or antidepressants if the pain is more characteristic of the nonlancinating type.

Phantom sensations occur in virtually all patients, whereas phantom limb pain occurs in 30% to 90% of amputees. It is usually described as cramping or squeezing, but may also be described as electric-like and is experienced in the phantom limb. The severity ranges from mild to incapacitating. One year after the amputation, 40% of patients no longer have phantom pain. The pathophysiology is complex and not completely understood, although it is likely that a peripheral mechanism of deafferentation, which ultimately helps produce spontaneous firing of spinal cord neurons and more rostral CNS centers (e.g., thalamus), may be an important factor.

Treatment is varied. One study showed evidence that preoperative analgesia with lumbar epidural bupivacaine or morphine reduced the incidence of phantom pain at 6 months' postamputation. Physical therapy, transcutaneous electrical nerve stimulation, nerve blocks, neurosurgical procedures, and neurostimulation are all used but unfortunately have had moderate and temporary effects, at best, in most patients. Parenteral calcitonin has recently been reported to produce good results in several individual cases. Medications are the mainstay of therapy but have variable benefits if symptoms last longer than 1 year.

INJURY TO THE DORSAL ROOT GANGLION

Acute Herpes Zoster

The herpes zoster virus involves both the DRG and the peripheral nerves. It stimulates an inflammatory process of the peripheral nerves with atrophy of large myelinated fibers and inflammatory changes in the dorsal and ventral horns of the spinal cord, implicating the DRG as the primary site of viral invasion. It has a characteristic acute distribution, with the thoracic dermatomes most commonly affected. Postherpetic neuralgia is most often located in the **thoracic region** (50%), followed by the ophthalmic division of the fifth cranial nerve (3% to 20%) and the cervical dermatomes (10% to 20%). It is infrequently bilateral (<1%) and may be recurrent (1% to 8%), usually in immunocompromised patients. Recurrences are frequently in the previous herpes zoster site (50%).

The incidences of acute disease, ophthalmic involvement, and postherpetic neuralgia **increase with advancing age**. Herpes zoster infections can be especially devastating in immunosuppressed and elderly patients, in that the infection may cause visceral and nervous system complications such as stroke. Pain typically follows dermatomal involvement and is described as an itching, burning, and sometimes lancinating sensation. The painful sensations that accompany acute herpes zoster typically are confined to the dermatomal distribution of the DRG involved as well as to the developing lesions. Thus the pain is usually well localized and usually described as sharp, burning, or aching paresthesia or dysesthesia. This is in contradistinction to the more diffuse and dull, or aching, quality of pain usually described in postherpetic neuralgia. The initial lesions in the acute herpes zoster usually heal completely by the fifth or sixth week. Most commonly, the intense stimulus-provoked pain at the lesion site begins to diminish in the second or third week as the lesions become encrusted. Paresthesia, likewise, improves with a diminution of the lancinating-like characteristics. The patient often continues to complain of an aching component, with residual sensory abnormalities resolving over months to an asymptomatic state in most patients.

One of the main goals of therapy is the prevention of postherpetic neuralgia, which occurs in up to 70% of patients. The incidence is especially high in the elderly. It seems clear now that the early treatment of acute herpes zoster not only effects the early resolution of the episode and decreases pain, but also aids in the prevention of postherpetic neuralgia. To our consternation, there are too many cases of acute herpes zoster that are not treated early enough and that eventually are complicated by the development of postherpetic neuralgia. Most patients referred to our unit come to us already carrying the diagnosis of postherpetic neuralgia. Steroids have been used successfully and have been shown to reduce acute and chronic manifestations when started within the first week. Care must be taken, however, in the elderly and immunosuppressed. Antiviral therapy begun within 72 hours may be effective and may also be used, particularly in immunosuppressed patients, as a preventive measure. Various anesthetic techniques, medication regimens, and topical agents have also been used.

We have had relative success at Massachusetts General Hospital with the use of **sympathetic blockade**, including epidural blocks using 0.25% bupivacaine during the first 2 weeks of acute herpes zoster onset. There are few side effects and the procedure is relatively simple and done on an outpatient basis.

Postherpetic Neuralgia

Postherpetic neuralgia has variable definitions. Because, in many cases, the hyperesthesia and hyperalgesia that accompanied the acute herpes zoster exists for several weeks after the lesions heal, we consider postherpetic neuralgia as pain that persists longer than 1 month after the complete healing of acute herpes zoster lesions.

The pain in postherpetic neuralgia is believed to result from deafferentation and hypersensitivity in the posterior horn of the spinal cord. All the same treatments used in acute herpes zoster have been used in postherpetic neuralgia, although with considerably less success. The mainstay of therapy is often the use of tricyclic antidepressants. Anticonvulsants, anxiolytics, and, less commonly, narcotic analgesics are also used. Some of our patients have benefited from 3 tablets of salicylate in a chloroform base ground to a paste and applied topically to the affected areas. Various other topical agents such as 2% lidocaine gel, have also been used with variable effects.

Antiviral therapy is not helpful in classic postherpetic neuralgia. In addition, we have not had much success with capsaicin, since most of our patients have been unable to tolerate the cutaneous side effects on already sensitive skin.

Dorsal root entry zone lesions have been used to treat some patients. This procedure involves laminectomy and electrocoagulation of the dorsal root entry zone adjacent to the intercostal nerve root affected by the herpes. Good results were reported by Nashold and Ostdahl (1979) in patients with intractable pain who failed all conservative measures. We have not had experience with this procedure in our patients. Implantable systems, both narcotic and electrical stimulation, have been praised for providing good results. However, the literature does not yet support the implantation of these devices as an early treatment option. Overall, since less than one third of patients with postherpetic neuralgia have severe pain persisting for longer than 1 year and most do improve over time, if there is no significant underlying medical problem such as decreased immunocompetence, we would reserve surgical treatment only as a last resort.

INJURY TO THE DORSAL HORN

Avulsion of the Brachial Plexus

Avulsion injuries to the brachial plexus may be termed the "motorcycle pain syndrome," since approximately 80% of these patients have been involved in a motorcycle crash. The pathophysiology is mechanical avulsion of afferent fibers, a deafferentation injury in the region of the dorsal root entry zone. This usually occurs in an abducted and hyperextended position of the arm. Avulsion is usually defined by myelography or MRI.

Brachial plexus avulsions present as severe burning, crushing, or paroxysmal shooting pain in isolation or in combination. In cases of avulsion, most patients will present with pain. Older patients suffer more. Many patients also have a flail arm that is usually numb. The pain is thought to result from aberrant and spontaneous firing of deafferented cells in the dorsal horn at the level of the injury. There may be secondary spread of abnormal firing at higher levels within the pain pathways. In approximately 30% of patients, the pain is lifelong. In the other 70% of patients, there is some clinical improvement, although this may be delayed for a number of years. Treatment is very difficult. Normal neuropathic medications are usually of limited benefit. Dorsal root entry zone lesions, described in the previous section, have been found to be efficacious, and in patients with flail arm, the risk of promoting motor deficits is not a major concern to the neurosurgeon and an aggressive approach may be taken.

INJURY TO THE SPINAL CORD

Trauma

Injury to the spinal cord causes various types of pain. Intractable pain will develop in 5% to 25% of patients with spinal cord trauma. The pathophysiology is that of deafferentation and compression of central sensory pathways involving both central tracts and gray matter specifically affecting neurons of the dorsal horn. At least six different types of pain are described in patients with spinal cord injury. Radicular pain is caused by injury of the dorsal roots at their level. Segmental pain is the most common type of pain and occurs at or just above the level of sensory loss. The combination of segmental pain and traumatic syringomyelia occurs with the development of spinal cysts, which cause compression of sensory pathways. Phantom pain occurs commonly in this spinal cord–injured population and is usually much more difficult to treat than in patients who had a limb amputation. Visceral pain also may accompany spinal cord trauma and occurs mostly in referred areas of the lower abdomen.

Treatment

Treatment of pain is primarily neurosurgical, though medications may offer some relief. At this time the operation of choice is the dorsal root entry zone operation. In some cases of traumatic syringomyelia, surgical drainage offers pain relief. Unfortunately, neither dorsal column stimulation nor deep brain stimulation has shown much promise in these patients.

INJURY TO THE BRAIN STEM

Syringobulbia

While there is some controversy regarding the exact pathophysiology of syringobulbia, we know the pain is caused by the expanding cystic structure and the pressure it exerts on the spinal pain pathways.

Treatment of pain is linked to the treatment of the underlying disorder. Neurosurgical drainage is the treatment of choice, though it is often limited by the inability to access the involved area.

INJURY TO THE THALAMUS

Central pain is exemplified by the thalamic pain syndrome originally described by Dejerine and Roussey in 1906. Pain of central origin remains mysterious in terms of the pathophysiologic alterations producing the pain syndrome: Not all patients with similar lesions have pain of central origin. This type of pain can be difficult to define clinically in its more subtle forms. Table 13-5 lists some of the most common clinical symptoms and signs of central pain. In the most clearly documented cases of central pain of various types, Bovie and Leijon showed that some of the symptoms are more common

Table 13-5. Clinical symptoms and signs of central pain

Symptoms

Known lesion of CNS causing sensory deficit

Deficit affects spinothalamic–cortical pathway important in temperature and pain sensibility

Sensory loss may fade

Painful/unpleasant sensory change located in area of sensory deficit

Pain is often delayed, usually seen within 1 year in 50% to 70% of patients

Burning, unpleasant tingling, pins-and-needles, numbness, tearing

Constant

Exacerbated by physical or mental stress and weather

Usually > 1 pain complaint

Signs

Loss of sensation to temperature or pinprick

Preservation of tactile sensation, vibration or kinesthetic

Spatial and temporal summation

Similar to sympathetically maintained pain

in lesions at different levels of the CNS. Thus, burning pain is more common in suprathalamic and brain stem lesions than in thalamic lesions, and lancinating pain is more common in patients with thalamic pain syndrome. Also, the intensity of pain is greater in patients with thalamic lesions compared to brain stem or suprathalamic lesions. Furthermore, thermal sense (warm and cold) was reduced in all patients, thermal sensibility was reduced in most patients, and vibratory sense was reduced in approximately 50% of patients. A majority of patients had hypersensitivity to various stimuli, and 50% of patients experienced radiation or aftersensations of pain. Less than 50% of patients had motor deficits. It is important to note that not all central pain syndromes produce classic findings. For example, in the thalamic pain syndrome there may be pain in only one extremity as opposed to the whole contralateral half of the body to the side of the lesion.

Stroke and Abscess

Patients with the thalamic pain syndrome described by Dejerine and Roussy present with unilateral burning pain, decreased sensation, dysesthesia, and hyperpathia on the side of the body opposite the thalamus involved. Although it is common for the whole contralateral half of the body to be involved, some patients present with partial syndromes. For example, only involvement of the foot may occur, which may be confused with SMP on first assessment. The syndrome is not present in all patients who suffer a stroke in the same thalamic region or in patients at risk for developing a stroke (those over 40 years of age).

Rarely is the pain present at the onset of stroke; rather, it usually occurs within the first year of stroke. It may, however, appear many years later. The pain is usually lifelong and very disabling, and patients are frequently depressed and even suicidal. The pain is of a classic neuropathic type associated with spontaneous, burning, constant, and sometimes intermittent stabbing qualities. This pain may be exacerbated by a number of non-noxious stimuli including heat, cold, touch, or movement. There is usually some motor deficit.

The major findings are sensory related, such as diminished light touch, allodynia, and hyperpathia. Vasomotor and pseudomotor changes make the syndrome akin to SMP in some cases.

Treatment

Thalamic pain syndrome is notoriously resistant to the usual medications. Recently, mexiletine, 200 mg qid up to 1200 mg/day, has been reported to be useful, and we have found this to be true in a few of our own patients. Other medications such as phenothiazine, tricyclic antidepressants, and anxiolytics have been tried with mixed success.

Recently there have been reports of thalamic pain produced by abscesses in the thalamus of patients with AIDS.

INJURY TO THE CORTEX

Seizures

There are rare cases of pain resulting from isolated damage of cortical structures. Also, unusual manifestations of seizures have produced pain in the appropriate somatotrophic areas, as determined by EEG correlation. The treatment of this form of central pain is found in the treatment of the underlying disorder.

INJURY TO THE SYMPATHETIC NERVOUS SYSTEM

Sympathetically Maintained Pain

SMP is defined as **a syndrome of sustained, diffuse, burning pain, allodynia (to touch, cold, or heat), or hyperpathia after traumatic (incomplete) nerve ablation or following minor injury, and often combined with vasomotor and sudomotor disturbances and later trophic changes**. Interruption of all sympathetic pathways early in the disease usually provides pain relief. SMP is perhaps the most severe of clinical pain syndromes. In one study using the McGill Pain Questionnaire, SMP levels were scored at 42 versus 25 for cancer pain and about 23 for postherpetic neuralgia.

Burning pain and continuous hypersensitivity may follow either major or minimal nerve injury, and these conditions have been termed **causalgia** and **reflex sympathetic dystrophy**, respectively. In either case there is increased sympathetic activity. It is essential to define SMP early and provide rigorous therapy. If this is not done the disease progresses and is essentially impossible to treat in the late stages.

Pathophysiology

This constellation of symptoms of SMP comprises what is thought to be a syndrome mediated primarily by the sympathetic nervous system. Descriptions of its common features have stood the test of time, but attempts to understand the primary pathophysiology more clearly have not been successful. Recent work has helped in our understanding of the multidimensional mechanisms of SMP, but without clearly defining its cause. Recently, Bennett and Xie created an animal model that re-creates most of the neuropathic and behavioral changes seen in causalgia in humans. Woolf, Roberts, Devor, and others have contributed to our understanding of the trauma-induced sensitization of spinal cord neurons by excessive afferent fiber activity, the resultant plasticity of afferent neurons, and the eventual sensitization of these neurons to light cutaneous stimuli, giving rise to allodynia. Campbell, Meyer, and Raja have postulated that alpha$_1$ adrenoreceptors become expressed on primary afferent nociceptors such that the release of norepinephrine by the postganglionic sympathetic terminals leads to activation of the nociceptors. Taken together, the evidence supports the concept that a stimulus produces afferent impulses to a primary nociceptor that lead to activation of preganglionic sympathetic neurons in the spinal cord. As a result, postganglionic neurons in the sympathetic ganglia are activated. This may then exert an effect on the primary afferent nociceptor by various means. Subsequently, both central (i.e., CNS neuroplasticity) and peripheral (i.e., ephaptic transmission or up-regulation of adrenoreceptors) mechanisms may sustain painful impulses in the absence of primary nociceptor activation.

Clinical Presentation

The pain is usually present immediately or relatively soon after the injury. Although the injury is sometimes easily defined, such as in direct nerve damage or a fracture, other times it is not easily traceable to a specific event. In most cases, the pain is in a peripheral portion of the arm or leg. Rarely the face and chest may be involved. The pain is constant, burning, and exacerbated by light touch and external stimuli such as temperature changes or even emotional stimuli. Table 13-6 lists clinical signs and symptoms of SMP. Significant findings include disuse atrophy, cool, clammy skin with hyperhidrosis, and sensory and motor loss. The motor findings may be profound, with dystonic limbs present in some cases (Table 13-7). One strange phenomenon of the syndrome is the fact that the same clinical manifestations may spread to a limb or, indeed, other limbs may become involved after the onset of the disease. The cause of this is not understood. This type of pain may persist indefinitely, particularly without treatment, although some cases remit spontaneously.

Table 13-6. Signs and symptoms of sympathetically maintained pain

Clinical
History
    Early onset of pain (within first week)
    Accidental injury, trauma, iatrogenesis
    Persistent pain
    Aggravated by physical and emotional factors
Physical signs
    Distal part of limb
    Usually superficial
    Vasomotor and sudomotor changes
    Trophic changes (usually progressive)
    Muscle weakness or atrophy
    Sensitivity to cold (acetone)
    Severity (stages 1, 2, and 3)

Diagnostic sympathetic block
Local anesthetic block of sympathetic chain
IV Phentolamine
Regional block (bretylium, guanethidine, labetalol)

Table 13-7. Motor signs in sympathetically maintained pain

Focal dystonia
Muscle weakness
Muscle spasms
Tremor
Increased tone and reflexes

Efforts have been made to define progression of the disease into various stages.

Although the diagnosis of SMP is facilitated by clinical evidence, the definitive diagnosis rests on the blockade of the sympathetic nervous system by either "needle" blockade of the system (stellate or lumbar blockade) or the "phentolamine test" (see Chap. 9). Table 13-8 lists the other tests that have been used in the assessment of patients with SMP, although we do not find these particularly useful clinically.

Treatment

Treatment usually involves sympathetic blockade and aggressive physical therapy. The **phentolamine test** (see Chap. 9) has proved to be very useful in diagnosing the disease. We have also found the use of repeated blocks or catheters placed at the sympathetic chain for continuous or intermittent blockade to be very useful.

Recent developments include the application of topical patches such as clonidine, an alpha$_2$-adrenergic agonist. The use of Bier blocks with labetalol or guanethidine has been useful in some patients. Ketorolac has also been useful in

Table 13-8. Diagnostic tests for sympathetically maintained pain

Assessment	Test
Sympathetic function	Sweat test
	Skin plethysmography
	Skin galvanic resistance
Skin blood flow	Xenon 133 clearance
	Skin thermoprobe
	Thermography
Radiologic examination	Plain x rays
	Bone scans
Sympathetic blockade	Sympathetic chain
	Phentolamine block
	Epidural infusion
	Intravenous regional block
Pain	Verbal analog scale
	McGill Pain Questionnaire

Table 13-9. Interventional treatment of sympathetically maintained pain

Sympathetic blockade
  Local anesthetic applied to sympathetic chain
  IV Phentolamine
  IV Regional
    Guanethidine
    Ketanserin (serotonin antagonist)
    Oral medications
Sympathectomy
Spinal cord stimulation
Physical therapy

some patients. The decision to go ahead with sympathectomy is not easy. Some patients do very well after the procedure, but others present with postsympathectomy pain, which may take months to resolve. Tables 13-9 and 13-10 list the interventional and pharmacologic approaches to the treatment of SMP. The earlier patients are seen in the course of their disease the more likely they will benefit from procedural approaches. We have found opioids particularly useful in the early stages of SMP.

Conclusions

The treatment of patients with neuropathic pain is a complex and challenging task. Understanding the pathophysiologic basis for the pain allows us to choose a better therapeutic approach. We still do not have the "ideal analgesic" for neuropathic pain, but great progress has been made in the past several years in understanding the basic mechanisms of neuropathic pain. A few simple rules, however, will facilitate treatment.

1. Develop with your patient an emphasis on **preventive treatment** or at least early aggressive therapy. This may involve something as clear-cut as good foot care of the diabetic patient or the use of psychobiologic treatment such as biofeedback in the highly anxious patient.
2. When using medications, remember that the **dose** of tricyclic antidepressant used to treat pain is usually lower than its dose for depression, and that anticonvulsants used to treat pain are usually used at their anticonvulsant dosages. When using these medications, it is usually advisable to begin with low doses and to proceed with dose escalation until either the therapy is beneficial or a side effect that limits treatment is noted.
3. Remember that **most patients in need of long-term care can indeed be helped**. Even those patients who do not have complete pain relief will have some relief, and in those cases your perseverance will be rewarded.
4. **Opioids** can be very useful in the treatment of neuropathic pain and SMP and should not be withheld from

Table 13-10. Pharmacologic treatment of sympathetically maintained pain

Class	Drug	Dose
Oral sympatholytics	Clonidine	0.1 mg tid
	Prazosin	2 mg bid
	Propranolol	80 mg tid
	Phenoxybenzamine	40–120 mg/day
Transdermal sympathectomy	Clonidine patch	0.1 mg every 3 to 7 days
Opioids	Slow release morphine sulfate	15–60 mg bid
	Immediate release or morphine elixir	5–20 mg q3h
Anticonvulsants	Carbamazepine	200 mg tid or qid
	Phenytoin	100 mg tid
	Clonazepam	3–8 mg/day
	Valproate	250 mg tid
Tricyclic antidepressants	Amitriptyline	10–150 mg/day
	Doxepin	10–150 mg/day
	Nortriptyline	25–200 mg/day

patients (see Chap. 22), particularly if these medications make a substantial difference in the ability of patients to be more active, return to work, etc.

Selected Readings

Clinical Neuropathic Pain

Asbury AK, McKhann GM, and McDonald WI (eds). *Diseases of the Nervous System—Clinical Neurobiology* (2nd ed). Philadelphia: Saunders, 1992. Pp. 858, 884.

Bovie J and Leijon G. Clinical Findings in Patients with Central Post-stroke Pain. In: Casey KL (ed). *Pain and Central Nervous System Disease: The Central Pain Syndromes*. New York: Raven Press, 1991. Pp. 65–75.

Campbell JN, Meyer RA, and Raja SN. Is nociceptor activation by alpha-1 adrenoreceptors the culprit in sympathetically maintained pain? *Am Pain Soc J* 1:3–11, 1992.

Casey KL (ed). *Pain and Central Nervous System Disease: The Central Pain Syndromes*. New York: Raven, 1991.

Dejerine J and Roussey G. Le syndrome thalamique. *Rev Neurol* 14:521–532, 1906.

Dellemijn PL, et al. The interpretation of pain relief and sensory changes following sympathetic blockade. *Brain* 117:1475–1487, 1994.

Fields HL. *Pain*. New York: McGraw-Hill, 1987.

Fields HL (ed). *Pain Syndromes in Neurology*. London: Butterworths, 1990.

Fields HL and Liebeskind JC (eds). Pharmacological Approaches to the Treatment of Chronic Pain: New Concepts and Critical Issues. In: *Progress in Pain Research and Management* (vol 1). Seattle: IASP Press, 1994.

Jensen TS and Rasmussen P. Phantom Pain and Other Phenomena after Amputation. In: PD Wall and R. Melzack (eds). *Pain* (3rd ed). New York: McGraw-Hill, 1994. Pp. 651–665.

Leijon G. Boivie J, and Johansson I. 1989. Central post stroke pain—neurological symptoms and pain characteristics. *Pain* 36:13–25, 1989.

McQuay HJ, et al. Dextromethorphan for the treatment of neuropathic pain: A double-blind randomised controlled crossover trial with integral n-of-1 design. *Pain* 59:127–33, 1994.

Nashold BS Jr., and Ostdahl RH. Dorsal root entry zone lesions for pain relief. *J Neurosurg* 51:59–69, 1979.

Richmond CE, Bromley LM, and Woolf CJ. Preoperative morphine pre-empts postoperative pain. *Lancet* 342:73–75, 1993.

Rowbotham MC, Davies PS, and Fields HL. Topical lidocaine gel relieves postherpetic neuralgia. *Ann Neurol* 37:246–253, 1995.

Treede RD, et al. The plasticity of cutaneous hyperalgesia during sympathetic ganglion blockage in patients with neuropathic pain. *Brain* 115:607–621, 1992.

Wall PD and Melzack R (eds). *Textbook of Pain* (3rd ed). Edinburgh: Churchill, Livingstone, 1994.

Basic Science Neuropathic Pain

Bennett GJ. An animal model of neuropathic pain: A review. *Muscle Nerve* 16:1040–1048, 1993.

Bennett GJ. Hypotheses on the pathogenesis of herpes zoster-associated pain. *Ann Neurol* 35:S38–41, 1994.

Bennett GJ and Xie YK. A peripheral mononeuropathy in rat that produces disorders of pain sensation like those seen in man. *Pain* 33:87–107, 1988.

Carlton SM, et al. Behavioral manifestations of an experimental model for peripheral neuropathy produced by spinal nerve ligation in the primate. *Pain* 56:155–166, 1994.

Gracely RH, Lynch SA, and Bennett GJ. Painful neuropathy: Altered central processing maintained dynamically by peripheral input. *Pain* 51:175–194, 1992.

Kajander KC and Bennett GJ. Onset of a painful peripheral neuropathy in rat: A partial and differential deafferentation and spontaneous discharge in A beta and A delta primary afferent neurons. *Neurophysiol* 68:734–744, 1992.

Koltzenburg M, Torebjork HE, and Wahren LK. Nociceptor modulated central sensitization causes mechanical hyperalgesia in acute chemogenic and chronic neuropathic pain. *Brain* 117: 579–591, 1994.

Luo L, Puke MJ, and Wiesenfeld-Hallin Z. The effects of intrathecal morphine and clonidine on the prevention and reversal of spinal cord hyperexcitability following sciatic nerve section in the rat. *Pain* 58:245–252, 1994.

Mao J, Mayer DJ, and Price DD. Patterns of increased brain activity indicative of pain in a rat model of peripheral mononeuropathy. *J Neurosci* 13:2689–2702, 1993.

Ochoa JL. Pain mechanisms in neuropathy. *Curr Opin Neurol* 7: 407–414, 1994.

Tal M and Bennett GJ. Dextrorphan relieves neuropathic heat-evoked hyperalgesia in the rat. *Neurosci Lett* 151:107–110, 1993.

Woolf CJ and Doubell TP. The pathophysiology of chronic pain—increased sensitivity to low threshold A beta-fiber inputs. *Curr Opin Neurobiol* 4:525–534, 1994.

Woolf CJ, Shortland P, and Coggeshall RE. Peripheral nerve injury triggers central sprouting of myelinated afferents. *Nature* 355:75–78, 1992.

Woolf CJ and Thompson SW. The induction and maintenance of central sensitization is dependent on N-methyl-D-aspartic acid receptor activation: Implications for the treatment of post-injury pain hypersensitivity states. *Pain* 44:293–299, 1991.

Woolf CJ and Walters ET. Common patterns of plasticity contributing to nociceptive sensitization in mammals and Aplysia. *Trends Neurosci* 14:74–78, 1991.

Postoperative Pain

Jane C. Ballantyne and David Borsook

> *"For all the happiness man can gain
> Is not in pleasure, but in rest from
> pain."*
>
> JOHN DRYDEN

Few Americans will go through life without having surgery, and those who undergo surgery will experience varying degrees of postoperative pain. In many cases this pain will be the worst of their lives. Postoperative pain is probably the most prevalent of all pain conditions, yet it tends to be inadequately treated. Physicians, nurses, and patients alike fear opioid drugs, although these remain the mainstay of acute pain treatment. Furthermore, because of the acute and finite nature of pain, there is a degree of complacency in treating it. Patients who have received exemplary pain management rate their surgical and hospital experience highly, and it may be important to optimize postoperative pain treatment for that reason alone. But there is also increasing evidence that the sequelae of undertreated pain are far reaching and often deleterious, which provides a greater impetus to improve pain treatment in postoperative patients. This chapter outlines the principles of postoperative pain management and briefly describes the treatments in everyday use at Massachusetts General Hospital (MGH).

Rationale for Active Treatment of Postoperative Pain

CONVENTIONAL VERSUS ACTIVE TREATMENT

Conventionally, pain has been treated by intramuscular opioids given intermittently, as needed. "Active" pain management implies a greater effort toward the goal of pain relief and entails preoperative preparation, patient choice of treatment, regular pain assessments, and the use of newer treatments such as epidural anesthesia, continuous nerve blocks, and patient-controlled analgesia (PCA). It will become clear later in this chapter that active pain management offers better pain relief than conventional treatment. Here we explore other reasons to support the use of active pain management.

ETHICAL AND HUMANITARIAN ISSUES

No one would argue against the ethical and humanitarian need to treat postoperative pain. But can the ethical and humanitarian argument be used to support active pain management? Do conventional methods satisfy the ethical need to treat pain, or should we improve on conventional methods? Perhaps the answer to these questions lies with individual physicians, who weigh the risks and benefits of each treatment, and, rightly or wrongly, use personal experience as well as scientific evidence to decide whether to use a treatment. But in weighing the risks and benefits, physicians should also assume the ethical responsibility of relieving pain and suffering. When treating pain, ethical and humanitarian issues are particularly important, since relief of suffering is the chief, and only undisputed, benefit of pain treatment.

PATIENT COMFORT AND SATISFACTION

Nothing satisfies operative patients more than having sailed through surgery with a minimum of pain and discomfort. Producing such a state of satisfaction is not, however, simply a matter of providing adequate doses of pain medication. Patients will be most satisfied if their therapy is properly tailored to their needs, with side effects titrated against efficacy. They are also more likely to be satisfied if they have been adequately prepared for the experience of postoperative pain; if they understand that they will need to tolerate a certain degree of pain at times, but that over the days the pain will abate; if they have been offered choices of methods of achieving pain relief; and if they know that their doctors and nurses are working with them to achieve the greatest possible relief.

DECREASED MORBIDITY AND RECOVERY TIME

Although some trials have demonstrated reduced recovery times and shorter lengths of hospital stay associated with the use of the more aggressive pain treatments (such as epidural therapy and PCA), other trials have not shown significant improvement. In addition, there is no true consensus on whether aggressive pain treatment can speed recovery after surgery. In a comprehensive meta-analysis of PCA trials, a 0.15-day reduction in hospital stay was found in patients treated with PCA compared to those treated with conventional therapy (intramuscular opioid, given on demand). The standard error (SEM) of this difference is .13 (p = .24), a nonsignificant finding. More specifically, morbidity has been studied in relation to various pain treatments, again with mixed findings. Pulmonary function is undoubtedly improved by epidural pain therapy. The incidence of deep venous thrombosis (DVT) is lower when epidural anesthesia is used, and the continuance of epidural therapy into the postoperative period also lowers the incidence of DVT. Whether mobility may be hastened by aggressive pain tratment or, conversely, ileus, confusion, and drowsiness may be worsened remains unclear. These are clinical impressions that have not yet been confirmed by controlled trials.

Turning now to the possible harmful sequelae of undertreated pain, there is increasing evidence that these sequelae are far reaching and may be deleterious. The fact that pain treatment can alter physiologic stress responses to surgery and trauma is well established. Whether these changes are desirable is less clear. However, evidence is now emerging that pain treatment can modulate immune responsiveness, thus lessening immune suppression (presumably a desirable effect). At the level of the spinal cord, genetic alterations in neurons in response to unmodulated sensory stimuli are being observed, which may account for long-term problems such as trauma-related chronic pain syndromes and phantom limb pain. Of particular interest was one study's finding that preoperative lumbar epidural blockade before lower limb amputation can lessen phantom limb pain.

Principles of Postoperative Pain Management

PSYCHOLOGIC PREPARATION

Patients who are well prepared psychologically for the experience of surgery and postoperative pain are markedly less anxious and easier to treat during the perioperative period than unprepared patients. Patients need reassurance from their surgeon, their anesthesiologist, and their nurses. If they have never had surgery before, they should be told about the process and about postoperative pain. They should be aware that some degree of postoperative pain is inevitable, and that their doctors and nurses will work with them to treat it. They should be familiar with the concept of pain assessment and the need to assess pain in order to modify treatments. They should also be told about the choices for postoperative pain management, and should discuss these options with their surgeon and anesthesiologist.

PREEMPTIVE TREATMENT

It is well known that established pain is more difficult to treat than new pain. People with recurring pain, such as headaches, know that if they treat their pain early, it is easier to abolish than if they allow it to mount. The same is true of postoperative pain. Patients who wake from anesthesia in pain appear to be more resistant to pain medication than those who are comfortable on awakening. A few, recently published trials have found that preemptive pain treatment reduces postoperative analgesic requirements. In another trial, a significant reduction in phantom limb pain was discovered after preoperative epidural blockade. The anesthesiologist has an important role in treating pain before and during surgery, and in using regional and local nerve blocks where appropriate.

ASSESSING PAIN

It is important to make the effort to assess pain and side effects regularly, for this is the only means of tailoring treatments to patients' real needs. The method chosen for assessments does not have to be elaborate; in fact, it is inappropriate to use complicated analog scales in the setting of postoperative pain. Simple questions such as "How bad is your pain?", "Do you have any nausea?", and "Do you feel like getting out of bed?" will often suffice. However, it is also necessary to have some means of quantifying pain that tells the patient's story, since doctors and nurses change shifts and are not always able to communicate with each other. For this reason, rudimentary pain scales are often used, and it is helpful if the scores are recorded in the patient's chart or on the vital signs record. A policy of regular assessment is also important, because it draws attention to the existence of pain and forces improved treatment.

Methods of Assessing Pain

CHOOSING A METHOD

Whatever method is chosen should be systematic and simple. Charting of pain levels is not essential, but it does help to ensure that systematic assessments are made and, at the same time, fosters communication. The regular assessment of pain is fundamental to good pain management, but it is essential to act on pain assessments, not simply to make them. Assessments of pain level and analgesic side effects are the tool by which analgesic regimens can be tailored to patients' needs.

VERBAL REPORTS

Verbal reports of pain are useful not only as an adjunct to the use of pain scales but also as the sole indicator of pain in many cases. In small institutions, where the individual patient is likely to be cared for by only a small group of people and where the need for communication is less of an issue, verbal reporting alone may be adequate. In some patients, verbal reports of pain are more meaningful than pain scores—the choice is a matter of clinical discretion.

VERBAL SCALES

At MGH, we use a numeric verbal scale for pain assessment in postoperative patients. We have chosen a 0 to 10 scale—0 being no pain and 10 being the worst pain imaginable. Any number of verbal scales can be devised. Many clinicians use a 0 to 100 scale. Others use a scale of words; for example, ranging from none, to mild and moderate, to severe. It is unimportant which scale is chosen, as long as it is standardized. MGH nurses and physicians record pain levels on the patient's vital signs record, as well as in the patient's charts.

VISUAL SCALES

Visual scales are the standard in some centers, and are particularly useful in children and in adults who are unable to comprehend a verbal scale. A visual scale can be extremely simple, such as a drawn scale with numbers or a printout of descriptive adjectives describing pain. In children, special scales that might be fun, or at least comprehensible to the child, are used. Examples are the "Oucher" scale, a series of unhappy and happy faces; the "Poker Chip Tool," using four red poker chips; and the "Thermometer," a giant cardboard thermometer.

OBJECTIVE MEASURES

Occasionally, objective parameters are the only available measure of pain. This is true for babies, the infirm elderly, the severely handicapped, and very sick patients, especially ventilated patients. It is easy to forget the issue of pain in these patients; yet, they suffer pain that is at least equal to that of conversant patients. Unfortunately, many objective measures are notoriously unreliable indicators of pain. There is no laboratory test that can measure pain, and efforts to find one have proved futile. Increases in heart rate, blood pressure, respiratory rate, and sweating may be indicators of pain, but are not specific and could indicate hypoxia, hypercarbia, pyrexia, or a full bladder just as readily. The most specific objective indicator of pain is patient posturing— grimacing, wincing, frowning, labored breathing, flexor posturing, rigidity, immobility, etc. All objective measures of pain may be difficult to interpret, and their interpretation requires experience and sound clinical judgment.

Methods for Achieving Pain Control

Table 14-1 summarizes pain control methods.

NONSTEROIDAL ANTI-INFLAMMATORY DRUGS

Some of the commonly used NSAIDs are listed in Table 14-2. NSAIDs act by a different mechanism than opioids, and for that reason are a useful alternative or adjunct to opioid therapy. Their action is mainly peripheral (not in the CNS) and their analgesic effect is secondary to their anti-inflammatory effect, which in turn is due to prostaglandin inhibition. Prostaglandin inhibition is also responsible for their chief side effects—namely, platelet dysfunction and gastritis. NSAIDs are useful as the sole treatment for mild to moderate postoperative pain. They also have an opioid-sparing effect when used in combination with opioids. Their use in postoperative patients may be limited by the fact that they are not injectable, so in patients who can take nothing by mouth, it is necessary to use suppositories. The exception is ketorolac, which is a relatively new, injectable, and extremely potent NSAID (equipotent with morphine). It has become a popular alternative to opioid therapy. There are drawbacks to its use, however. It is expensive (about 20 times more costly than morphine) and, because of its potency, applying equally to side effects and efficacy, it can only be safely used for 1 or 2 days (manufacturers' recommendation). NSAIDs are contraindi-

Table 14-1. Methods for achieving pain control

Intervention	Comments
NSAIDs	
Oral (alone)	Effective for mild to moderate pain. Begin preoperatively. Relatively contraindicated in patients with renal disease and risk of, or actual, coagulopathy. May mask fever.
Oral (adjunct to opioid)	Potentiating effect resulting in opioid sparing. Cautions as above.
Parenteral (ketorolac)	Effective for moderate to severe pain. Expensive. Useful where opioids are contraindicated, especially to avoid respiratory depression and sedation. Cautions as above.
Opioids	
Oral	As effective as parenteral in appropriate doses. Use as soon as oral medication tolerated.
IM	Has been the standard parenteral route, but injections painful and absorption unreliable. Hence, avoid this route when possible.
SQ	Preferable to IM for low-volume continuous infusion. Injections painful and absorption unreliable. Avoid this route for long-term repetitive dosing.
IV	Parenteral route of choice after major surgery. Suitable for titrated bolus or continuous administration (including PCA), but requires monitoring. Significant risk of respiratory depression with inappropriate dosing.
PCA	IV or SQ routes recommended. Good, steady level of analgesia. Popular with patients but requires special infusion pumps and staff education. Cautions as for IV opioids (above).
Epidural and intrathecal	When suitable, provides good analgesia. Expensive if infusion pumps are employed. Significant risk of respiratory depression, sometimes delayed in onset. Requires careful monitoring.
Local anesthetics	
Epidural and intrathecal	Limited indications. Expensive if infusion pumps are employed. Effective regional analgesia. Opioid sparing. Addition of opioid to local anesthetic may improve analgesia. Risks of hypotension, weakness, numbness.
Peripheral block	Limited indications. Limited duration unless catheters are employed. Effective regional analgesia. Opioid sparing.
TENS	Effective in reducing pain and improving physical function. Requires skilled personnel and special equipment. Useful as an adjunct to drug therapy.
Education/instruction	Effective for reduction of pain. Should include procedural information and instruction aimed at reducing activity-related pain. Requires staff time.

NSAIDs = nonsteroidal anti-inflammatory drugs; TENS = transcutaneous electrical nerve stimulation; IM = intramuscular; SQ = subcutaneous; IV = intravenous; PCA = patient-controlled analgesia.

cated in patients with bleeding disorders, patients who are therapeutically anticoagulated, patients with a history of peptic ulcer disease or gastritis, and patients with renal dysfunction. At the MGH, NSAIDs are used for the following indications:

1. Mild to moderate postoperative pain, as sole therapy
2. In combination with opioids for moderate postoperative pain, particularly when weaning from stronger medication; proprietary compounds (e.g., oxycodone/acetaminophen compound [Percocet], codeine/acetaminophen compound [Tylenol #3]) commonly used
3. Particularly in the pediatric population under 6 months of age; careful titration of opioids is essential
4. Ketorolac is reserved for cases where opioids are contraindicated (e.g., respiratory depression) or when other treatments have failed

SYSTEMIC OPIOIDS

Systemic opioid treatment has long been the conventional postoperative pain treatment and is the standard by which other treatments are measured. This does not, in any way, make it inferior to other pain treatments. In fact, as long as the principles of postoperative pain management (above) are adhered to, this form of treatment provides satisfactory pain control and, in many cases, is the treatment of choice. It remains the mainstay of postoperative pain treatments for moderate to severe pain.

Routes of administration and their indications are summarized in Table 14-1. Conventionally, the intramuscular route was chosen for use in postoperative patients, because the intravenous route was believed to be unsafe (because of the risk of respiratory depression), the subcutaneous route less reliable than the intramuscular, and the per rectum route undesirable. The oral route is, of course, unusable in nil per os patients, and the sublingual route is limited by lack of availability of sublingual preparations. It is unnecessary to subject patients to painful intramuscular injections, and judiciously administered intravenous opioids (i.e., given as small boluses while monitoring pain level, respiratory effort, and alertness) are just as safe and preferable. The intravenous route is also ideal for PCA, which is discussed below. Most postoperative patients receive bolus administrations of opioids, although continuous intravenous or subcutaneous therapy may sometimes be useful—for example, in ventilated patients in whom there is no danger of respiratory depression.

Commonly used opioids and their doses are summarized in Table 14-2. Morphine is the first choice of opioid at MGH. We usually prescribe a dose range so that nurses can select a dose according to the patient's need. Morphine is a naturally occurring opioid and is the oldest, best tried, and cheapest of all the opioid drugs. It is a simple agonist at mu, kappa, and delta receptors, and its actions are not complicated by partial agonism or mixed agonism/antagonism. Its effects and side

Table 14-2. Analgesics and related drugs: Dosages for adults

Generic name	Proprietary name	Oral dose (mg)	Parenteral dose (mg)
Nonsteroidal anti-inflammatory drugs			
Aspirin[a]	—	650 q6h	—
Trisalicylate	Trilisate	500–1500 bid	—
Ibuprofen[a]	Motrin, Advil	200–800 q6h	—
Naproxen	Naprosyn	250–500 q12h	—
Ketorolac	Toradol	—	30 (load) + 15–30 q6h
Acetaminophen[a,b]	Tylenol	500–1000 q3–4h	—
Opioids			
Propoxyphene	Darvon	65 q3–4h	—
Codeine	—	15–60 q4–6h	30–60 q4–6h
Butorphanol	Stadol	—	2–4 q3–4h
Buprenorphine	Buprenex	—	0.3–0.6 q6–8h
Oxycodone	In Tylox, Percocet, Percodan; also available as elixir	5–10 q4–6h	—
Morphine[a]	—	10–20 q2–3h	5–10 q3–4h
Slow release	MS-Contin, Roxanol	10–30 q12h	—
Meperidine	Demerol	50–150 q3–4h	100–150 q2–3h
Hydromorphone	Dilaudid	2–4 q4–6h	2–4 q4–6h
Methadone	Dolophine	2.5–10.0 q6–8h	2.5–10.0 q6–8h
Naloxone	—		0.2–1.2 bolus

Antiemetics, major tranquilizers			
Metoclopramide	Reglan	10 tid	10 q6h
Prochlorperazine	Compazine	5–10 tid	5–10 q4–6h
Droperidol	Inapsine	5–15 q8H	1.25–5.0 q6h
Antihistamines, anxiolytics			
Diphenhydramine	Benadryl	25 q4h	—
Hydroxyzine	Vistaril	50–100 qid	25–100 qid
Laxatives			
Senna	Senokot	1–2 tablets tid	—
Docusate	Colace	100 tid	—

[a] Also available as a suppository.
[b] Acetaminophen is not an anti-inflammatory, but is efficacious in acute pain.
Dosages and intervals are initial estimates for an average 70-kg adult and may need to be adjusted according to the individual patient's weight, preference, or tolerance.
This list is not comprehensive. Other classes of drugs not listed here may be beneficial in postoperative pain for individual cases.

effects are well known and understood. Morphine may be contraindicated in patients with biliary spasm because it is believed that it can worsen the spasm, but this issue is still debated. Opioid drugs other than morphine may be indicated in some other incidences, such as in the patient who expresses a preference for another drug, in the patient who is allergic to morphine, or in the patient in whom morphine proves ineffective. Meperidine has been widely used in the United States as the opioid of first choice for acute pain. We discourage the use of this drug as a first-line treatment because of its known toxicity (excitatory effects in the CNS due to the metabolite normeperidine), which may be especially marked in patients with compromised renal function. Meperidine has traditionally been used in woefully deficient doses. A 50-mg bolus is inadequate for severe pain in most adults, and 100–150 mg should be considered as the standard adult dose. Bolus administration should be given every 3, not 4, hours to avoid re-emergence of pain, since meperidine is a relatively short-acting drug.

The side effects of opioid drugs occasionally limit their use. Respiratory depression is a true risk of opioid treatment, and patients receiving opioids should always be monitored for adequacy of ventilation. Monitoring for adequacy of ventilation comprises observing the patient's respiratory rate, depth and pattern of breathing, skin color and mucous membranes, and state of arousal. Monitors such as the pulse oximeter are useful in the immediate postoperative period, and in patients at risk (e.g., neonates and patients with baseline ventilatory compromise), but are not necesssary or even useful later in the postoperative course in most patients. Ventilation monitors are useful in neonates, especially premature neonates, and in patients with known sleep apnea. Severe respiratory depression should be treated with naloxone (IV boluses of 0.1 mg in adults, until the desired effect is reached).

Development of addiction is the other undesirable effect of opioids that has a major impact on the use of opioid treatment. Addiction is extremely rare in patients, however. Nevertheless, fear of addiction is widespread among physicians, nurses, and patients and often results in inappropriate avoidance of opioid treatment. We can only try to reassure our colleagues and patients and inform them of the negligible risk of developing addiction in the acute pain setting.

Other side effects are usually more of a nuisance than a barrier to treatment and can most often be treated—nausea with antiemetics, pruritus with antihistamines, constipation with laxatives (see Table 14-2). Occasionally it is necessary to lower the dose of opioid, especially if oversedation is a problem, or even to withdraw treatment (supplement it with an NSAID). Ketorolac is a useful alternative when opioids need to be withdrawn.

EPIDURALS

For certain well-chosen indications, a functioning epidural produces superior pain relief. The problem with epidurals is that technical expertise is needed to place the epidural catheters and, even in the best hands, they do not always work. Thus, a promise of superb pain relief is not always fulfilled. Nevertheless, if an epidural is indicated, we always recommend it to our patients, with a warning that it may fail. At MGH, we recommend epidurals for postoperative pain therapy primarily as follows (discussion of when to use epidurals intraoperatively is beyond the scope of this chapter).

1. Patients having thoracic or upper abdominal surgery
2. Patients having thoracic, upper, or lower abdominal surgery and who have significant pulmonary or ventilatory disease
3. Patients having lower limb surgery, in whom early mobilization is important (early active or passive mobilization)
4. Patients having lower body vascular procedures, in whom a sympathetic block is desirable

The use of epidurals postoperatively in patients having thoracic and upper abdominal surgery, in particular, has transformed a period of severe discomfort and uncontrollable pain, with slow recovery due to breathing difficulties, to one of relative comfort (some patients with epidurals are actually pain free) and improved pulmonary function.

Postoperative epidural pain therapy should always be in the charge of the anesthesiologist or the anesthesia department. The anesthetist should administer or prescribe all medications given through the epidural and should visit the patient at least once a day to check the catheter for slippage or kinking and the catheter site for inflammation or tenderness. Anesthesia personnel should also monitor the effectiveness of the epidural treatment and make changes, if necessary. At the end of treatment, anesthesia personnel should be responsible for pulling the catheter and ensuring that it is removed intact.

The role of the nursing staff is also important in caring for patients with epidural catheters, and nurses should be appropriately trained before they are expected to look after these patients. They need to know the appropriate medications for epidural administration, the normal appearance of the catheter and catheter site, how pumps operate, and which side effects can be treated by them and which should prompt a call to the physician in charge.

The standard infusion for postoperative epidural therapy at MGH is a mixture of 0.1% bupivacaine with 10 μg/ml of fentanyl. The 0.1% bupivacaine is merely a carrier for fentanyl and has little effect on its own (except in the frail, including the neonate), although it does have a synergistic effect with fentanyl. Fentanyl is chosen because of its relatively short duration of action and its lipophilicity, which contributes to its tendency to bind locally to spinal cord receptors, rather than float cephalically toward the vital centers in the brain. (A high incidence of delayed respiratory depression is associated with the use of epidural morphine, due to its hydrophilicity and its tendency to reach the medullary respiratory center.) In infants under 1 year of age we do not use fentanyl, since this age group is particularly sensitive to the respiratory depressant effects of opioids. In children aged 1 to 7 years we use a lower fentanyl dose (3 μg/ml). Recommended adult and pediatric doses are presented in Table 14-3. We use a standard form for epidural orders (Fig. 14-1), which includes orders for alternative treatment should the epidural fail and orders for the treatment of side effects.

The most troublesome side effect of epidural fentanyl is probably pruritus, which usually responds either to lowering of the infusion rate or to an antihistamine (see Table 14-2). Sedation may also be a problem, especially in the elderly, and will only respond to lowering of the infusion rate or discontinuance of epidural fentanyl. Nausea rarely occurs with epidural fentanyl. Epidural therapy may affect gut mobility and delay recovery from ileus, and some surgeons prefer not to use epidurals postoperatively for that reason.

PATIENT-CONTROLLED ANALGESIA

PCA is simply a form of opioid therapy (usually systemic), but instead of relying on nurses for each bolus of pain medication, the patient can dose him- or herself. An additional advantage that stems from the ease with which the patient gets each dose of medication is that it becomes feasible to administer frequent small doses, rather than large doses every 3 to 4 hours, so that dosing more closely matches the needs of the patient (Fig. 14-2). The PCA device consists of a microprocessor-controlled pump that allows programming of dose, dose intervals, maximum dose per set time, and background infusion rate. The pumps became popular after the advent of the microprocessor, which allowed the pump to be reduced to a reasonable size. Patients tend to like PCA because of the control they gain over their own treatment. Moreover, because it avoids delay in administration of pain medication by busy nurses, as well as inappropriate dosing (because of variations in narcotic need and unpredictable absorption from depot injections), PCA may offer better pain control than traditional methods.

The successful use of PCA depends first and foremost on the appropriate selection of patients. Patients who are too old, too confused, too young, unable to control the button, or who do not want the treatment are not suitable candidates. Patients who have mild to moderate pain, or in whom the duration of pain is expected to be short, are also unsuitable for PCA. Success also depends on the cooperation of patients. Ideally, patients should be educated about PCA before undergoing surgery, because many of them will otherwise be incapable of using the method properly in the early postoperative period. In the first few hours after surgery, it may be necessary to supplement the PCA with carefully monitored, nurse-controlled boluses. It is tempting to think that once patients are hooked up to PCA pumps, they do not need pain treatment. But if the pain is neglected in the early postoperative period, it may be more difficult to treat later.

Table 14-3. Suitable regimens for epidural infusions in adults and children

Solutions

<1 yr—0.1% bupivacaine *without* fentanyl

1–7 yr—0.1% bupivacaine with 3 μg/ml fentanyl

>7 yr or adult—0.1% bupivacaine with 10 μg/ml fentanyl

Special indications—fentanyl without bupivacaine

Rate of infusion

Adults

Starting rate—2–7 ml/hr

For increasing pain—increase in increments up to 9.9 ml/hr

For decreasing pain or for side effects—decrease in increments down to 0.5 ml/hr

Children

Starting rate—0.1 ml/kg per hour of appropriate solution (see above)

For increasing pain—Increase in increments up to 0.3 ml/kg per hour

For bolusing catheter—≤6 kg 1 cc of 1% lidocaine with 1:200,000 epinephrine

      6–15 kg 2 cc of 1% lidocaine with 1:200,000 epinephrine

      >15 kg 5 cc of 1% lidocaine with 1:200,000 epinephrine

Pediatric mixtures of bupivacaine/fentanyl may be indicated for adult patients in special circumstances.

CONTINUOUS EPIDURAL ANALGESIA

DATE

1. Prepare epidural mixture:
   (bupivacaine 0.1%, fentanyl 10 µg/ml)
   Infuse via:
   catheter at _____ ml/hr

2. Heparin lock with flush if no IV

3. Tylenol 1–2 PO q4h prn, for pain;
   _____ mg IM q4h prn, for nausea;
   Benadryl 25 mg PO q4h prn, for itching

4. NO PARENTERAL OR PO NARCOTICS
   OR SEDATIVES UNLESS ORDERED
   BY THE PAIN SERVICE

5. For side effects (nausea, vomiting, itching/
   pruritus, urinary retention):
   a) reduce infusion rate to _____ ml/hr
   b) if problems persist, notify Pain Service

6. For decreasing pain:
   titrate dose down as low as _____ ml/hr

7. For increasing pain:
   a) increase infusion rate to _____ ml/hr
   b) if pain persists after 1 hour, call Pain
   Service

8. If epidural infusion (catheter or pump) is
   not functioning or is ineffective, stop infusion
   and give:
   _____ mg _____ prn
   or if patient-controlled analgesia (PCA)
   would be preferable, call Pain Service and
   confirm the following PCA orders:
   a) PCA demand dose
   b) delay (lock out)
   c) basal setting
   d) hourly limit

   _____ , MD

MONITORING

1. Record RR q2h, HR and BP q4h

2. Record pain and sedation levels, verbal and
   motor response q4h while awake. (Refer to
   EPIDURAL ANALGESIA SCORING
   GUIDE on reverse side of this form.)

3. With initiation or an increase in rate:
   a) record RR every hour for 4 hours, then
   q2h.
   b) record pain and sedation levels every
   hour for 4 hours (while awake), then
   q4h as in No. 2

4. If bolus dose is given, record RR, HR and
   BP, pain and sedation levels, verbal and
   motor response 15 minutes after dose, then
   as in No. 3

5. If RR < 10, evaluate state of consciousness
   and contact the Pain Service.

6. If HR < _____ or systolic blood pressure
   (SBP) < _____ contact the Pain Service.

7. Notify the Pain Service if the catheter is no
   longer in use.

8. IN AN EMERGENCY, IF UNABLE TO
   CONTACT PAIN SERVICE, CALL:

   _____

   Insert the names and telephone numbers of
   the staff:

   _____

   _____

   _____

   _____

   _____

Fig. 14-1. The Massachusetts General Hospital Pain Center's continuous epidural analgesia guidelines.

At MGH, we use the intravenous route exclusively for PCA in postoperative patients. The form we use for PCA orders is shown in Figure 14-3, and includes orders for alternative treatment should the intravenous route fail, plus orders for the treatment of common side effects. In Tables 14-4 and 14-5, recommended PCA regimens for both adults and children are displayed. Morphine is the drug of choice for PCA; hydromorphone and meperidine are reserved for patients in whom morphone has failed or is contraindicated (see p. 252).

The side effects of and precautions for PCA opioids are the same as those of any systematically administered opioid (see p. 252). In general, PCA is extremely safe because patients who are oversedated will not be able to press the PCA button, and therefore will not receive the additional dose that may push them into obtundation. This safety feature will be bypassed if anyone other than the patient attempts to control the PCA, and that practice should be discouraged. The exception to the general safety of PCA is its use by elderly and confused indi-

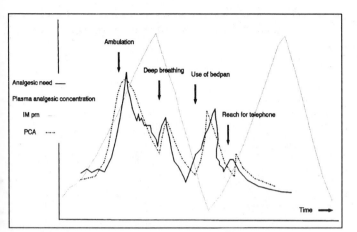

Fig. 14-2. Theoretical comparison between postoperative analgesic need and plasma analgesic concentration attained during a conventional analgesic regimen (IM prn) or patient-controlled analgesia (PCA).

viduals, who, despite confusion and early obtundation (or maybe because of it), will sometimes overdose themselves.

INTRAOPERATIVE NEURAL BLOCKADE

Nerve blocks performed before or during surgery provide excellent pain control during the early postoperative period if they last through the operative period. Infiltration of wounds with local anesthetic by surgeons can also contribute significantly to the control of early postoperative pain. Intraoperative neural blockade can reduce postoperative analgesic requirements and, in some cases, negate the need for postoperative analgesia. Intraoperative nerve blocks are particularly useful in children, who tolerate analgesics poorly and in whom pain is particularly distressing.

PROLONGED NEURAL BLOCKADE—
USE OF CATHETERS

Occasionally, prolongation of neural blockade is indicated. Neural blockade can only be prolonged beyond the life of the chosen local anesthetic by using continuous infusions of local anesthetic via catheters. (Neural cryotherapy and direct severance of nerves used to be done to produce prolonged nerve blockade, but these practices are now condemned because they are known to result in an unacceptably high incidence of chronic pain.) Continuous infusion of local anesthetic into the pleural space via an intrapleural catheter is effective for thoracotomy and upper abdominal incisional pain, but has yet to prove its worth in comparison to thoracic epidural therapy. Brachial plexus catheter therapy can be useful after hand surgery when physical therapy is needed.

PATIENT-CONTROLLED ANALGESIA

DATE

1. DISCONTINUE PREVIOUS PAIN MEDICATIONS

2. NO SYSTEMIC NARCOTICS TO BE GIVEN EXCEPT BY ORDER OF PAIN SERVICE

3. DRUG: _____ mg/ml

4. PCA pump settings:
   PCA dose from _____ to _____ ml
   begin with _____ ml
   delay time _____ minutes
   basal rate _____ ml/hr
   night basal _____ ml/hr, 11 PM–7 AM, prn
   hour limit range _____ ml/hr

5. Loading dose:
   _____ ml every 5 minutes until patient is comfortable. Maximum total loading dose: _____ ml

   Loading dose can be repeated 2qh during the first 12 hours after surgery, if indicated.

6. Infuse D_5W to keep vein open (KVO) via Y-set if no maintenance IV solution is ordered.

7. In the event of pump failure or nonpatent IV, give _____ mg IM, every _____ hr, prn, for pain

8. For obtundation or respiratory rate < __/min:
   a) give Narcan _____ mg (_____ ml of _____ mg/ml solution)
   b) reduce infusion rate to _____ ml/hr
   c) give 100% oxygen by mask

MONITORING

1. Record baseline HR, BP, RR.

2. Record HR, BP, RR 15 minutes after starting pump or giving loading dose.

3. Record RR, analgesia, and sedation levels every 4 hours (refer to Scoring Guide on reverse side of this form). If vital signs, mental status, or sedation problems appear, record RR and BP every hour until stable.

4. Discontinue PCA and call Pain Service if:
   a) HR < _____
   b) BP < _____
   c) RR < _____
   d) There is excessive sedation

5. Refrain from pushing the button for the patient, other than to demonstrate its use.

6. IN AN EMERGENCY, IF UNABLE TO CONTACT PAIN SERVICE, CALL:

   _____

   Insert the names and telephone numbers of the staff:

   _____
   _____
   _____
   _____
   _____

_____, MD

Fig. 14-3. The Massachusetts General Hospital Pain Center's patient-controlled analgesia guidelines.

TRANSCUTANEOUS ELECTRICAL NERVE STIMULATION

TENS is useful for postoperative pain in selected patients. The device consists of a series of electrodes that are placed on the site of the pain (either side of the surgical incision in the case of postoperative pain) and through which a low-voltage electrical stimulus is passed. The treatment is theoretically based on the gate-control theory of pain of Melzack and Wall. Randomized, controlled trials have confirmed its efficacy in postoperative pain compared with controls (no TENS), but have not shown it to be better than sham TENS (electrodes with no current); likewise, sham TENS is also better than no TENS. It is likely, therefore, to have a predominate placebo effect. It does not stand up against drug therapies as a sole treatment for anything other than mild postoperative pain, but it may be useful in reducing analgesic requirements and possibly improving pulmonary function in selected patients. At MGH we do not offer TENS routinely for postop-

Table 14-4. Adult patient-controlled analgesia

Requirements	Drug		
	Morphine	Dilaudid	Meperidine
mg/ml	1	0.5	10
Demand dose (ml)	1	0.5	1
Range (ml)	0.5–2.0	0.5–2.0	0.5–2.0
Lockout interval	6 min	10 min	6 min
Basal rate (ml/hr)			
Day	0	0	0
Night	0.5	0.5	0.5
Hourly limit (ml)	<12	<6	<10
Loading dose (mg) (every 5 min until comfortable)	2 mg	0.5 mg	2.0 mg
Maximum loading dose (mg)	10–15 mg	2–4 mg	75–150 mg

These suggested dosages are based on those required by a healthy, 55–70-kg, opioid-naive adult; adjustments must be made according to the condition of the patient, his or her prior opioid use, and the recent (preoperative) use of opioids.

erative pain, but a few patients do request it, and they can obtain it through our physical therapy department.

BEHAVIORAL THERAPY

The goal of behavioral therapy is to provide patients with a sense of control over their pain. All patients are benefited by being well prepared psychologically for the experience of surgery and postoperative pain (see Psychologic Preparation above). Simple relaxation strategies and imagery techniques can help those patients who find such interventions appealing. Relaxation strategies and imagery techniques do not need to be complex in order to be effective. Simple strategies, such as brief jaw relaxation, music-assisted relaxation, and recall of peaceful images, have been found to be effective in reducing anxiety and analgesic requirement. They take only a few minutes to teach, although they may require reinforcement at times. Patients who wish to practice simple relaxation exercises can be given information and recommended techniques. Elaborate behavioral therapy has no place in the treatment of postoperative pain, unless the pain is likely to be prolonged or to recur.

Postoperative Pain in Special Populations

CHILDREN

There are many differences between adults and children that make pain treatment in children a particular challenge. It is

Table 14-5. Patient-controlled analgesia or continuous infusion of morphine for pediatric cases

Children Under 7 Years of Age (Use dilute solution—0.2 mg/ml.)		
Requirements	Dose (mg/kg)	Example: for a 10-kg child, using 0.2 mg/ml
Basal rate (per hour)	0.01–0.05	0.1 mg = 0.5 ml
Hourly limit	0.03	0.3 mg = 1.5 ml
Initial bolus (every 5 min until comfortable)	0.02	0.2 mg = 1 ml
Maximum bolus	0.1	1 mg = 5 ml
For increasing pain	2 to 3 times basal	
For nonfunctioning IV, if morphine needed, give 0.05–0.10 mg/kg		

(These children can usually cope with patient-controlled dosing; use dilute solution—0.2 mg/ml.)

Children 7 to 11 Years of Age		
Age Range (yr)	Approximate weight (kg)	PCA setting using 0.2 mg/ml
7–8	20	1/6/0
9–11	30	2/6/0

(These children cope well with PCA; use standard solution—1 mg/ml; over 15 yr treat as adults.)

Children 12 to 15 Years of Age		
Age range (yr)	Approximate weight (kg)	PCA setting using 1 mg/ml
12–14	40–50	0.5/6/0
15	>50	1/6/0

not as easy to assess pain in children. Children, particularly babies and infants, do not handle drugs as well as adults. Also, children hate needles. Epidurals are technically more difficult to place and more difficult to maintain. And the sight of a child in pain is particularly distressing, especially to the child's parents.

Appropriate methods of pain assessment in children will differ at different ages. Broadly, there are three stages of a child's development, when different means of pain assessment are suitable. Infants, babies, and very young children (birth to about 4 years of age) cannot realistically provide reliable reports of pain. The mother's or father's instinct is often the best indicator in these very young patients. Nurses and doctors need to listen to the parents, as well as use other objective measures of pain (see Objective Measures above). Assuming developmental normality, older children (from 4 years to 7 or 8 years) can provide reliable self-reports of pain using assessment tools designed for young children (see Visual Scales above), by communicating via their parents, and often by direct communication with doctors and nurses. Children over the age of 7 or 8 years and who understand the concept of numeric order can use a verbal or visual numeric scale such as those used in adults (see p. 246).

Drug handling in infants and babies is less efficient than in adults due to the immaturity of their kidneys, liver, and brain. Babies and infants are particularly sensitive to the depressant effects of opioids, especially premature babies. Differences in drug handling will affect the choice of analgesic and treatment, the need for intensive monitoring, and drug dosages. For severe pain in babies and young children (under 7 years of age) who have not had an epidural placed intraoperatively, continuous intravenous infusion of morphine is the treatment of choice at MGH (see Table 14-5 for dosages). However, we always carefully monitor these patients due to the danger of respiratory depression in this population (see Systemic Opioids above). As soon as the period of severe pain has passed, we change to an oral or rectal regimen (commonly 10 mg/kg acetaminophen, with or without 0.5 mg/kg codeine). Young children are particularly tolerant of rectal medication and averse to injections. For severe pain in older children (over 7 years of age), PCA morphine is our treatment of choice (see Table 14-5 for dosages), switching to an oral or rectal regimen as soon as indicated. For mild to moderate postoperative pain in babies and children, an oral or rectal regimen (as above) is suitable from the outset.

Epidural therapy can be very useful for severe postoperative pain located below the shoulders in the young. It can produce excellent pain relief, but, as in adults, there may be failure due to technical difficulties. Also, catheter placement can be difficult in small patients. The caudal route of entry is often chosen in infants and babies because of the relative ease of catheter placement. Unfortunately, this choice may limit the useful life of the catheter because of soiling and contamination within the diaper area. Recommended dosage regimens are presented in Table 14-3. Because of the risk of respiratory depression in neonates and babies, we omit fentanyl from the infusion in babies under 1 year of age. When fentanyl is included in the mix, pediatric patients need to be carefully monitored (see p. 261).

The treatment of pain in pediatric patients is not easy. A certain level of experience and understanding is needed to treat these patients safely and effectively. It may be simpler to undertreat children's pain, and the temptation is to do so, especially since the very young are unable to communicate their pain. However, effective pain management in children goes a long way toward improving their hospital experience, has the longer-term benefit of minimizing fear of medical treatment, and is known to have the immediate benefit of minimizing stress responses.

THE ELDERLY

The elderly often appear to be stoical, and it is not clear whether they have a different threshold of pain, whether past experience has altered their attitude toward pain, or whether they truly do not feel pain to the same extent as younger adults. As with babies and children, it is tempting to undertreat pain in the elderly, because these patients do not always communicate pain very clearly. Moreover, the elderly may not metabolize drugs efficiently, so this is an additional consideration when using opioids. The elderly are more likely to become sedated and confused when given opioids. We find the best approach is to offer structured treatment to the elderly. For severe pain, small, intermittent doses of morphine (2–6 mg q4h) or other opioids are suitable. Epidural therapy can be helpful and circumvents the use of systemic opioids, although even epidural fentanyl can cause confusion in the elderly (see p. 254).

THE MENTALLY AND PHYSICALLY HANDICAPPED

These patients present a challenge because they may be unable to communicate pain in a normal way. As with the very young and the very old, effective pain management may involve time and patience in an effort to learn what the patients are experiencing and how best to help them. The cooperation of those adults who normally care for handicapped patients is indispensable. Drugs are metabolized normally in most of these patients, although individuals with baseline breathing difficulty may be sensitive to the respiratory depressant effects of opioids.

DRUG ABUSERS

How to treat drug abusers who have acute or postoperative pain is largely a matter of philosophy. At MGH, we believe that these patients, like any others, should be given the benefit of good control of acute pain, and that the treatment of addiction should be postponed until after the period of acute pain. In narcotic abusers, we use large doses of opioids to treat postoperative pain if it is necessary to abolish pain. We consider PCA an effective modality for drug abusers, since it provides an element of control and lessens the anxiety associated with trying to obtain medication. Several basic considerations apply to the drug abuser.

First, find out what recreational substances are being used, approximately how much is being used, and how recently the substances were used. (This information is often unreliable but should at least be sought.) Is the patient in withdrawal, and is it necessary to treat the withdrawal? In the case of narcotic abuse, opioid drugs may be continued to treat pain, and withdrawal symptoms may still manifest if the patient has been consuming large quantities of recreational narcotic. A clonidine patch is useful in this situation. Never use an opioid antagonist (naloxone) in opioid addicts. This could result in an immediate and extreme withdrawal response with a sympathetic outpouring, cardiac dysrhythmias, and even cardiac arrest and death.

It may be advantageous to minimize opioid requirement by supplementing treatment with opioid-sparing therapies (NSAIDs, epidurals, local nerve blocks). On the other hand, total reliance on these therapies and total withdrawal of opioids from a narcotic abuser are ill advised, partly because they will result in an unnecessarily severe withdrawal syndrome, and partly because pain will be very difficult to control without opioids. Is the patient on a methadone program? If so, our policy is to continue the preadmission dose of methadone and prescribe additional medication to treat pain, as needed.

Finally, once arrangements have been made for the patient's discharge, or when the period of acute pain is over, refer him or her for rehabilitation.

INTENSIVE CARE PATIENTS

These patients form a special population because, in many cases, they are unable to communicate pain, either because of severe illness or because they are ventilated and sedated (sometimes paralyzed). Options for pain treatment may be extended because ventilated patients are not at risk of respiratory depression. Although these patients are often unable to communicate, it is important to treat their pain to reduce distress and anxiety and to attenuate stress responses. In fact, in certain patients, notably those with cardiac disease, high-dose opioids are indicated to minimize stress responses. Assessment of pain may necessarily be a matter of judging how much pain the patients are likely to have, according to the amount of surgical or other trauma they have undergone. Opioids can also be used in the intensive care unit (ICU) to sedate ventilated patients, independent of their use as analgesics. Standard opioid therapy for ventilated ICU patients is continuous intravenous infusion. Morphine is chosen for infusion at MGH (starting at 0.1

mg/kg per hour), but many centers prefer the limited accu mulation offered by shorter-acting opioids such as fentany and alfentanil. Alert or unventilated ICU patients can b treated as normal patients, with the proviso that sick pa tients may handle drugs inefficiently. Epidurals are usefu even in ventilated patients, especially if the need for venti lation is likely to be short lived.

Conclusions

Effective postoperative pain management involves adherence to certain basic principles. First and foremost, pain must be assessed systematically and regularly, so that pain treatmen can be modified according to need. Pain that is treated preemptively or early is easier to treat than established or severe pain. In this respect, treatment during the operative and early postoperative period is important. Patients should be involved with their treatment, educated about surgery and postoperative pain and about the options for treating pain and offered choices of treatment. Finally, patients in specia populations need special consideration. The actual choice o treatment is of secondary importance, once the principles o postoperative pain management are adhered to. Postopera tive pain has often been inadequately treated in the past, due in part to complacency and in part to fear of analgesic side effects. But today's patients expect better pain control, and exemplary pain management goes a long way toward im proving patients' satisfaction with their hospital care. Fo this reason, and because good pain control is humane and reduces morbidity, we should endeavor to treat pain to the best of our ability.

Selected Readings

Ballantyne JC, et al. Postoperative patient-controlled analgesia meta-analyses of initial randomized control trials. *J Clir Anesth* 5:182–193, 1993.

Carr DB, et al. Appendix B. Acute Pain Management: Operative or Medical Procedures and Treatment. *Clinical Practice Guide line*. AHCPR Pub. No. 92-0032. Rockville MD: Agency fo Health Care Policy and Research, Public Health Service, U.S Department of Health and Human Services, 1992.

Cousins M. Acute and Postoperative Pain. In: PD Wall and R Melzak (eds). *Textbook of Pain* (3rd ed). Edinburgh: Churchill Livingstone, 1994. Pp. 357–385.

Guinard JP, et al. A randomized comparison of intravenous ver sus lumbar and thoracic epidural fentanyl for analgesia afte thoracotomy. *Anesthesiology*, 77:1108–1115, 1992.

McQuay HF, Carroll D, and Moore RA. Postoperative orthopaedic pain—the effect of opiate premedication and local anesthetic blocks. *Pain* 33:291–295, 1988.

Porter J and Jick H. Addiction rare in patients treated with narcotics. *N Engl J Med* 302:123, 1980. Letter.

Ready LB, et al. Postoperative epidural morphine is safe on surgical wards. *Anesthesiology* 75:452–456, 1991.

Scherer R, et al. Complications related to thoracic epidural analgesia: A prospective study in 1071 surgical patients. *Acta Anaesthesiol Scand* 37:370–374, 1993.

Pain in Burn Patients

Andreas Dauber and Bucknam McPeek

> *"There is physical pain and there is mental pain and scarring. You can see the outside, but what a lot of people don't see is that we are truly burned on the inside as well."*
>
> BURN SURVIVOR

More than 2 million burn injuries occur annually in the United States, thermal burns being most prevalent. Chemical and electrical burns are the least common burns in patients. Approximately 1 in 20 burn patients requires extended hospitalization. Burn injuries result in physical and psychologic injury. Pain is a major component of burn injury.

Patient-centered outcome surveys of burn pain are rare. A number of authors have reported widespread underestimation and undertreatment of burn pain. Between 35% and 50% of burn survivors report woefully inadequate pain control. The **average** reported pain intensity during burn treatment procedures is characterized as "excruciating."

Types of Burn Injury

Burns vary in **extent** from less than 1% of the body surface area to 100%. Burns vary in **depth** from superficial to full thickness, perhaps with massive destruction of muscle or bone.

In **first-degree burns**, the injury is superficial, is characterized by erythema, and involves only the epidermis. The victim usually suffers mild to moderate discomfort and healing occurs within a week.

Second-degree burns are deeper, partial-thickness injuries that destroy the epidermis and variable amounts of dermis as well as epidermal appendages. Second-degree burns are extremely painful. Most of the pain is due to the damage of sensory nociceptive receptors that are preferentially sensitive to tissue damage. In addition to direct damage from the burn, second-degree burns leave the protective layer of skin damaged, with normally covered nerve endings exposed to stimulation. These lesions heal slowly with nerve regeneration, some tissue contraction, and the occasional need for skin grafting.

Third-degree burns destroy the skin completely. They are, by definition, full thickness. Regions of third-degree burns may be painless after the initial injury for a period due to destruction of cutaneous nociceptors. Although the central part of the initial wound may be analgesic, almost every third-degree burn is surrounded by painful areas of second-degree injury. These areas heal by epidermal regeneration, since some of the epidermal appendages remain intact. This healing process can be painful. With inadequate cleansing and debridement, a surface pseudomembrane comprised of wound exudate and necrotic eschar accumulates. As long as the eschar and pseudomembrane exist, the center of a third-degree burn is painless. Of course, unremoved eschar and membrane serve as a nidus for infection, the major life-threatening factor in burn victims.

Types of Burn Pain

There are different components of burn injury pain, including acute and chronic pain. In the acute postburn state, the most severe pain is the result of therapeutic procedures such as dressing changes. There is also a continuous background pain at rest, which may persist from weeks to months.

Pain related to burn injury may worsen with time due to a number of factors: increase in anxiety and depression; sleep disturbance and deconditioning; and regeneration of nerve endings (possible neuroma formation), which is known as postburn neuralgia.

Chronic pain may result from contractures, neuropathic pain, or subsequent nerve and tissue damage that may follow surgical procedures.

Acute Treatment for Burn Pain

See Chapter 14 for additional information. The main goal of treatment for serious burns is to clean the burn area by debridement or surgical excision, thus removing necrotic tissue and other sources of infection. Retained necrotic tissue is quickly colonized by microorganisms that release exotoxins and endotoxins that exacerbates the inflammation already present in burns. After removal of necrotic tissue by cleaning or surgical excision, the next step is to promote coverage of the open wound wherever possible by a skin graft from unburned areas of the patient's own body. In very large burns, autologous skin grafts or artificial skin can provide temporary coverage.

Patients suffer continual shifts from moderate, or even low, background discomfort to excruciating pain associated with treatments such as burn dressing changes, manual debridement of open wounds, and physical therapy. In addition, there are frequent surgical operations, excisions of eschar, and harvesting of large areas of normal skin for grafting. Skin donor sites often give rise to severe pain. Treatment of burn pain thus involves pain of the primary injury as well as pain from repeated therapeutic procedures. Burn dressing changes and debridements may occur twice a day, physical therapy once or twice a day, and surgical interventions several times a week.

Pain therapy must address not only background pain but also repeated episodes of severe incident pain occurring during treatment, perhaps as often as three to six times a day. Because of this variation in the intensity of pain from hour to hour or even minute to minute, burn pain treatment for patients suffering from acute burns requires repeated assessments, treatment, and titration of analgesic drugs.

Opioid analgesics are the mainstay for the treatment of acute pain. Various routes of administration have been described and tested in the burn population. **Morphine** is the most widely used drug in burn centers. Because it can be used in different routes and formulations for administration, it is most suitable for this purpose. **Hydromorphone** (Dilaudid) is an opiate similar to morphine. We use it for the occasional patient who finds the side effects of morphine too distressing or who is hypersensitive to morphine. **Meperidine** has no advantages over morphine. When given to burn patients it has been shown to cause the accumulation of its toxic metabolite, normeperidine, which can produce cerebral irritation ranging from dysphoria, to agitation, and even to seizures. Meperidine is not recommended in burn patients for more than brief, acute, prehospital treatment of burn pain. Continuous **fentanyl** administration by infusion leads to a rapid development of tolerance and to excessively high dose regimens to control pain. Fentanyl, if used at all, should be reserved for special procedures such as burn dressing changes. Bolus administration of the phenylpiperidines (fentanyl, alfentanil, sufentanil) can produce chest wall rigidity. This factor makes it advisable to have general anesthesia with muscle relaxation available for its use in nonintubated burn patients.

For most patients probably the best route of administration is intravenous patient-controlled analgesia. This technique allows a patient to self-administer an analgesic drug, usually morphine or hydromorphone, by pressing a button that causes a machine to deliver a measured dose of the drug intravenously. Most patients, even children as young as 6 or 7 years, learn to control the pain themselves by pushing the button only when they are in pain. The onset of analgesia with morphine is approximately 6 to 10 minutes, so patients can pretreat themselves or be pretreated by a physician or nurse just before a painful therapeutic procedure. Or they can receive measured doses of the analgesic drug during the procedure and when the pain of the procedure has passed they are comfortable and, usually, not oversedated.

Psychologic Treatments of Burn Pain

Burn patients need continuing psychologic support in both the acute and chronic phases of burn treatment. One of the most important points made by many burn survivors is the presence of fear, depression, nightmares, and hallucinations. In addition to pharmacologic interventions (e.g., sedatives and antidepressants) ongoing psychosocial support is absolutely necessary, since most burn patients come from a previously healthy population, and the burn injury not only results in short-term changes and severe pain but also prolonged changes of health, chronic pain, and perhaps permanent disfigurement.

Relaxation, imagery, distraction through music, and biofeedback can be used in addition to pharmacologic measures to reduce the patient's pain. Patients, both adults and children, should be carefully advised about treatment plans, their needs, scheduling, and exactly what to expect and when, all with the aim of giving the patient as much of a sense of "being in control" as possible.

Transcutaneous electrical nerve stimulation is another modality that can sometimes provide effective pain relief in selected patients.

Selected Readings

Atchinson NE, Osgood PF, Carr DB, and Szyfelbein SK. Pain during burn dressing change in children: Relationship to burn area, depth, and analgesic regimens. *Pain* 47;41–45, 1991.

Carr DB, Osgood PF, and Szyfelbein SK. Treatment of Pain in Acutely Burned Children. In: NL Schechter, CB Berde, and M. Yaster (eds), *Pain in Infants, Children, and Adolescents*. Baltimore: Williams & Wilkins, 1993.

Choiniere M, Auger FA, and Latarjet J. Visual analogue thermometer: A valid and useful instrument for measuring pain in burned patients. *Burns* 20:229–235, 1994.

Choiniere M, Grenier R, and Paquette C. Patient-controlled analgesia: A double-blind study in burn patients. *Anesthesia* 47; 467–472, 1992.

Dauber A, Carr DB, and Breslau A. Burn survivors' pain experiences: A questionnaire-based survey. Presented at the Seventh World Congress on Pain, International Association for the Study of Pain, Paris, 1993.

Osgood PF and Szyfelbein SK. Management of Pain. In: JAJ Martyn (ed), *Acute Management of the Burned Patient*. Philadelphia: Saunders, 1990.

Perry S and Heidrich G. Management of pain during debridement: A survey of U.S. burn units. *Pain* 13;267–280, 1982.

Herman RA, et al., Pharmacokinetics of morphine sulfate in patients with burns. *Burn Care Rehabil* 15:95–103, 1994.

16

Headache

Michael Cutrer

> *"I have a pain upon my forehead here."*
>
> OTHELLO — ACT 3, SCENE 3 —
> WILLIAM SHAKESPEARE

Headache is an ancient affliction. Therapeutic incantations and treatments can be found in pre-Christian Sumerian and Egyptian writings. Aretaeus of Cappadocia in second-century Turkey writes of headache sufferers who "hid from the light and wished for death."

Headache is a common affliction. In 1985, a large-scale, survey-based study reported the prevalence of headache in the United States to be 78% of women and 68% of men. It has been estimated that 40% of adults in North America have experienced a severe debilitating headache at least once in their lives.

Despite their ancient predecessors and seeming omnipresence in emergency rooms and clinic waiting rooms, headache patients must still contend with widespread indifference and suspicion of their complaints as well as haphazard and sometimes even inappropriate treatment. This is unnecessary and can even be tragic because (1) headache can be the presenting symptom for a serious or life-threatening abnormality, and (2) the majority of patients with recurrent headache show a good response to therapy.

Anatomy of Head Pain

Over 50 years ago, epilepsy surgery performed on the brains of awake patients under local anesthesia indicated that brain tissue itself was relatively insensate to electrical or mechanical stimulation, whereas electrical stimulation of the meninges or meningeal blood vessels produced a severe, boring headache. The meninges and meningeal vessels are richly supplied with small-caliber pain fibers called **C fibers**, which are likely to be the key structures involved in the generation of headache. The C fibers from the meninges converge into the trigeminal nerve and project to the trigeminal nucleus caudalis in the lower medulla, where they synapse. From the caudal brain stem, fibers carrying nociceptive signals project to more rostral trigeminal subnuclei and the thalamus (ventral posterior medial, medial, and intralaminar nuclei). Projections from the thalamus ascend to the cerebral cortex, where painful information is localized and reaches consciousness.

Pathogenic Theories of Headache

Many of the difficulties encountered by headache sufferers arise from our still primitive understanding of the pathophysiology that produces headaches in most patients. Head pain results from the activation of the pain fibers that innervate intracranial structures, regardless of the activating stimulus (Fig. 16-1). In a small number of patients, an identifiable structural or inflammatory source for the headache can be found using neuroimaging or other laboratory investigations. In these patients, treatment of the primary abnormality results in resolution of the headache. However, the overwhelming majority of patients that one encounters in clinical practice suffers from primary headache disorders like migraine or tension headache, in which physical examinations and laboratory studies are unrevealing. Research into the pathophysiology of headache has been limited by the subjective nature of the complaints and the paucity of animal models with which to test hypotheses. Theories of migraine pathogenesis fall roughly into two categories—vasogenic theory and neurogenic theory.

VASOGENIC THEORY

In the late 1930s investigators observed the following:

1. Cranial vessels appeared to be important in the generation of headache.
2. In many patients, extracranial vessels became distended and pulsated during a migraine attack.
3. Vasoconstrictive substances like ergot alkaloids could abort headache, and vasodilatory substances like nitrates could provoke an attack.

Based on these observations, they theorized that:

1. Intracranial vasoconstriction is responsible for the aura of migraine.
2. Headache results from a rebound dilation and distention of cranial vessels.
3. Head pain is enhanced by vasoactive polypeptides.

NEUROGENIC THEORY

The alternative hypothesis holds that:

1. Migraine is caused by a dysfunction of the brain itself, involving a lowered cerebral threshold to migraine attacks.
2. When precipitating factors exceed this threshold, a migraine attack occurs.
3. While the vascular changes may occur during a migraine attack, they occur as a result rather than the cause of the attack.

Proponents of the neurogenic theory pointed to the broad range of neurologic symptoms associated with a migraine attack that cannot be explained on the basis of vasoconstriction within a single cerebrovascular distribution, as well as to pro-

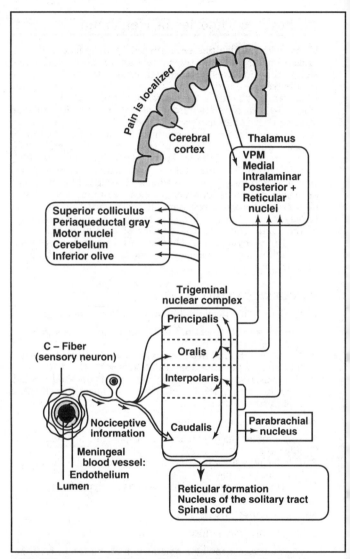

Fig. 16-1. Overview of the mechanism leading to headache pain perception after activation of trigeminovascular nociceptive neurons (VPM = ventral posterior medial.)

dromal symptoms such as euphoria, hunger, thirst, or fluid retention, which precede the headache in many people by as much as 24 hours.

SENSORY NEUROPEPTIDES IN HEADACHE

There is increasing experimental evidence that once activated, C fibers release neuropeptides (i.e., substance P, neurokinin A, calcitonin–gene-related peptide) that generate a neurogenic inflammatory response within the meninges. This response consists of (1) increased plasma leakage from meningeal vessels, (2) vasodilation, and (3) activation of mast cells and endothelial cells.

Once set into motion, this process may act to lower the threshold of the C fibers to further activation and, as a result, prolong and intensify the headache attack. Drugs known to be effective in ending a migraine attack, such as dihydroergotamine mesylate or sumatriptan succinate, have been shown to act at serotonin (5-HT) receptor subtypes to block the release of neuropeptides and the development of neurogenic inflammation.

Clinical Approach to Acute Headache

When faced with a patient in the emergency department whose primary complaint is that of a severe headache, the first question to be answered is: **Is this headache symptomatic of a potentially serious underlying abnormality requiring rapid and appropriate treatment?**

In the vast majority of cases the headache will represent a particularly severe episode in a primary headache disorder. However, the distinction between primary and secondary (symptomatic of another cause) headaches must be made as rapidly and accurately as possible. The setting is often not optimal. The emergency ward is usually a busy place and there may be pressures to deal with the patient quickly. The patient is often in distress. Family members are often alarmed, making it difficult to obtain a complete history. However, it is crucial to use the history and physical examination to determine the patient's risk level, to order diagnostic tests, and to provide therapy accordingly. Laboratory tests and imaging studies ordered without strong clinical indication are usually unrevealing, may further cloud an already confused picture, and often place an unnecessary financial burden on the patient.

Several points in the history and physical examination are valuable in making these distinctions, as outlined below.

IMPORTANT QUESTIONS TO ASK

1. **Is this headache the first of its kind?** If the headache is unlike anything experienced previously, the risk in-

creases. If it is similar (even if of greater intensity) to attacks experienced over many months or years, it is more likely to be a benign process. This question becomes increasingly important after the age of 40 years, as the incidence of the first attack of migraine decreases and the incidence of neoplasm and other intracranial pathology increases.

2. **Was this headache of sudden onset?** A persistent headache that begins and reaches its maximal intensity within a few seconds or minutes is more suggestive of an ominous cause. Migraine tends to start small and gradually intensifies over 30 minutes to 1 hour. Cluster headaches can intensify rapidly, but attacks typically resolve within an hour or two.

3. **Has there been any alteration in mental status during the course of the headache?** Generally, a family member or friend who has been with the patient must answer this question. While migraineurs can appear fatigued, especially after prolonged vomiting or analgesic use, obtundation and confusion are more suggestive of meningitis, encephalitis, or subarachnoid hemorrhage.

4. **Has there been recent or coexistent infectious disease?** Infection in other locations (i.e., lungs, paranasal or mastoid sinuses) may have preceded meningitis. Fever is **not** a feature of migraine or a primary headache disorder. Fever may also occur in association with subarachnoid hemorrhage, although usually 3 to 4 days after the actual hemorrhage.

5. **Did the headache begin in the context of vigorous exercise or seemingly trivial head or neck trauma?** While effort-induced migraine or coital migraine certainly exists, the rapid onset of headache with strenuous exercise, especially when minor trauma has occurred, increases the possibility of carotid artery dissection or intracranial hemorrhage.

6. **Does the head pain tend to radiate posteriorly?** Pain radiation between the shoulders or lower is not typical of migraine and may indicate meningeal irritation from subarachnoid blood or infection.

7. Other important points not to be overlooked in a careful history:

   A. **Do other family members have similar headache?** Migraine has a strong familial tendency.

   B. **What medications does the patient take?** Certain medications can cause headache. Anticoagulants and oral antibiotics place the patient at a higher risk for hemorrhage or partially treated CNS infection.

   C. **Does the patient have any other chronic illness or a history of neurologic abnormality?** These may confuse the neurologic examination.

   D. **Is the headache consistently in the same location or on the same side?** Benign headache disorders tend to change sides and locations, at least occasionally.

IMPORTANT PHYSICAL FINDINGS

When approaching the neurologic examination in a headache patient, it is important to remember that findings can be subtle and can change from the time the patient initially presents in the emergency department. Therefore, it is crucial to examine each patient carefully, especially when there are atypical elements in the history. A basic neurologic examination that addresses the following six components should be performed.

1. **Mental status:** What is the patient's level of consciousness? Is the patient able to maintain normal attention during the examination? Are language and memory normal?
2. **Cranial nerves:** Each cranial nerve should be tested separately. Are there asymmetries? Is there papilledema?
3. **Motor involvement:** Are motor strength and muscle tone symmetrical and within the normal range? Are there any abnormal involuntary movements?
4. **Sensory involvement:** Are there asymmetries of pain, temperature, or proprioceptive sensation?
5. **Coordination:** Is there dysmetria or gait ataxia?
6. **Reflexes:** Is there asymmetry of reflexes in either the upper or lower extremities?

Three findings on examination should be considered **Red Flags**:

1. **Nuchal rigidity** can be an indicator of either meningitis or subarachnoid hemorrhage.
2. **The toxic-appearing patient.** Is there a low-grade fever or persistent tachycardia? Does the patient appear more acutely ill than most migraine patients?
3. **Any previously unnoticed neurologic abnormality.** Subtle findings such as a slight pupillary asymmetry, a unilateral pronator drift, or extensor plantar response markedly increase the level of risk.

WHEN TO ORDER LABORATORY TESTS OR IMAGING STUDIES

Laboratory tests should be obtained to confirm the presence of abnormalities suspected from the history and physical examination and should be appropriate for the pathology suspected. Laboratory, electroencephalographic, or neuroimaging "fishing trips" are discouraged because they rarely provide useful information, can delay treatment, and can divert attention from more relevant findings.

At present, the CT scan is the imaging study most likely to be available in the acute setting. There are three major indications for an urgent CT scan: (1) the presence of papilledema, (2) any impairment of consciousness or orientation, and (3) the presence of localizing or lateralizing findings on neurologic examination.

CT scanning is most useful for identifying recent intracerebral and extracerebral hemorrhages, hydrocephalus and brain abscesses, or other space-occupying lesions.

A large review of published articles on the use of CT and MRI scanning in patients presenting with headache, conducted by the Quality Standards Subcommittee of the American Academy of Neurology, revealed that abnormalities were found in 2.4% of the patients who had normal neurologic examinations. Pathology was found in 0.4% of the patients who had normal neurologic examinations and whose headaches were identified as migraine.

Differential Diagnosis of Secondary Headaches

Headache can be symptomatic of many underlying abnormalities. The relative frequency of secondary headaches is low compared to that of primary headache disorders. However, it is vital that these headaches are diagnosed quickly and treated appropriately.

VASCULAR ETIOLOGY

Subarachnoid hemorrhage is usually the result of leakage from an aneurysmal vessel. It is a neurosurgical emergency and can be identified by CT scan. The aneurysm itself can be localized by an arteriogram. The **clinical features** of subarachnoid hemorrhage are as follows:

1. Sudden, explosive onset with maximal intensity in seconds.
2. Extreme intensity, often described as "the worst headache of my life."
3. Nuchal rigidity or stiff neck. Blood acts as a chemical irritant in the subarachnoid space, causing activation of pain fibers and muscle spasm.
4. A precipitous decrease in the level of consciousness as the brain stem becomes compressed.

If one or more of these features is present, urgent evaluation with CT or lumbar puncture, or both, is indicated. Other important, but less specific, features include photophobia and vomiting.

Sometimes patients may experience "sentinel bleeds" or small, warning leaks of the aneurysm, which are similar in quality to but less intense than full-blown hemorrhage. These warnings must be evaluated promptly, since they can be followed by a larger hemorrhage in 2 to 14 days.

Subdural Hematoma

Subdural hematoma, a collection of blood between the dura mater and the brain substance, can present as a dull, continuous headache. Subdural hematomas can occur after minor head trauma or spontaneously and should be considered in elderly patients or in patients on anticoagulants.

Cerebellar Hemorrhage

Cerebellar hemorrhage can present as a headache followed rapidly by signs of brain stem compression (i.e., altered mental status, pupillary or eye movement abnormalities, or focal weakness). Cerebellar hemorrhage is a neurosurgical emergency. It is one of the few hypertensive hemorrhages associated with a good prognosis for recovery **if the hematoma is recognized and evacuated quickly**.

Arteriovenous Malformations

Arteriovenous malformations (AVMs) are vascular abnormalities that shunt blood directly from arterial to venous structures, bypassing the capillary beds. AVMs can cause ipsilateral headache with a migraine-like quality. Occasionally an AVM can be detected by listening for a bruit over the orbit or head. AVMs can also hemorrhage, resulting in a more precipitous headache and focal neurologic deficits.

Intracerebral Arterial Occlusions

Intracerebral arterial occlusions with infarction can sometimes be accompanied by headache. In general, though, the clinical picture is dominated by a persistent neurologic deficit.

Cerebral Venous Sinus Occlusions

Occlusion of cerebral venous sinuses can also be associated with headache and neurologic deficits. **Cavernous sinus thrombosis** is associated with severe ocular pain and injection combined with abnormalities of cranial nerves III, V_1, V_2 and VI. **Sagittal sinus thrombosis** can manifest as headache, seizures, and focal neurologic findings.

Carotid Artery Dissection

Carotid artery dissection occurs as blood separates muscular layers of the carotid artery following endothelial damage. It can follow seemingly minor head or neck trauma and can cause severe head and neck pain often referred to the brow, eye, orbit, or mastoid area. Associated neurologic signs may occur, including (1) tongue paralysis, if cranial nerve XII is affected, and (2) Horner's syndrome, if sympathetic fibers traveling with the carotid artery are involved.

INFECTIOUS ETIOLOGY

Meningitis

Inflammation of the meninges secondary to infection is a neurologic emergency and must be dealt with quickly and correctly. CNS infection can be due to bacterial, viral, mycobacterial, or fungal organisms. Meningitis can follow a brief systemic illness or may appear without an antecedent infection. A patient with meningitis may present with (1) severe headache, (2) fever, (3) neck pain and stiffness, (4) photophobia, (5) seizures, and (6) rash.

When faced with this clinical picture, an emergent evaluation for meningitis is crucial. To evaluate for meningitis, a lumbar puncture must be performed. If there are focal findings on neurologic examination (i.e., unilateral or focal weakness, eye movement abnormality, pupillary abnormality, or altered mental status) an emergent CT should be performed, if possible, to rule out the presence of a posterior fossa tumor, abscess, or hematoma, which would make a lumbar puncture risky. However, if bacterial meningitis is suspected, **do not delay antibiotic treatment while waiting for a CT scan**. Nor should lumbar puncture be inordinately delayed for this reason.

Meningoencephalitis

Meningoencephalitis is present when both the meninges and brain parenchyma are involved. It can result from viral infections, with the most ominous cause being herpes meningoencephalitis. The presentation of meningoencephalitis can be similar to meningitis but is sometimes less sudden in onset and follows a brief, mild flu-like illness. The presence of seizures or mild mental status changes in the days before presentation can be suggestive of meningoencephalitis. Cerebrospinal fluid examination is necessary in these patients and MRI or CT can confirm temporal lobe involvement.

Brain Abscess

Brain abscess is a focal collection of pus within the brain substance secondary to bacterial infection after direct or hematogenous spread of the organism (most commonly *Streptococcus, Staphylococcus*, and anaerobes). Headache, vomiting, focal neurologic signs, and depressed mental status may occur as the result of mass effect. Surgical or antibiotic treatment of the lesion usually brings improvement in the headache. Subdural empyema is a collection of pus between the brain parenchyma and the dura mater, which can manifest as headache, vomiting, altered mental status, and focal neurologic deficits. Treatment consists of surgical drainage and antibiotic therapy.

Acute Sinusitis

Acute sinusitis can be associated with frontal headache. Sphenoid sinusitis can mimic migraine and maxillary sinusitis can be mistaken for migraine. Patients tend to assume that any frontal headache is sinusitis. Before making this diagnosis and treating with antibiotics, it is appropriate to look for the features of sinusitis (i.e., sinus opacification on x-ray studies or illumination, fever, or purulent nasal discharge).

Upper Respiratory or Systemic Viral Infection

Upper respiratory or systemic viral infection can be the cause of a mild to moderate headache. These minor infections are not associated with neck stiffness, photophobia, or changes in mentation.

AIDS

Headache can be a prominent clinical feature of acute and chronic HIV infection as well as AIDS-related opportunistic infections such as *Cryptococcus* and *Toxoplasma gondii.*

NEOPLASTIC ETIOLOGY

Intracranial Tumors

Most patients who present for evaluation of severe, recurrent headaches have at least some concern that their headaches are the result of an undiagnosed intracranial tumor. Fortunately, the majority of patients with headache does not have an underlying structural cause. However, it is important to identify those who do.

Forsythe and Posner (1992) examined 111 consecutive patients with brain tumor identified by either CT or MRI scans. Headaches were present in 48% of the patients. Based on this population, the characteristics of tumor-associated headaches were as follows:

1. Headaches were usually described as dull and pressure-like and were similar in quality to tension-type headache in 77% of cases (only 9% of headaches were similar to migraine).
2. Headaches were usually bifrontal but worse ipsilateral to the tumor.
3. Nausea was associated with the headache in about half of the cases.
4. Headaches were intermittent (62%) and of moderate to severe intensity (median of 7 on an intensity scale of 1 to 10).
5. The classic brain tumor headache (i.e., one that was progressive and started in the morning) occurred only 17% of the time.
6. Headaches in patients with increased intracranial pressure tended to be resistant to common analgesics.

No headache type is specific for a brain tumor. Factors that should increase suspicion of an intracranial tumor include (1) papilledema, (2) the presence of neurologic deficits, (3) prior history of a malignancy, and (4) evidence of cognitive abnormality or altered mental status.

The treatment of headaches associated with intracranial tumors is outlined as follows. If headaches are **mild to moderate**, then simple analgesics are often effective. If surgical intervention is likely, aspirin and other nonsteroidal anti-inflammatory drugs should be avoided. If the pain is **severe** opiates may be useful. If there is evidence of significant **edema** surrounding the tumor, intravenous steroids may improve the headache by decreasing the swelling. **Surgical or radiotherapeutic treatment** of the tumor may improve the headache.

INFLAMMATORY ETIOLOGY

Temporal Arteritis

Temporal arteritis is an inflammatory vasculitis affecting primarily the temporal arteries. It typically affects individuals over the age of 60 years and can result in rapid and permanent loss of vision. Five features are associated with temporal arteritis. (1) The headaches are orbital or frontotemporal in location and are described as a dull, constant pain with superimposed jabbing sensations. (2) The head pain can be aggravated by cold temperatures. (3) Jaw or tongue pain can occur with chewing. (4) Transient visual symptoms can occur (inferior altitudinal defect). And (5) accompanying constitutional symptoms can include weight loss, anemia, mononeuropathy, and elevated liver function tests.

Transient visual symptoms can rapidly progress to permanent visual loss. The erythrocyte sedimentation rate is elevated in 95% of cases. Definitive diagnosis is based on positive findings in a temporal artery biopsy, which can still be obtained within 48 hours of the initiation of treatment with steroids. When the diagnosis is suspected, prompt treatment with steroids is necessary to avoid visual loss (which becomes bilateral in 75% of cases in which there is unilateral loss).

Autoimmune Inflammatory Process

Headache can be a feature of collagen vascular disorders like systemic lupus erythematosus and autoimmune angiopathies like isolated angiitis of the CNS.

HYPERTENSIVE ETIOLOGY

It is unlikely that moderate elevations in blood pressure are causative of headache. Extreme elevations in blood pressure (diastolic pressures >120 mm Hg) are associated with headache. These headaches are often diffuse and tend to peak in intensity in the morning with gradual resolution over several hours.

The International Headache Society Classification recognizes four categories of headache associated with severe hypertension.

1. **Acute pressor response to an exogenous agent.** Headache occurs in temporal association with a rise in blood pressure due to specific toxins or medications and resolves within 24 hours of normalization of blood pressure.
2. **Pheochromocytoma,** an adrenal tumor that secretes epinephrine. Headache occurs with increases in blood pressure, is of long duration (minutes), and is often accompanied by sweating, anxiety or palpitations.
3. **Malignant hypertension** (including hypertensive encephalopathy), in which headache is associated with grade 3 or 4 retinopathy and often with altered mental status. The headache is temporally related to the hypertensive

episode and disappears within 2 days of reduction of blood pressure.

4. **Preeclampsia or eclampsia.** Headache is associated with elevated blood pressure, proteinuria, and edema in pregnant and peripartum women. Headache resolves within 7 days of reduction of blood pressure or termination of the pregnancy.

OCULAR ABNORMALITY—GLAUCOMA

Two forms of glaucoma present with headache: **Pigmentary glaucoma**, a form of secondary open-angle glaucoma, occurs when pigment from the iris is liberated into the aqueous during exercise and subsequently blocks outward flow through the trabecular meshwork. The patients, frequently young myopic males, present with exercise-induced headache and blurred vision.

Acute-angle closure glaucoma, in which there is no free flow of aqueous through the pupil, results in forward bulging of the iris with obstruction of the trabecular meshwork. Episodes can be precipitated by dilation of the eye (either physiologic or pharmacologic). It presents with visual blurring; severe ocular pain, sometimes radiating to the forehead or teeth; red injected eye; cloudy cornea; dilated, unresponsive pupil; and marked elevation in intraocular pressure.

Urgent ophthalmologic referral is appropriate in either type of glaucoma. For acute-angle closure glaucoma, laser iridotomy is often necessary. Glaucoma is sometimes confused with cluster headache. In **cluster headache**, the pupil is small rather than dilated and ptosis is often present.

SUBSTANCE-INDUCED HEADACHE

Various substances are known to induce headaches in susceptible individuals. Headache can occur with both acute exposure and as a result of withdrawal after chronic intake of the substance (Tables 16-1 and 16-2).

BENIGN INTRACRANIAL HYPERTENSION (PSEUDOTUMOR CEREBRI)

Increased intracranial pressure can occur in the absence of hydrocephalus or intracranial mass. The resulting syndrome is characterized by (1) headache, (2) papilledema, (3) absence of localizing neurologic signs, (4) normal cerebrospinal fluid composition, and (5) transient visual blurring.

The diagnosis is made by lumbar puncture (CSF pressure >250 mm Hg; normal CSF composition) after neuroimaging has excluded a mass lesion. In adults, females have a higher incidence (between 3 and 10 times) than males. Visual field testing often reveals an enlarged blind spot. The prototypical patient is an overweight woman of child-bearing age. Spon-

**Table 16-1. Substances that induce headache
with acute exposure**

alcohol
carbon monoxide
cimetidine
cocaine/crack
danazol
diclofenac
estrogen/birth control pills
indomethacin
monosodium glutamate
nifedipine
nitrates/nitrites
ondansetron
phenylethylamine
ranitidine
tyramine

**Table 16-2. Substances that induce headache on
withdrawal after chronic use**

alcohol
caffeine
ergotamine
opiate analgesics

taneous recovery is characteristic, but therapy geared toward
prevention of visual loss is usually instituted.

Differential Diagnosis of
Primary Headaches

In clinical practice, the vast majority of patients investigated
because of head pain will ultimately prove to have a primary
headache disorder (i.e., recurrent headaches for which no underlying structural, infectious, or other systemic abnormality
can be found). Migraine and tension type headaches comprise
the bulk of this population, but cluster headache and other
less common syndromes are occasionally seen. To classify and
investigate primary headaches, the International Headache
Society (IHS) has developed Classification and Diagnostic
Criteria for Headache and Facial Pain. These criteria are invaluable for clinical research and are presented below, with
the caveat that many patients do not fall neatly into any one
diagnostic category.

MIGRAINE

It is estimated that approximately 16% of women and 6% of
men in the United States meet the diagnostic criteria for mi-

graine. Migraine sufferers frequently have family members who also have recurrent headaches. Migraine falls into two categories: (1) migraine without aura (previously called common migraine) and (2) migraine with aura (previously called classic migraine). Patients with migraine often report prodromal symptoms that begin 24 to 48 hours before a headache attack. These symptoms can include hyperactivity, mild euphoria, lethargy, depression, cravings for certain foods, frequent yawning, and other atypical symptoms. Prodromal symptoms should not be confused with the migraine aura, which occurs within 1 hour of the onset of the headache and consists of specific neurologic symptoms.

Migraine without Aura

To meet the IHS's diagnostic criteria for migraine without aura a patient must have had at least five attacks that fulfill each of the following categories:

1. Headache attacks lasting 4 to 72 hours (untreated or treated unsuccessfully)
2. Headache has at least two of the following characteristics:

   A. Unilateral location
   B. Pulsating quality
   C. Moderate or severe intensity (inhibits or prohibits daily activity)
   D. Aggravation by walking stairs or similar routine physical activity

3. During headache, at least one of the following:

   A. Nausea and/or vomiting
   B. Photophobia and phonophobia

4. Headaches not correlated to another physical abnormality

Migraine with Aura

For the diagnosis of migraine with aura, in addition to fulfilling the criteria of migraine without aura, patients must have experienced at least two attacks with three of the four following characteristics.

1. Attacks are associated with reversible aura symptoms indicating focal cerebral cortical and/or brain stem dysfunction.
2. At least one of the aura symptoms develops gradually over 4 minutes or two or more symptoms occur in succession.
3. No aura symptom lasts for more than 1 hour. (If more than one aura symptom is present, accepted duration is increased accordingly.)
4. Headache follows resolution of aura symptoms within 1 hour or less. (Headache can sometimes begin simultaneously with the aura.)

Neither the headache nor the aura symptoms can be correlated to another physical abnormality.

Typical migraine aura symptoms include:

1. Homonymous visual disturbance, classically a scintillating scotoma
2. Unilateral paresthesias and/or numbness, often affecting the distal extremities or the perioral region of the face
3. Unilateral weakness
4. Aphasia or other language disturbance

The aura symptoms in some patients localize to the brain stem. These include:

1. Visual symptoms in the temporal and nasal fields of both eyes
2. Dysarthria
3. Vertigo
4. Tinnitus
5. Decreased hearing
6. Double vision
7. Ataxia
8. Bilateral paresthesias
9. Bilateral weakness
10. Decreased level of consciousness

Basilar Migraine

Patients in whom brain stem symptoms predominate are generally given the diagnosis of basilar migraine. One must bear in mind that many of these symptoms are subject to misinterpretation, since they can occur with anxiety and hyperventilation. In many patients, basilar attacks are intermingled with typical attacks. Dizziness is frequently reported as a feature of an otherwise typical attack of migraine with aura.

Migraine with Prolonged Aura or Complicated Migraine

During these migraine attacks the aura symptoms persist for more than 1 hour, but less than 1 week, and neuroimaging studies are normal.

Familial Hemiplegic Migraine

Migraine with aura, including hemiparesis, where at least one first-degree relative has identical attacks. This form of migraine has been localized to chromosome 19 in several families.

TENSION-TYPE HEADACHE

Tension-type headache is probably the most common primary headache disorder. It has been referred to by many names in the past, including muscle contraction headache, essential headache, stress headache, and psychomyogenic headache. The exact pathogenesis of tension-type headache and the importance of muscle contraction to its generation are still poorly understood. Pericranial muscle spasm or tenderness may or may not be present. Tension-type headache occurs in both episodic and chronic forms.

To meet the IHS's diagnostic criteria for tension-type headache patients must have had at least 10 headaches fulfilling each of the following categories:

1. Headache lasting from 30 minutes to 7 days
2. Headaches that have at least two of the following pain characteristics:

   A. Pressing/tightening (nonpulsatile) quality
   B. Mild or moderate intensity (does not prohibit normal routine)
   C. Bilateral location
   D. No aggravation by routine physical activity

3. No associated nausea or vomiting
4. Either photophobia or phonophobia, but not both
5. Headaches not correlated with any other physical abnormality

CLUSTER HEADACHE

Cluster headaches are much less common than migraine or tension-type headaches. They afflict men 5 to 6 times more often than women and the age of onset is typically 20 to 40 years. The syndrome derives its name from the fact that attacks occur in series lasting for weeks or months (the so-called cluster periods) separated by remissions that usually last for months or years. During cluster periods, headache attacks are provoked by alcohol, histamine, or nitroglycerine. The pain is very severe and throbbing and, at times, sharp in quality. During a cluster headache a patient is often agitated and frequently paces, unlike a migraine patient who prefers to avoid movement in a quiet, dark room. **In some instances the clustering pattern of the episodic form can change into the chronic form in which there is no remission.**

To meet the IHS's diagnostic criteria for cluster headache the patient must have experienced at least five attacks fulfilling each of the following criteria:

1. Severe unilateral orbital or supraorbital and/or temporal pain lasting 15 to 180 minutes untreated
2. Headache associated with at least one of the following signs on the ipsilateral side:

   A. Conjunctival injection
   B. Lacrimation
   C. Nasal congestion
   D. Rhinorrhea
   E. Forehead and nasal sweating
   F. Miosis
   G. Ptosis
   H. Eyelid edema

3. Attacks occur with a frequency of at least one attack every other day to eight attacks per day
4. Headaches not correlated with any other physical abnormality

Chronic Paroxysmal Hemicrania

Chronic paroxysmal hemicrania is a relatively rare syndrome in which attacks are similar in character of pain and associated signs to cluster headache. It differs from cluster headache in the following ways:

1. Attacks occur with greater frequency (>5 per day for more than half the time).
2. Attacks tend to be very brief (5 to 20 minutes).
3. Prolonged remissions do not occur.
4. Females are affected more frequently than males.
5. Attacks are very responsive to indomethacin (150 mg or less per day).

MISCELLANEOUS BENIGN HEADACHES

Several headache syndromes are not associated with a structural cause but are distinct from migraine, tension-type, or cluster headaches. The following is a brief listing and description of these syndromes.

Hemicrania continua is a syndrome consisting of severe, sharp, localized pain lasting 15 to 30 minutes and occurring 10 to 20 times per day. It is more common in women and can be provoked by certain head movements.

Idiopathic stabbing headache is a series of icepick-like jabbing pains, occurs often in migraineurs on the side frequently affected by migraine attacks. Attacks often respond to oral indomethacin (25 mg tid)

Benign exertional headache can be precipitated by any form of exercise. It is generally bilateral in location and can last from several minutes to 24 hours.

Cold-induced headaches can result from either exposure of the head to low ambient temperatures or passage of a cold liquid or solid material over the palate or posterior pharynx (i.e., "ice-cream" headache).

Orgasm-induced headache can occur in susceptible individuals with masturbation or sexual intercourse. The headache is usually bilateral at onset and can be prevented by ceasing sexual activity before orgasm. A rarer form, a secondary headache, is associated with cerebral aneurysm.

Benign cough headache is bilateral at onset, reaches maximal intensity in seconds, and persists for less than 1 minute after being precipitated by coughing. This diagnosis may be made only after a structural lesion has been excluded by neuroimaging.

Refractory Headaches

CHRONIC DAILY HEADACHE

The IHS classifies headaches that are present for at least 15 days per month during at least 6 months per year as chronic

Patients usually describe these headaches as being tension type in quality, although more severe attacks similar to migraine may be interspersed. The typical features of chronic daily headache include:

1. Pressing or tightening quality
2. Mild or moderate severity
3. Bilateral location
4. No aggravation with routine physical exertion
5. No vomiting
6. Possible nausea, photophobia, or phonophobia

In some patients, migraine is gradually transformed into chronic daily headache, but more frequently episodic tension-type headache evolves into a chronic form. In both instances overuse of analgesic or ergotamine-containing medications can have an important role in perpetuating and aggravating the condition. Prophylactic therapy in patients taking daily analgesic or ergotamine-containing medications is often ineffective. Discontinuation of daily analgesic or ergotamine use often results in improvement.

STATUS MIGRAINOSUS

Migraine attacks that persist for longer than 72 hours despite treatment are classified as status migrainosus. During status migrainosus headache, free periods of less than 4 hours (sleep not included) may occur. Status migrainosus is usually associated with prolonged analgesic use. It requires in-patient treatment. (See Therapy for Status Migrainosus, page 290.)

Rational Approach to Pharmacologic Treatment of Primary Headaches

Pharmacologic treatment of headache patients can be divided into two broad categories: (1) acute therapy given during an attack to end it, and (2) prophylactic treatment given daily to decrease the frequency and severity of future attacks.

TREATMENT OF MIGRAINE

Acute Therapy for Mild to Moderate Attacks

Acetaminophen

Occasionally patients will have some mild attacks that, when caught early, will respond to over-the-counter analgesics like acetaminophen (650–1000 mg). In migraine patients this is usually not the case. Mild to moderate attacks during pregnancy should be treated with acetaminophen. The use of chronic high doses of acetaminophen over long periods can lead to liver damage.

Nonsteroidal Anti-inflammatory Drugs

NSAIDS, including aspirin (900–1000 mg), ibuprofen (1000–1200 mg), naprosyn (500–825 mg), and ketoprofen (100–200 mg), can be used to treat mild to moderate attacks. The main side effects are gastrointestinal irritation and prolonged bleeding times.

Midrin

Midrin is a combination medication containing acetaminophen, isometheptene mucate (a mild vasoconstrictor), and dichloralphenazone (a mild sedative). In a certain percentage of patients, moderate attacks will respond to midrin. Two tablets should be taken at the onset of headache followed by one tablet each hour until relief occurs, or until a maximum of 5 tablets within a 12-hour period has been ingested. Side effects include dizziness and occasional skin rash. It has been my experience that midrin seems to be less likely than many of the other combination medications to generate a rebound headache syndrome, although daily use of any of these treatments is not recommended.

Acute Therapy for Severe Attacks

Butalbital

Butalbital is a barbiturate combined with caffeine, acetylsalicylic acid, and/or acetaminophen in several medications (including fiorinal, fioricet, phrenilin, and esgic). Other preparations have codeine as well. The recommended dosage is 2 tablets every 4 hours not to exceed 6 per day. These medications are best suited for the treatment of moderate to severe, infrequent headaches. When used infrequently they can be quite effective. If used to treat headaches occurring more than twice per month, patients often overuse them and begin to have rebound headaches. In prescribing these drugs, physicians should be wary of escalating use. Side effects include sedation, dizziness, and gastrointestinal disturbance.

Oral Opiate-containing Medications

Oral opiate-containing medications have little place in the treatment of chronic recurrent primary headaches and should be avoided until all other treatment alternatives have been considered. If under certain conditions they are the only viable option (i.e., pregnancy, severe vascular disease), the physician should use the medications with caution and discuss risks of rebound headache syndromes and dependency with the patients before prescribing the drug.

Ketorolac Trimethamine

Ketorolac trimethamine is a potent NSAID that is available in injectable form. It can be given intramuscularly for the treatment of severe migraine attacks with early and prominent vomiting. A single preliminary report indicates that it is less effective than dihydroergotamine with metoclopramide. Also, it is costly treatment. However, some patients appear to respond well to it, and it may be a viable alternative if intravenous access is a problem or if vasoactive agents (i.e., dihydroergotamine or sumatriptan) are contraindicated. Side effects include gastrointestinal disturbance, hypertension, rash, bronchospasm, and increased bleeding with short-term usage. As with any NSAID, there is a risk of renal damage with long-term chronic use.

Ergotamines

Ergotamine-containing medications are available in oral, sublingual, and suppository formulations in the United States. Ergotamines are the classic antimigraine agents and can be effective if patients can tolerate the side effects of nausea and peripheral vasoconstriction. They are typically most effective if given early in the migraine attack. Another potential problem is overuse, which can result in a chronic daily headache syndrome and, in extreme cases, the gangrene-like complications of ergotism. If prescribing the suppository form, physicians should instruct patients to cut the suppository in half or into quarters to find the lowest effective dose and thereby reduce ergotamine-induced nausea. Contraindications include coronary artery disease, angina, peripheral vascular disease, Raynaud's phenomenon, uncontrolled hypertension, and severely impaired renal or hepatic function.

Dihydroergotamine

Dihydroergotamine (DHE) is an injectable hydrogenated ergot that, until recently, was the mainstay of nonopioid treatment of acute headache attacks. It has less potent peripheral arterial vasoconstrictive effects and can be effective even when given well into the attack. It can be given intravenously with somewhat less nausea than ergotamine; however, an antiemetic given prior to intravenous treatment is still usually required. At present, an intranasal formulation is awaiting approval by the Food and Drug Administration (FDA).

The following are guidelines for administering DHE in the acute setting:

Early in the attack: Administer DHE 1–2 mg IM or SQ. A total dose of up to 3 mg may be given within 24 hours.

Well into a severe attack: Administer prochlorperazine 5 mg IV, or metaclopramide 10 mg IV, followed in 5 to 10 minutes by DHE 0.75–1.0 mg IV given over 2 to 3 minutes.

If the attack has not subsided **after 30 minutes**, an additional 0.5 mg IV of DHE may be given.

Side effects of DHE include nausea, vomiting, tingling, transient tachycardia, and bradycardia. The use of prochlorperazine can sometimes be associated with extrapyramidal side effects.

Contraindications are similar to ergotamine tartrate.

Sumatriptan

Sumatriptan is a relatively selective 5-HT 1B/D agonist that exerts both direct vasoconstrictor and antineurogenic inflammatory effects on dural vessels. In large-scale, double-blinded clinical trials, 6 mg injected subcutaneously significantly reduced headache at 1 hour in over 80% of patients (versus 22% after placebo). Sumatriptan treatment is also associated with improvement in the nausea, vomiting, photophobia, and phonophobia that accompany many migraine attacks. It has also been shown to be equally effective when given up to 4 hours after the onset of a headache attack. Oral and intranasal formulations are presently awaiting FDA approval.

Side effects are usually brief and transient and include pressure-like sensations in the head, neck, and chest, tingling in the neck or scalp, and occasional dizziness.

Contraindications include definite or suspected ischemic heart disease, pregnancy, vasospastic angina, or uncontrolled hypertension.

Neuroleptics

Neuroleptics have been used as an alternative to Demerol or vasoactive medications in the emergency department setting for the treatment of severe migraine attacks. In one small parallel, double-blind study, pain relief with chlorpromazine did not reach statistical significance. In two larger blinded comparison studies chlorpromazine was significantly more effective than intravenous meperidine. The necessity for an intravenous line and the side effects of hypotension, sedation, and akathisia limit its use. If administered, an intravenous line should be started and 500 ml of normal saline should be administered before chlorpromazine. Chlorpromazine can then be administered in a 10-mg dose, which can be repeated in 1 hour. Patients should have repeated blood pressure measurements and should have at least an hour of bed rest after dosing. Alternatively, prochlorperazine 10 mg IV can be given without the prior saline infusion and repeated in 30 minutes.

Meperidine

Meperidine is an opioid analgesic that—especially in combination with an antiemetic—is frequently administered intramuscularly in the emergency department to treat severe migraine attacks. There are actually no good double-blind, placebo-controlled clinical trials of its effectiveness. The published reports of open trials do not indicate efficacy, although the dosages studied were rather low. In one double-blind comparison study, it was found to be inferior to chlorpromazine. Its main beneficial effect may be that of induction of sleep with resultant resolution of the attack. With the alternatives now available, the use of parenteral opioids should be limited to patients with infrequent attacks or patients in whom other treatments are contraindicated such as severe peripheral or cerebral vascular disease, coronary artery disease, or pregnancy.

Therapy for Status Migrainosus

If efforts to end a migraine attack in the emergency department are unsuccessful and the patient requires hospitalization, intravenous treatment with DHE is the treatment of choice, provided there are no contraindications (pregnancy, angina, coronary artery disease).

Raskin (1990) has established a protocol for the administration of intravenous DHE:

1. Metoclopramide 10 mg IV plus DHE 0.5 mg IV given over 2 to 3 minutes.
2. *If headache stops but nausea develops,* no DHE is given for 8 hours, then 0.3 or 0.4 mg of DHE plus 10 mg of metoclopramide is given every 8 hours for 3 days.
3. *If head pain persists and no nausea develops,* 0.5 mg of DHE is repeated in 1 hour; if headache is relieved but nausea develops, administer DHE 0.75 mg IV q8h for 3 days plus metoclopramide 10 mg; if headache is relieved and no nausea develops, administer DHE 1.0 mg q8h plus metoclopramide 10 mg for 3 days.
4. *If headache stops and no nausea develops,* administer DHE 0.5 mg plus metoclopramine 10 mg IV q8h for 3 days.

DHE should be given undiluted through an intravenous heplock.

Diarrhea is a common side effect of the DHE protocol and can be controlled with oral diphenoxylate.

Contraindications to intravenous DHE include Prinzmetal's angina, pregnancy, coronary artery disease or uncontrolled hypertension, peripheral vascular disease, and severe renal or hepatic disease.

When patients are hospitalized and given intravenous DHE, special attention should be given to the amount of analgesic medications they were taking prior to admission. Status migrainosus is frequently associated with overuse of abortive medications, and patients should be watched carefully for evidence of barbiturate or opiate withdrawal.

If no prophylactic regimen has been instituted in a patient with episodes status migrainosus, then initiation of prophylactic therapy is appropriate.

Prophylactic Therapy

Acute drug treatment of headache is largely symptomatic and has no benefit beyond the single attack. In the many patients who have infrequent attacks, an effective abortive agent is sufficient. However, the frequent use of abortive agents rapidly becomes a part of the problem. Once a patient has slid into the insidious cycle of analgesic rebound, prophylactic therapy may be futile and the headaches just keep getting worse.

If attacks occur more than once or twice per month, if they are sufficiently severe to prohibit normal activities, or if the patient's dread of the attacks is intrusive to his or her daily life, then prophylactic therapy should be considered (Table 16-3).

Table 16-3. Prophylactic medications useful in migraine

Drug	How supplied (mg)	Daily oral dosage (mg)
Beta-blockers		
Propranolol (Inderal)	10, 20, 40, 80	40–240
Nadolol (Corgard)	20, 40, 80, 120, 160	20–80
Atenolol (Tenormin)	25, 50, 100	50–150
Timolol (Blocadren)	5, 10, 20	20–60
Metoprolol (Lopressor)	50, 100	50–300
NSAIDs		
Naproxen sodium (Aleve, Anaprox)	220, 275, 550	480–1100
Naproxen (Naprosyn)	250, 500	750–1000
Ketoprofen (Orudis)	25, 50, 75	150–300
Aspirin	375	1000–1300
Antidepressants		
Amitriptyline (Elavil)	10, 25, 50, 75, 100, 150	10–120
Calcium-channel blockers		
Flunarizine	Not available in U.S.	
Verapamil (Calan)	40, 80, 120	120–480
Anticonvulsants		
Divalproex sodium (Depakote)	125, 250, 500	250–1500
Serotonin antagonist		
Methysergide (Sansert)	2	4–8
Monoamine oxidase inhibitor		
Phenelzine (Nardil)	15	30–60

The choice of a prophylactic agent should be individualized to the patient. Other medical problems are often contraindications to certain prophylactic medications, and occasionally the same prophylactic medicine can be used to treat migraine as well as a preexistent illness.

Prophylactic medications are empiric treatments. Thus far, the mechanism of action of the prophylactic medications is not known. Most of these medications were originally used for other indications and their antimigraine effects were found coincidentally. It is likely that in many cases their effect on migraine is unrelated to the action for which they were originally prescribed.

Most prophylactic agents are associated with increased appetite. Patients should be warned about potential weight gain.

Prophylactic medications fall into a two-tiered hierarchy. First-line agents are those that are likely to be effective without intolerable side effects. Second-line agents may be effective when the first-line agents have failed, but carry with them the risk of more frequent or potentially serious side effects.

First-Line Agents

BETA-ADRENOCEPTOR BLOCKERS. These medications were originally prescribed as antihypertensive agents. The beta blockers that have been shown to be effective migraine prophylactic agents in clinical trials include (1) propranolol, (2) nadolol, (3) atenolol, (4) timolol, and (5) metoprolol.

The antimigraine activity of these medications **does not** depend on CNS penetration, their cardioselectivity, or 5-HT binding. The only common pharmacologic property that separates the beta-blockers that are effective in migraine prophylaxis from those that are ineffective is the lack of partial sympathomimetic activity. Owing to differences in pharmacologic properties among the various agents, failure of one agent is not an indicator of failure of the rest.

Side effects occur in 10% to 15% of patients and include hypotension, fatigue, dizziness, gastrointestinal disturbance (diarrhea, constipation), depression, insomnia, and memory disturbance. Contraindications include asthma, congestive heart failure, chronic obstructive pulmonary disease, peripheral vascular disease, cardiac conduction defects, and brittle diabetes.

NONSTEROIDAL ANTI-INFLAMMATORY DRUGS. NSAIDs exert analgesic, anti-inflammatory, and antipyretic effects through their inhibition of cyclo-oxygenase. Cyclo-oxygenase inhibition blocks the formation of proinflammatory prostaglandins as well as the aggregation of platelets. Thus far, it has been difficult to correlate prophylactic efficacy with inhibition of platelet function.

NSAIDs that have been shown to exhibit prophylactic effects in controlled clinical trials include (1) aspirin, (2) naproxen/naproxen sodium, (3) tolfenamic acid, (4) ketoprofen, (5) mefenamic acid, and (6) fenoprofen.

Side effects of NSAIDs are mainly referable to the gastrointestinal tract (dyspepsia, diarrhea, gastritis) but can also include increased bleeding and, with long-term high-dose use, renal abnormalities. With toxic levels tinnitus can occur.

Contraindications include peptic ulcer disease, hypersensitivity to other NSAIDs, chronic anticoagulation therapy, renal or liver disease, or age under 12 years.

There have been no trials to compare the efficacy of different NSAIDs.

Naproxen sodium is the only agent that has been shown to be effective in controlled studies for the treatment of **menstrually associated migraine**. This, coupled with its proven efficacy in double-blind studies, makes it the first choice among the NSAIDs in migraine prophylaxis.

ANTIDEPRESSANTS. The only antidepressant with significant evidence of efficacy in migraine prophylaxis is the tricyclic antidepressant, amitriptyline. Other antidepressants sometimes prescribed to treat migraine include fluoxetine, imipramine, clomipramine, and femoxetine, but evidence supporting their use is not well established.

Amitriptyline inhibits reuptake of both noradrenaline and 5-HT; however, reuptake inhibition does not appear to correlate with efficacy in migraine. Clinical trials also indicate that amitriptyline's antimigraine activity is unrelated to its antidepressant activity. In fact, the doses generally useful in the treatment of migraine are well below those required to treat depression.

Side effects include sedation, dry mouth, weight gain, photosensitivity of the skin, tachycardia, constipation, or urinary retention.

Contraindications include narrow-angle glaucoma, urinary retention, pregnancy, and cardiovascular, renal, or liver disease.

CALCIUM-CHANNEL ANTAGONISTS. These drugs block the transmembrane influx of calcium ions through slow, voltage-dependent channels. They were first introduced for use in the treatment of migraine based on their presumed blockade of the vasospastic phase in a migraine attack. Since at this point in time, cerebral arterial vasospasm appears unlikely to occur in migraine, and flunarizine, the most effective of the calcium-channel blockers, exerts minimal calcium-channel blockade on cerebral arteries at therapeutically relevant doses, it would seem that their vasodilatory effects are not important in migraine therapy.

Flunarizine, which is probably the most effective of these agents, has a beneficial effect similar to propranolol. However, flunarizine is not available in the United States. Of those remaining, only verapamil has sufficient evidence of efficacy from double-blind clinical trials to warrant its use in the treatment of migraine.

Verapamil has been shown in two small placebo-controlled, double-blind trials to be superior to placebo. In a third trial, no significant difference was seen. In general, verapamil can be tried when other well-established agents have not been effective or well tolerated.

Side effects include hypotension, edema, nausea, constipation, and, in some cases, headache.

Contraindications include bradycardia, cardiac conduction defects, sick sinus syndrome, and use of beta-blockers.

Second-Line Agents

VALPROIC ACID. This anticonvulsant, which is known to inhibit gamma-aminobutyric acid aminotransferase, has been shown in recent double-blind clinical trials to affect a significant reduction in headache frequency and severity. It is included as a second-line agent because it is associated with a 1% to 2% incidence of neural tube defects in infants born to women taking it during the first trimester of pregnancy.

Other side effects include nausea, sedation, tremor, transient hair loss, weight gain, inhibition of platelet aggregation factor, and minor elevations in liver function tests.

Contraindications include hepatic disease, pregnancy, and clotting abnormality.

METHYSERGIDE. This ergot derivative was one of the first drugs used for migraine prophylaxis. For years it was thought to work via inhibition of 5-HT$_2$ receptors. However, recent evidence that potent, selective 5-HT$_2$ antagonists are weak or ineffective in migraine makes this unlikely. Double-blind clinical trials have demonstrated methysergide to be effective in reducing the frequency, severity, and duration of migraine attacks. Unfortunately, it is associated with the serious complications of retroperitoneal, pericardial, or pleural fibrosis. Because of the risk of these potentially fatal side effects, it should be reserved for only severe cases that are refractory to the other prophylactic regimens. Since the fibrotic complications are reversible early in the process, methysergide should be discontinued for 6 to 8 weeks every 6 months. The early symptoms of retroperitoneal fibrosis include decreased urine output and leg or back pain.

Other potential side effects are nausea, vomiting, depression, edema, sedation, dizziness, lightheadedness, peripheral edema, and vasoconstrictive effects.

Contraindications include uncontrolled hypertension, cardiovascular disease, pregnancy, peripheral vascular disease, history of thrombophlebitis, history of fibrotic disease, and impaired liver or renal function.

PHENYLZINE. This monoamine oxidase inhibitor has been shown in an open trial to be effective in 20 of 25 patients with severe migraine. The potential for a hypertensive crisis after dietary intake of tyramine-containing foods should limit its use to patients with severe migraine who have been refractory to other treatments and who are committed to strict dietary monitoring.

Other side effects include orthostatic hypotension, urinary retention, gastrointestinal disturbance, hepatotoxicity, and failure of ejaculation.

TREATMENT OF TENSION-TYPE HEADACHE

Acute Treatment

The majority of tension-type headaches are of mild to moderate severity and many patients employ nonprescription medications effectively.

Nonsteroidal Anti-inflammatory Drugs

NSAIDS are the mainstay of the acute treatment of tension-type headaches (Table 16-4). For side effects and contraindications, see p. 293.

Acetaminophen

Acetaminophen, in both 650 and 1000 mg doses, has been reported to be superior to placebo in the treatment of headache. Gastric side effects are much less prominent than in the nonsteroidals. Severe headaches are less likely to respond to acetaminophen.

Muscle Relaxants

Muscle relaxants are sometimes used to treat tension-type headache. Theoretically, these agents relax pericranial muscles and thereby affect pain. In practice, results of these treatments are usually disappointing. Such agents include diazepam, baclofen, dantrolene sodium, and cyclobenzaprine hydrochloride. Clinical trials of these medications in the treatment of acute tension-type headaches are nonexistent; therefore, their use is largely empiric.

Prophylactic Treatment

Tricyclic antidepressant medications are generally considered the first-line agents in the prophylactic treatment of tension-type headache. Of these, amitriptyline is the drug of choice. The tricyclic antidepressants inhibit reuptake of 5-HT and norepinephrine, although their exact mechanism of action in tension-type headache is not known. Other types of medications sometimes used include NSAIDs, atypical antidepressants, and valproate.

Medications Useful in Prophylaxis of Tension-Type Headache

Amitriptyline

Amitriptyline, a tertiary amine, has been shown to effect headache improvement in double-blind, placebo-controlled

Table 16-4. NSAIDs commonly used in tension-type headache

Medication	Initial dose (mg)	Repeat dose (mg)
Aspirin (325 mg)	650–975	975
Ibuprofen	600–800	600
Ketoprofen	50–75	50
Naprosyn	500–750	500
Naproxen sodium	550	275
Ketorolac (oral)	20	10
Indomethacin (suppository)	50	—

studies. Dosages range from 10 to 100 mg/day, or higher if tolerated. In some patients, its use is somewhat limited by its anticholinergic side effects (i.e., sedation, dry mouth, tachycardia, constipation, or urinary retention). To minimize the sedation, it should be given in a single dose 1 to 2 hours before bedtime. It should be started at a low dose (10 mg/day) and slowly increased over several weeks (10-mg increments at intervals of 1 to 2 weeks). Patients should be told that any beneficial effects may not be seen for 4 to 6 weeks. Other tricyclic antidepressants, such as nortriptyline, desipramine, and imipramine, may be useful; however, at present, evidence of their efficacy is scant.

Doxepin

Doxepin, another tricyclic antidepressant, improved tension-type headaches, as reflected in a headache score in a small double-blind study. Dosages from 10 to 150 mg/day have been used. Side effects are similar to amitriptyline.

Maprotiline

Maprotiline, a tetracyclic antidepressant, may be useful in chronic tension-type headache. In a small double-blind, placebo-controlled trial it decreased headache severity by 25% and increased headache-free days by 40%. Dosages from 25 to 150 mg/day are used to treat depression. Low doses should be tried in headache patients.

Fluoxetine

Fluoxetine, an atypical antidepressant, was reported in a small open study to be effective in tension-type headache.

Nonsteroidal Anti-inflammatory Drugs

NSAIDs are clearly first-line agents in the acute treatment of tension-type headaches; however, at present, there are no studies of their effectiveness in prophylaxis.

TREATMENT OF CLUSTER HEADACHE

Acute Treatment

Oxygen Inhalation

Oxygen inhalation is a safe and effective treatment for individual attacks of cluster headache in many patients. The patient who is most likely to respond to oxygen treatment is the one with episodic-type cluster headaches and who is under the age of 50 years.

Oxygen therapy is given as follows: 100% oxygen is delivered at a rate of 8 L/min for 15 minutes via a loose-fitting face mask. Nasal biprongs are unlikely to be effective. Patients who respond to oxygen usually do so within 10 minutes.

Unlike ergotamine, oxygen does not cause nausea and is not contraindicated in patients with coronary artery disease or peripheral vascular disease. The mechanism of its effect is unknown.

Ergotamine Tartrate

Ergotamine tartrate has been used since the 1940s to treat cluster headache attacks. The sublingual and inhalational routes appear to be superior to tablets taken orally. Ergotamines are an effective and well-tolerated treatment in many patients. DHE may also be of use in the acute treatment of cluster headaches. A double-blind, crossover study using intranasal DHE showed an effect on severity of the attacks but no significant effect on the duration. (See p. 289 for side effects and contraindications.)

Sumatriptan

Sumatriptan (5-HT$_{1D}$ agonist) was found to be effective in markedly reducing both the pain and conjunctival injection of cluster headache within 15 minutes in about three quarters of patients in a double-blind, controlled study. Thus far it appears to be very well tolerated in cluster headache patients. However, it should be remembered that sumatriptan is contraindicated in patients with coronary artery disease, which is common among middle-aged males, who make up the majority of cluster headache sufferers. (See p. 290 for side effects and contraindications.)

Prophylactic Treatment

In general, prophylactic treatment for cluster headache is given only during the cluster period. Once remission is established, in most cases within 3 to 6 weeks, the prophylactic agent is tapered and withdrawn.

Verapamil

Verapamil is frequently used in cluster headache with good results in many patients and few side effects. The recommended dose is 240–480 mg/day. One open-labeled trial reported a response rate of 69% in cluster headache. Another double-blind comparison trial found it to be equal to lithium in effect. (See p. 294 for side effects and contraindications.)

Ergotamine Tartrate

Ergotamine tartrate is the traditional agent used in the prophylactic treatment of cluster headache. In doses of 2–4 mg/day in either oral or suppository form, ergotamine is an effective, well-tolerated medication for many cluster headache patients. (See p. 289 for side effects and contraindications.)

Methysergide

Methysergide prophylaxis is efficacious in about 70% of cases of episodic cluster headache. The development of retroperitoneal, pleural, or pericardial fibrosis, which limits its use in migraine, is not as likely to occur in cluster headache, because the length of use is shorter. In cluster headache patients, methysergide should be discontinued for 4 to 6 weeks after 2 to 3 months of treatment. (See p. 295 for side effects and contraindications.)

Lithium Carbonate

Lithium carbonate has been shown in over 20 open clinical trials to be effective in the treatment of chronic cluster headache. There is also evidence that it can have a beneficial effect in the episodic form. Because of its rather narrow therapeutic window, it is important to monitor serum lithium levels during periods of treatment. The serum level should be obtained 12 hours after the last dose and should not exceed 1.0 mmol/L (therapeutic range is usually from 0.3 to 0.8 mmol/L). It is important to remember that certain medications can interact with lithium to increase the serum level; these include NSAIDs and thiazide diuretics. Average daily doses range from 600 to 900 mg, but should be titrated according to serum concentrations.

Steroids

Steroids are widely used in the treatment of both the episodic and chronic forms of cluster headache, even though documentation of their effect is largely limited to open trials. Prednisone, in doses of 60–80 mg/day for 1 week and then tapered over 1 to 2 weeks, is a frequently used protocol. Doses should be determined on an individual basis and should be geared toward brief courses and low but effective doses to avoid side effects (i.e., hyperglycemia, hypertension, psychiatric symptoms, and weight gain).

TREATMENT OF OTHER HEADACHES

Indomethacin-sensitive Headaches

There are several headache syndromes that frequently respond to prophylactic treatment with indomethacin. Indomethacin, a potent NSAID, is not effective in migraine and has significant gastrointestinal side effects. These syndromes include (1) chronic paroxysmal hemicrania, (2) hemicrania continua, (3) benign cough headache, (4) effort and coital migraine, and (5) idiopathic jabbing headaches.

It is not known why these headaches respond to indomethacin when others do not. Clinical features of indomethacin-sensitive headaches are (1) a tendency to be provoked by certain movements or activities, (2) a relatively brief duration, and (3) severe intensity.

To treat these syndromes, an initial dose of 25 mg tid is increased over several days until the attacks cease (sometimes requiring up to 150–250 mg/day). After relief is stable for several days, the dose should be titrated downward to the lowest effective maintenance dose (usually 25–100 mg/day). There is great variation between individuals in the maintenance dose required. The headaches often return after maintenance is discontinued, but prolonged remissions can occur.

Indomethacin can have potentially serious gastrointestinal side effects when given over long periods of time. These include dyspepsia, peptic ulcer, and gastrointestinal bleeding. Other potential side effects include dizziness, nausea, and purpura. Because of these side effects, it is important to find the minimum effective dose. The elixir and suppository forms appear to be better tolerated than tablets in most patients.

Nonpharmacologic Treatment of Headache

Nonpharmacologic treatments include very old therapies such as application of pressure, heat, or cold directly to the head, as well as electrical stimulation, dental treatment, acupuncture, hypnosis, relaxation training, biofeedback, and cognitive therapy. All of these techniques have proponents, but the inherent difficulties in designing and carrying out blinded, unbiased studies make it almost impossible to make blanket statements regarding their efficacy. It is impossible to predict whether an individual patient will benefit. If a patient obtains relief with one of these therapies, why argue with success?

Six Hints for Successful Headache Management

1. **Less is more.** In prescribing prophylactic therapy, start with a small dose and titrate upward using small increments at 1- to 2-week intervals. This will allow you to determine the lowest effective dose. Large initial doses and rapid dose increases will result in intolerable side effects, and effective drugs can be wrongly branded as failures. Even if side effects do not appear, patients should not be on more medicine than is necessary.

2. **Don't abandon ship.** If a prophylactic medication does not work at a modest dose, titrate upward slowly and systematically. Listen to the patient and let side effects be your guide. Give the medication an adequate amount of time to work and push to the maximum tolerable dose before giving up. Jumping to another drug too soon can result in denying your patient adequate treatment, when 10 mg more might have been effective.

3. **Pregnancy and prophylaxis can potentially precipitate problems.** Women who intend to become pregnant should be withdrawn from prophylactic treatment because the effects of many of these drugs on the fetus (especially in the first trimester) are not known. In many cases, pregnancy induces a remission in migraine attacks.

4. **All headaches are not created equal.** Just because a patient has intermittent severe migraine attacks does not mean that every headache he or she has is a migraine requiring aggressive abortive therapy. Many migraineurs have frequent simple tension-type headaches intermixed and the frequent use of ergotamines, analgesics, or barbiturate-con-

taining medications can become a part of the problem. The resulting iatrogenic rebound syndrome creates headaches for the patient and doctor alike. Treatment of mild headaches should be correspondingly mild. Patients depend on their physician to advise them of appropriate treatment.

5. **Prophylaxis is not a life sentence.** Once a patient has been headache free for 6 to 12 months, begin to talk with him or her about tapering the medications. If the attacks return immediately, you can almost always escalate the dose again. In many cases the headaches do not return. Even when they do return, prolonged periods of remission can intervene, during which the patient has been without headaches or medications.

6. **Have a plan.** One of the best therapeutic interventions is to give the patient a predetermined set of actions to take in response to his or her headaches. The patient should leave with a sense of what he or she can do in response to a mild, moderate, or severe headache. In addition, it is often good to tell those patients on prophylactic therapy what the next step will be if their present medication does not work. The lives of many patients are dominated by either their headaches or the dread of their headaches, and having a good plan begins to give them back a sense of control, which can be therapeutic in and of itself.

Selected Readings

Braam MJ, et al. Survey of analgesia regimens in burns centres in the UK. *Burns* 20:360-362, 1994.

Edmeads J. Emergency management of headache. *Headache* 28; 675–679, 1988.

Forsyth PA and Posner JB. Headaches in patients with brain tumors: A study in 111 patients. *Ann Neurol* 32;289, 1992.

Gabai IJ and Spierlings ELH. Prophylactic treatment of cluster headache with verapamil. *Headache* 29;167–168, 1989.

Mathew NT, Stubits E, Nigam MP. Transformation of episodic migraine into daily headache. *Headache* 22;66–68, 1982.

Medina JL and Diamond S. Cluster headache variant: Spectrum of a new headache syndrome. *Arch Neurol* 38;705–709, 1981.

Olesen J, ed. IHS Classification and Diagnostic Criteria for Headache Disorders, cranial neuralgias and Facial pain. *Cephalalgia* 8(Suppl 7);9–92, 1988.

Olesen J, Teelft-Hansen P, and Welch KMA, eds. *The Headaches*. New York: Raven, 1993.

Quality Standards Subcommittee of the American Academy of Neurology. Practice parameter: The utility of neuroimaging in the evaluation of headache in patients with normal neurologic examinations (summary statement). *Neurology* 44;1353–1354, 1994.

Raskin HN. *Headache*. New York: Churchill-Livingstone, 1988.

Raskin NH Treatment of status migrainosus: The American experience. *Headache* 30(Suppl 2);550–553, 1990.

Sjaastad O and Spierings ELH. "Hemicrania continua"—another headache completely responsive to indomethacin. *Cephalalgia* 4;65–70, 1984.

Taylor H, ed. *The Nuprin Report*. New York: Louis Harris & Associates, 1985.

Thomas JE, Rooke ED, and Kvale WF. The neurologist's experience with pheochromocytoma. *JAMA* 197;754–758, 1966.

Welch KMA. Drug therapy in migraine. *N Engl J Med* 329; 1476–1483, 1994.

Pain Management in Sickle Cell Crisis

Roberto Feliz

> *"As to pain, I am almost ready to say the physician who has not felt it is imperfectly educated."*
>
> S. WEIR MITCHELL

Sickle cell disease, which affects 0.15% of black children in the United States, is due to a substitution of valine for glutamic acid in the sixth position of the beta chain of hemoglobin. The exact reason why this amino acid substitution causes sickling is not known. When red blood cells containing beta chains with this amino acid substitution are exposed to conditions of decreased oxygen tension (i.e., deoxyhemoglobin), a process of microtubular polymerization and polymer aggregation is initiated. As an end product of this process a distorted sickle red blood cell is produced. Initially, the sickling process affects only the nuclear and internal milieu of the cells, which ordinarily is an oxygen-reversible process. However, when a cell sickles and unsickles repeatedly, the membrane is affected in that it loses potassium and water, and the cell becomes irreversibly sickled. It remains so even when the oxygen tension is increased.

Infarctive Crisis

Patients with sickle cell disease manifest periods of comparative well-being interspersed with periods of vaso-occlusive crisis. Once sickling has occurred red blood cells lose their pliability and become rigid. Increased blood viscosity results in vascular stasis, further sickling, sludging in the microcirculation, and vascular obstruction with tissue hypoxia and infarction. Tissue death is clinically experienced by the patient as a painful crisis.

ETIOLOGY

A number of inherited and acquired factors determine the frequency and severity of the sickle cell crisis. These include amounts of hemoglobin S in the red blood cell, nature of other hemoglobin in the red blood cell, interaction of sickling with thalassemia and glucose-6-phosphate dehydrogenase deficiency, hypothermia, dehydration, hypoxia, exertion, acidosis, and infections. These associated factors lead to a wide variability in clinical presentation among different patients as well as in an individual patient.

DISEASE PROCESS

Acute pain from the infarctive crisis may affect any tissue. The pain occurs especially in the bones, chest, and abdomen. It is important to distinguish the abdominal pain originating from an infarctive crisis (i.e., kidneys, spleen) and the pain originating from an acute surgical abdomen such as cholecystitis, appendicitis, or bowel perforation. Fever and myalgia are often present, even in the absence of demonstrable infection. This has recently led several investigators to the belief that, in addition to being a vaso-occlusive phenomena, a sickle cell crisis is also an acute inflammatory process. Pulmonary infarctions are common and may lead to repeated episodes of acute pleuritic chest pain, dyspnea, elevation of white blood cell count, and typical or atypical pneumonias. The combination of fever and anemia may result in tachycardia, which, if severe, may lead to angina. Acute arthritis with synovial effusion can occur; fluid examination may be required to distinguish a crystal from a septic arthritic joint. Bone pain is a frequent complaint. This may be difficult to differentiate from osteomyelitis or osteoarthritis. Men may develop painful priapism requiring surgical decompression.

Patients with sickle cell disease and long-standing symptoms often experience chronic pain. The recurring episodes of vaso-occlusion and subsequent infarctive crisis may lead to chronic neuropathic or central pain (i.e., thalamic pain after a cerebrovascular accident, chronic headache, neuralgias, and painful paresthesias are not uncommon in these patients).

Myofascial pain is extremely common yet often goes undiagnosed. Orthopedic pathologies, including osteomyelitis often caused by *Salmonella*, as well as vertebral compression fractures and aseptic necrosis of the femoral head, may occur.

Chronic leg ulcers are a particularly common feature in sickle cell patients. Finally, chronic cholecystitis attributable to chronic hemolysis and formation of pigmented gallstones are also frequently experienced by these patients.

TREATMENT

If pain is the most urgent of symptoms, then a sickle cell crisis demands from the physician the most prompt and involved attention. Despite the severity of the pain, many of these patients frequently go untreated. This appears to stem from several factors:

1. The complexity of objective means of pain assessment, requiring the physician to rely on the patient's report to treat the pain.
2. The lack of a specific treatment and the fear of causing addiction.
3. Frequent encounters between the health care provider and the patient often lead to the attitudes and impression that these patients are manipulative and drug seekers. The patient perceives the staff as uncaring and punitive. This

mutual distrust can lead to an atmosphere of hostility and confrontation.

Once a small blood vessel is totally obstructed by sickle cells, the obstruction is probably irreversible, and, in fact, it has been stated that a painful crisis represents an event that has already happened.

Oxygen Therapy

The role of oxygen therapy in the treatment of infarctive crisis is poorly defined. Hyperbaric oxygenation has been found to be ineffective in relieving the pain. It is generally believed that little therapeutic advantage is gained by administering oxygen when the arterial Po_2 is above 80 mm Hg. Despite this long-standing recognition, physicians continue to provide oxygen in an attempt to "unsickle" the red blood cells. Although oxygen therapy may have negative effects on erythropoiesis, it seems doubtful that it does any harm. Moreover, the presence of a small amount of additional dissolved oxygen in the plasma may be of some help.

Pharmacotherapy

Pharmacotherapy for the management of an infarctive crisis represents a particularly difficult problem for the physician. The standard recommendation for the treatment of a painful crisis of sickle cell anemia has been hospitalization, keeping the patient warm, oxygenation, intravenous hydration, and parenteral narcotics given as needed by the intramuscular or subcutaneous route. The repeated administration of intravenous fluids and parenteral analgesia, however, may result in abscess formation and peripheral nerve palsies in these patients.

In an attempt to remedy the problems encountered with recurrent admissions and treatment of sickle cell crisis, several emergency rooms now have established protocols for the management of painful sickle cell crisis based on oral therapy.

Systemic therapy using sedatives, non-narcotic analgesics, and opioids alone or in combination is usually required. The route of administration—orally, epidurally, intramuscularly, intravenously, or by patient-controlled analgesia—depends on whether the hospital emergency room has an established protocol for triage and treatment of painful sickle cell crisis (Fig. 17-1).

If no protocol exists, most hospital emergency rooms routinely begin treatment with a combination of intramuscular or subcutaneous meperidine, 75 mg, combined with hydroxyzine (Vistaril), 25 mg, given every 3 to 4 hours on an as-needed basis. The patient is then admitted to the hospital for the duration of the crisis, usually 3 to 7 days. It has become increasingly popular to use morphine, meperidine (Demerol), or hydromorphone (Dilaudid) in either continuous intravenous infusion or patient-controlled analgesia.

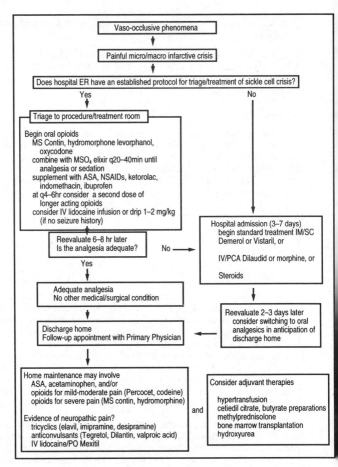

Fig. 17-1. Approach to patients with sickle cell anemia. (ASA = acetylsalicylic acid; NSAIDs = nonsteroidal anti-inflammatory drugs; PCA = patient-controlled analgesia.)

For reasons that are unclear, meperidine is the most commonly prescribed analgesic to patients with sickle cell disease. Meperidine use in this population can give rise to three major problems. First, it has a short half-life, approximately 3 hours. Second, as the patient improves, the drug administration is typically converted from parenteral to oral, but the low oral bioavailability is often not considered, and thus an ineffective dose of oral medication may be prescribed, resulting in increased pain. Third, in humans, meperidine is metabolized to normeperidine, which is renally excreted. CNS excitation and seizures have been linked directly to its accumulation. This may be a worrisome side effect, particularly in the case of sickling associated renal dysfunction.

In most instances, the painful manifestation of infarctive crisis gradually disappears over a period of hours to days with symptomatic management. At this time, depending on the severity of residual pain, the patient may be converted to oral analgesics and sedatives. This may involve a combination of acetaminophen or a nonsteroidal anti-inflammatory drug (ibuprofen, ketorolac). Nonsteroidal anti-inflammatory drugs must be used with caution in this patient population because they may cause renal failure in patients with possible borderline renal function. Frequently, however, opioids for mild to moderate pain must be prescribed (i.e., oxycodone, propoxyphene).

Pregnant women whose labor is superimposed on sickle cell pain may be candidates for a continuous epidural infusion (1–10 ml/hr) 0.1% bupivacaine in combination with 2 μg/ml of fentanyl.

Home Maintenance

Management of chronic pain in sickle cell disease can be difficult. Some patients may only require aspirin or acetaminophen between periods of acute infarctive crisis. Others may require more potent analgesics. Recently, it has been found that treating sickle cell pain like cancer pain is an effective analgesic approach for long-term management in these patients. This approach has been found to reduce hospital use by adult patients with sickle cell pain. Depending on the diagnosis, a nonsteroidal anti-inflammatory drug in combination with a sedative/anxiolytic and/or a longer-acting opioid (slow release morphine sulphate, morphine sulphate elixir) may suffice. Occasionally, chronic sickle cell pain may be opioid resistant, particularly if the pain is neuralgic or neuropathic in origin. This type of pain may respond better to treatment with tricyclics (amitryptiline [Elavil], imipramine, or desipramine) or anticonvulsants (carbamazepine, phenytoin [Dilantin], or valproic acid, clonazepam, intravenous lidocaine, or oral mexiletine). These patients are then usually discharged home, where, as outpatients, these medications are titrated to an analgesic effect unless intolerable side effects are present.

ADJUNCTIVE THERAPY

In an attempt to prevent or ameliorate the severity of the vaso-occlusive crisis, several adjunctive therapies have been tried. Hypertransfusion may be considered as an approach to get a patient through a limited period of risk such as anticipated surgery. The risk of HIV, hepatitis, and iron overload should deter this mode of therapy. Cetiedil citrate has been shown to shorten the duration of an acute painful crisis and reduce the number of painful sites. A short course of high-dose methylprednisolone has been shown to decrease the duration of severe pain in children and adolescents; however, these patients have more rebound attacks after therapy is discontinued. Other strategies aimed at preventing vaso-occlusive episodes and subsequent infarctive crisis include the use of butyrate preparations, bone marrow transplantation, and hydroxyurea aiming to decrease intracellular hemoglobin polymerization and erythrocyte sickling by increasing the levels of fetal hemoglobin.

DRUG ADDICTION

The risk of drug addiction is a constant hazard among sickle cell patients. Addictive behavior should not be rewarded. At the same time, addicted patients should never be made to suffer for fear of reinforcing their addiction. The physician must control the dose and the time of administration of narcotics. The usual approach is to give the patient a maintenance dose (e.g., methadone) as well as a dose of narcotics that will be effective in covering the painful crisis in a typical nontolerant patient.

Recurrent Crisis

If the hospital emergency room has an established protocol for triage and treatment of typical bouts of infarctive crisis, and no other acute medical or surgical problems are identified, these patients may be rushed to a procedure/treatment room in the emergency room where the patient is kept warm, aggressive intravenous (at times oral) hydration is begun, oxygen administration is provided, and the protocol for the management of sickle cell crisis based on oral therapy is started. This usually involves providing an initial loading dose of a long-acting opioid, usually 30–60 mg of MS Contin, or an equal dose of hydromorphone, oxycodone, or butorphanol. An immediate-acting narcotic is then provided, usually 10–20 mg of MS Elixir, or immediate release morphine sulfate (MSIR) given every 20 to 40 minutes until adequate analgesia or sedation is achieved. Subsequently, a second dose of the longer-acting opioid may be provided or the immediate-acting opioid may be given every 2 hours for breakthrough pain. Analgesia narcotics may be supplemented with acetaminophen or a nonsteroidal medication, usually ketorolac.

Patients who develop nausea are treated with an antiemetic medication, usually prochlorperazine (Compazine), metoclopramide, or odansetron (Zofran)/granisitron (Kytril). These patients are then re-evaluated 6 to 8 hours later. Patients who respond to treatment may be discharged home, usually on an opioid for mild pain (i.e., Percocet, codeine) and a nonsteroidal antiinflammatory drug, along with a follow-up appointment with the primary care physician. Nonresponders are admitted to the hospital where analgesia is provided using the more standard approach, as already described.

Conclusions

Painful crisis is the primary reason why sickle cell patients seek recurrent medical attention. Yet, despite the disabling nature of a painful crisis, these patients are frequently undertreated because of the unfounded assumption that they are malingerers or drug seekers. This stereotype and the mutual distrust that has developed between the patient and caregiver can be overcome if the suspicions are set aside and the disease is treated for what it is—a true medical emergency that, at times, may even be aborted if treated early.

Selected Readings

Beutler E. The Sickle Cell Diseases and Related Disorders. In: DW Williams, et al. (eds.). *Hematology* (4th ed.). New York: McGraw-Hill, 1990. Pp. 613–644.

Brookoff D, and Polomeno R. Treating sickle cell like cancer pain. *Ann Intern Med* 116:364–368, 1992.

Carache S. Treatment of sickle cell anemia. *Annu Rev Med* 32: 195–206, 1981.

Cole TB, et al. Intravenous narcotic therapy for children with severe sickle cell pain crisis. *Am J Dis Child* 12:1255–1259, 1986.

Finer P, et al. Epidural analgesia in the management of labor pain and sickle cell crisis—case report. *Anesthesiology* 68: 799–800, 1988.

Friedman, et al. Oral analgesia for treatment of painful crisis in sickle cell anemia. *Ann Emerg Med* 15:7;787–791, 1986.

Gil KM, et al. Observation of pain behaviors during episodes of sickle cell disease pain. *Clin J Pain* 10:128–132, 1994.

Griffin TC, et al. High-dose intravenous methylprednisolone therapy for pain in children and adolescents with sickle cell disease. *N Engl J Med* 330:734–737, 1994.

Rosenbloom BE and Tanaka KR. Treatment of pain in sickle-cell crisis. *N Engl J Med* 331:335, 1994.

Schechler NL, et al. PCA for adolescents in sickle-cell crisis. *Am J Nurs* 719–722, 1988.

Serjeant GR, et al. The painful crisis of homozygous sickle cell disease: Clinical features. *Br J Haematol* 87:586–591, 1994.

Shapiro BS, Cohen DE, and Howe CJ. Patient-controlled analgesia for sickle-cell-related pain. *J Pain Symptom Manag* 8: 22–28, 1993.

Sporrer KA, et al. Pain in children and adolescents with sickle cell anemia: A prospective study utilizing self-reporting. *Am J Pediatr Hematol Oncol* 16:219–224, 1994.

Pain in the Terminally Ill

Elon Eisenberg, David Borsook, and Alyssa A. LeBel

> *"Pain, whose unchecked and familiar speed*
> *Is howling, and keen shrieks day after day."*
>
> PERCY BYSSHE SHELLEY

Cancer Pain Can and Must Be Treated

Recent studies have shown that more than one third of patients with cancer have pain at the time of diagnosis of their cancer, and that more than two thirds of patients with advanced cancer have at least moderate to severe pain. It is well accepted among pain specialists that pain can be treated and relieved in the vast majority (>80%) of these patients. Both the knowledge and the means for the treatment of cancer pain are available, but, paradoxically, often underutilized. Several factors are believed to contribute to undertreatment of cancer pain—the most prevalent being poor medical education in the wide clinical spectrum of cancer pain syndromes and their therapeutic strategies, "myths" regarding opioids and their use (e.g., fear of opioid addiction by both patients and physicians and nurses), and undue concerns about respiratory depression. Effective cancer pain management requires the recognition of the nature of cancer pain and the appropriate ways to assess the pain, the pharmacology of opioid and nonopioid analgesics, and advanced pain management techniques (patient-controlled analgesia [PCA], spinal opioids, and anesthetic and neurosurgical interventions). This chapter summarizes those issues and emphasizes the concept that cancer pain can and must be treated.

The Nature of Cancer Pain

Pain in patients with cancer can originate from the tumor itself (e.g., chemical inflammation, mechanical pressure on nerves), remote effects of the tumor (e.g., paraneoplastic painful neuropathy), diagnostic procedures (e.g., bone marrow biopsy), treatment of the cancer (e.g., irradiation-induced mucositis), or pain unrelated to the patient's malignancy.

Cancer pain, like other types of pain, can be classified in a number of different ways:

1. Time course—acute versus chronic
2. Etiology—nociceptive versus neuropathic (deafferentation)
3. Location—somatic versus visceral

Patients with cancer may experience any of these pain classes. Cancer patients, particularly those in advanced stages, are prone to develop new types of pain as time goes by due to either the progressive nature of their illness or to diagnostic and therapeutic interventions that are often required. Furthermore, these patients often experience two or more pains simultaneously, e.g., multiple pains from multiple bone metastases. It is important to note that a single lesion can sometimes present itself in more than one type or location of pain. A classic example would be thoracic spinal cord compression due to spinal metastasis with a clinical presentation of an interscapular nociceptive pain and a different radicular neuropathic pain.

Patients with cancer frequently experience "breakthrough pain," which is an acute pain exacerbation that may be related to a certain factor (usually mechanical) such as position changes or may not be associated with any recognized precipitating factor (Portenoy and Hagan, 1990). Breakthrough pain usually requires special treatment considerations, as discussed subsequently.

To summarize, **cancer pain is multifactorial and dynamic in nature and therefore necessitates a continuous and consistent assessment.**

Assessment of Cancer Pain

DEFINING THE PAIN

A definition of pain is critical in the management of cancer pain. Specific factors to determine include:

Temporal nature of the pain
Localization—focal, generalized, and referred
Etiology—specific pain syndromes
Pathophysiology—somatic, visceral, and neuropathic
Concurrent problems—physical, psychologic, and social

Pain may be described as acute or chronic. **Acute pain is first pain.** It has a well-defined onset, is temporary, is provoked by injury and subsides with healing, is usually associated with autonomic signs, and is transmitted by normal sensory activity. Examples in cancer patients include mucositis, pathologic fractures, ileus, and urinary retention.

Chronic pain occurs in the absence of a detectable tissue-damaging process or persists at least 1 month beyond healing, is not associated with autonomic signs, and may be associated with peripheral and CNS dysfunction (neuropathic pain). In the patient with cancer, both temporal categories usually exist simultaneously.

Localization of pain is straightforward if its origin is cutaneous and it corresponds to a dermatomal map. Visceral pain is frequently difficult to localize, is perceived in an area larger than the affected structure, and may be felt in a body region remote from the pathologic site.

Pain syndromes in patients with cancer are associated with direct tumor infiltration in approximately 75% of cases, frequently presenting as bony (base of skull syndromes, vertebral body syndromes) or neuropathic (peripheral neuropathy, plexopathy, leptomeningeal metastases) pain. Pain syndromes associated with cancer therapy—surgery, chemotherapy, radiation—occur in approximately 20% of patients. Pain syndromes not associated with cancer or cancer therapy occur in approximately 5% of patients and include such problems as osteoarthritis, diabetic neuropathy, aortic aneurysm, and herpes zoster infection, which is five times more common in cancer patients than in the general population.

Pathophysiologic characterization of cancer pain directly dictates appropriate therapy. **Somatic pain** occurs as a result of tissue injury, is aching or gnawing in quality, is generally well localized, and is initiated by nociceptive activation in cutaneous and deep tissues. It is usually manageable with anticancer therapy (radiation therapy) and common analgesics (morphine, nonsteroidal anti-inflammatory drugs [NSAIDs]). Examples include bone metastases, fractures, and postsurgical pain.

Visceral pain is also associated with tissue injury, specifically infiltration, compression, distention, or dilatation of thoracic and abdominal viscera. Surgical resection of the viscera does not usually result in persistent pain. Visceral pain is aching, poorly localized, and often referred to distant cutaneous sites.

Neuropathic pain results from injury to the peripheral or central nervous system, or both, from tumor, surgery, radiation, or chemotherapy. Severe or dull pain is frequently associated with sensations of shooting or electrical pains superimposed on a background of burning and aching sensations. Pain is often felt in a region of sensory deficit, and mild stimuli may be perceived as painful (allodynia). Possible mechanisms of neuropathic pain include spontaneous hyperactivity of deafferented spinal pain transmission neurons, ectopic impulse generation in damaged nociceptive primary afferent fibers, and CNS plasticity with the development of activation of aberrant inputs to deafferented central pain transmission neurons, from spinal centers to the cerebral cortex.

The psychosocial assessment of the patient with cancer pain should address the following issues: the meaning of the pain to the patient and the family (i.e., severe pain implies a terminal state); the patient's typical coping response to stress and pain (i.e., would relaxation techniques, increased patient education, individual or group support, or cognitive therapy be helpful?); the patient's concerns about using controlled substances such as opioids, anxiolytics, or stimulants; changes in mood such as depression and anxiety; and the economic effect of pain and its treatment.

The definition of pain is further enhanced by asking patients to assess the intensity of their present pain as well as pain at its least and worst. The most reliable and valid pain intensity scales are the simple descriptive scale, the 0 to 10 numeric scale, and the visual analog scale (VAS).

CLINICAL ASSESSMENT

Clinical assessment naturally includes a thorough medical and neurologic examination and the use of appropriate diagnostic tools, within the framework of the evaluation just described, to ultimately identify the source of pain or a specific cancer pain syndrome. However, unidentified cancer pain syndromes or prolonged diagnostic processes should not deter adequate pain treatment.

Some common pain syndromes defined by physical examination include bone metastases, spinal cord compression, plexopathies, and mucositis. Bone metastases commonly occur with cancer of the lung, breast, and prostate and are found most frequently in the spine, pelvis, femur, and skull. The most common presenting symptom is pain, which is usually dull, aching, and aggravated by movement. Pain is typically somatic in character, well localized but possibly in multiple sites, and occasionally accompanied by neuropathic pain due to adjacent neural compression or invasion. Pathologic fractures and hypercalcemia may accompany the syndrome.

Spinal cord compression due to epidural spinal metastases is a medical emergency. In general, patients who are ambulatory when they begin treatment remain so; about one half of patients who have paraparesis before treatment regain ambulation, and patients who are paraplegic rarely recover motor control. Symptomatic vertebral body metastases occur in 5% to 10% of all cancer patients. In 8% of patients, symptomatic spinal metastases are the presenting symptom. In patients with epidural spinal cord compression, back pain is the presenting symptom in 90% of cases. Dull, aching midline back pain is usually the first symptom of epidural metastases. It is often progressive and may be associated with sharp radicular pain, suggesting nerve root involvement. Generally, neurologic deficits develop 7 weeks after initial symptoms. Treatment includes high-dose steroids, radiation therapy, and occasionally surgical intervention.

Cervical, brachial, and lumbosacral plexopathies may result from direct tumor infiltration or compression by fibrotic tissue after radiation therapy. In general, the pain of plexopathy due to tumor precedes neurologic deficits by weeks to months, whereas radiation plexopathy presents with a nonpainful loss of function. In brachial plexopathy, the lower plexus is most commonly involved, and the pain is described as a moderate to severe ache in the medial upper extremity radiating to the fourth and fifth fingers.

Mucositis may be present in patients receiving cytotoxic chemotherapy or radiation therapy to the head and neck. Pain intensity is due to the extent of tissue damage and the degree of local inflammation. It is described as a burning sensation, and it is often associated with erythema. Management includes the aggressive use of potent analgesics (opioids) and appropriate antimicrobial agents.

The desired outcome of a comprehensive pain assessment is a practical treatment plan, which should consider the following factors: the treatment setting (inpatient or outpatient), the therapeutic strategy (primary therapy of the cancer, medications, anesthetic blockade, or neurosurgical strategies), adjuvant therapies (social service, physical therapy, psychologic support), a system for monitoring the pain and its side effects (patient diary, VAS scores, bedside vital sign sheets), and scheduled follow-up (primary care physician, emergency contacts, pain clinic) (Fig. 18-1).

Cancer Pain Management

The most effective therapy for cancer pain is primary treatment of the tumor with radiation therapy, surgery, and chemotherapy. However, medical therapy with the use of analgesics is a frequent adjuvant to primary therapy, especially during painful antitumor procedures, and is the treatment of choice for chronic cancer pain, such as pain as a sequela of antitumor therapy and secondary to metastases (Fig. 18-2). Opioids are the mainstay of treatment for severe cancer pain. In 1982, the World Health Organization (WHO) declared that morphine was the drug of choice for cancer pain. This choice is based on several factors, including the availability of this agent (except in some developing countries); a bioavailability rate of 35% to 75%; a half-life of 2 to 3 hours, which is equal to the duration of analgesia; linear pharmacokinetics with repeated dosing; and multiple routes of administration.

PHARMACOTHERAPY

The three major classes of analgesics are aspirin and NSAIDs, opioids, and adjuvant agents. WHO has outlined guidelines for the use of these agents for cancer pain:

1. The use of the three-step analgesic ladder according to pain severity. For mild to moderate pain, NSAIDs or other weak analgesics (acetaminophen) are chosen. For moderate to severe pain, weak narcotics such as codeine and oxycodone are added. For severe pain, potent opioids such as morphine and hydromorphone are used. Adjuvant agents, which generally act centrally in specific pain states, may be added at each step for specific indications, such as the use of anticonvulsants for neuropathic pain and antidepressant agents for mood disturbance, insomnia, and neuropathic pain. Not all patients "climb" up all three ladder steps. For example, a patient presenting with severe pain due to bony metastases is started on opioids (third step) as the initial therapy, with or without NSAIDs and adjuvants. The guiding principles of

---

Step 1: Primary and pharmacologic therapy

Drug therapy
  opioids, e.g., morphine, levorphanol, Dilaudid
  neuropathic medications, e.g., clonazepam, mexiletine, Tegretol, Dilantin,
    amitryptiline
  anti-inflammatory medications, e.g., NSAIDs, steroids
  antianxiety medications, e.g., Ativan
  antidepressants, e.g., amitryptiline, nortryptiline, Prozac
  other medications, e.g., droperidol, haloperidol
Radiation therapy
Chemotherapy

Step 2: Alternate routes for opioid therapy

Systemic
  intravenous
  subcutaneous infusions
  transdermal
  rectal
Epidural (percutaneous)
  morphine, fentanyl–bupivacaine mix, clonidine
Intrathecal (percutaneous)
  morphine
Intraventricular (neurosurgically placed)
  morphine

Step 3: Nerve blocks

Anesthetic
  e.g., sympathetic block for acute onset of herpes zoster
Lytic
  e.g., celiac plexus block in patients with pancreatic cancer

Step 4: Neurosurgical approaches

Pituitary ablation
Intraventricular catheter
Permanent epidural/intrathecal catheter, i.e., subcutaneous
Cordotomy
Myelotomy
Rhizotomy

Fig. 18-1. The "four-step" approach to the medical treatment of cancer pain patients at Massachusetts General Hospital.

care are individualization of therapy, frequent reassessments of the patient, and balancing beneficial and adverse effects.

2. Medications are administered orally whenever possible. Tolerance to opioids will develop more slowly with this route and painful intramuscular injections will be avoided.

3. Analgesics are administered around the clock rather than as needed.

4. Side effects are anticipated and vigorously treated.

5. Placebo treatment is never appropriate care.

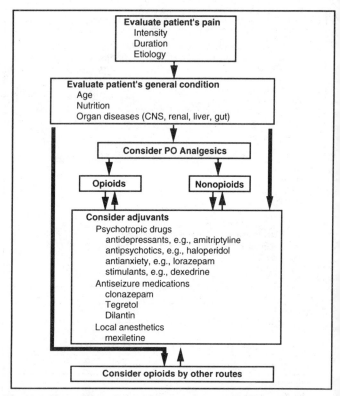

Fig. 18-2. Approach to pharmacotherapy in cancer pain patients at Massachusetts General Hospital.

Nonopioid Analgesics

The nonopioid analgesics (aspirin, acetaminophen, and NSAIDs) are used for mild to moderate pain and are a heterogeneous group of substances with different chemical properties but some similar pharmacologic properties. They have antipyretic, antiplatelet, and anti-inflammatory effects, the last due to the inhibition of cyclo-oxygenase with subsequent blockage of prostaglandin (PG) synthesis. PGE_2 and the leukotrienes are potent activators of peripheral and, possibly, central nociceptive neurons. The mechanism of acetaminophen remains obscure, but a central mechanism is likely, possibly involving CNS excitatory amino acid receptors. All nonopioids are not associated with tolerance, and all have a ceiling effect. Greater than 1300 mg of aspirin will not provide increased efficacy—only toxicity. In general, the maximal recommended dose of these medications is 1.5 to 2 times the starting dose. Side effects are common and dose dependent and include bleeding diathesis due to platelet antiaggregation and gastroduodenopathy. Also renal impairment is a hazard of morphine. Less common side effects are confusion, dysphoria, and exacerbation of heart failure and hypertension. In cancer patients with compromised blood clotting, the preferred agents are acetaminophen and choline magnesium trisalicylate (Trilisate). For all these agents, careful monitoring of blood count, fecal blood, and hepatic and renal function is suggested.

One useful effect of the nonopioids is their synergism with opioids, allowing one to use lower doses of each type of agent with minimal toxicity and maximal efficacy.

Opioid Analgesics

These agents are used to treat moderate to severe cancer pain. Morphine is the best studied opioid and is usually the drug of choice. Other opioids with different properties may be selected, however. The factors that influence this choice are analgesic potency, receptor-binding affinity, medication half-life, route of administration, dosage, and drug toxicity.

Traditionally, opioids are classified as weak and strong, a distinction based on customary use rather than significant pharmacologic differences. Weak opioids include codeine, oxycodone, hydrocodone, and propoxyphene. Of note, oxycodone and morphine have equal oral potency. However, oxycodone is usually commercially available in fixed dose combinations with aspirin or acetaminophen, limiting the upward titration of the opioid component. Using oxycodone (5-mg tablets) alone, when available, will obviate this problem. Strong opioids are available in noncombination formulations with no ceiling effect and unlimited upward titration. For example, if a cancer patient presents with mild pain, based on the WHO ladder approach, initial treatment with an NSAID such as choline magnesium trisalicylate is appropriate. The starting dose for this drug is usually 750 mg tid, increasing to a maximum of 2000 mg bid if pain persists over several days. If the patient then complains of moderate pain, the next addition is a weak opioid, alone or as a combination drug. One could choose 5 mg of oxycodone and 325 mg of acetaminophen (Percocet), 1 to 4 tablets every 4 to 6 hours, being careful not to exceed the acetaminophen "ceiling" of 4000 mg. If analgesia is still not achieved, one would add a strong opioid, such as 60–80 mg of oral morphine in divided doses, around the clock.

The choice of appropriate opioid is also influenced by its receptor-binding affinity. The pure agonist opioids, such as morphine, oxycodone, and hydromorphone, have a high affinity to mu receptors and a low affinity to kappa receptors. Activation of mu receptors results in potent analgesia as well as sedation, euphoria (with acute use), respiratory depression, bowel hypomotility, dependence, and tolerance. Of interest has been the characterization of two populations of mu receptors, mu_1 and mu_2, the latter possibly unassociated with the nonanalgesic effects of opioids. The agonist–antagonist opioids, such as pentazocine, produce analgesia, predominantly by activating kappa receptors, antagonizing mu receptors, and limiting adverse effects such as respiratory depression. These agents have a ceiling effect, however, and may not be given to patients receiving full opioid agonists, since mixed agents will likely produce opioid withdrawal and increased pain. Therefore, these agents are rarely indicated for treatment of cancer pain.

Opioids may also be selected according to the length of their half-lives. Morphine, hydromorphone, meperidine, oxycodone, and codeine have short half-lives of 3 to 4 hours. Levorphanol, methadone, and slow-release morphine (MS Contin) have half-lives of 8 to 12 hours. Of note, with the chronic use of methadone, the plasma half-life may increase to 24 to 48 hours, with the duration of analgesia remaining at 8 to 12 hours. A similar discrepancy between analgesic duration and plasma half-life, with chronic use, is noted for levorphanol. Therefore, these medications are best considered second-line opioids and are most frequently used in patients with prior opioid exposure. Repetitive doses of opioids with long half-lives may lead to drug accumulation and adverse effects, necessitating careful drug titration, especially in the elderly population. If delirium and confusion present difficulties, the use of an opioid with a short half-life is preferred.

Regarding meperidine, repetitive dosing may lead to the accumulation of its toxic metabolite, normeperidine, which has a half-life of 12 to 16 hours and is associated with CNS stimulation with subsequent tremor, delirium, and seizures. Normeperidine is two times more potent as an anticonvulsant and half as potent as an analgesic than meperidine. This toxic metabolite rapidly accumulates in patients with renal failure. In general, cancer patients with chronic pain require both a long-acting opioid for constant, chronic pain and a short-acting agent for breakthrough pain.

Route of administration is also an important consideration in the choice of an opioid. Opioids are administered by the simplest, safest, and least invasive route that will provide adequate analgesia. The oral route is preferred during the early stages of cancer. In the terminal stages, two routes of administration are required in 60% of patients, and three routes in 25%.

Most opioids are available in oral preparations, as tablets or in liquid form. For chronic cancer pain, the general practice is to combine an opioid with a long half-life around the clock with an immediate-release form, as needed, for breakthrough pain. For example, sustained-release morphine (MS Contin, Oramorph SR), which provides 8 to 12 hours of analgesia, is combined with an immediate-release or short half-life opioid (MSIR tablets, MSO_4 elixir, hydromorphone, oxycodone).

Rectal opioid preparations are available for morphine, oxymorphone, and hydromorphone and are used in patients who are sedated and confused, have gastrointestinal obstruction, or are unable to tolerate parenteral medication. The dose is equivalent to the parenteral dose of an opioid with a short half-life. The intravenous route is the fastest way to achieve analgesia and is used in patients who have rapidly escalating or otherwise uncontrolled pain or who are unable to swallow (severe nausea, mucositis). The intramuscular route is contraindicated due to pain with injection, a possible variable rate of absorption, and potential abscess formation or injection site fibrosis. Onset of analgesia after an intravenous bolus is within minutes. The duration is short, and prolonged analgesia requires continuous infusion. PCA offers the compliant patient the possible combination of a basal, continuous infusion with rapid delivery, as needed, of preselected bolus doses. This technique is most useful for patients with chronic and incident pain. The subcutaneous route is applicable for either PCA or continuous infusion and provides an alternative to the intravenous route in the home setting. The subcutaneous needle is changed every 3 days and generally is placed in the abdominal tissue. An external pump supplies a preselected dosage of medication. Dosing is equivalent to the intravenous route, as are blood levels at steady state. Bolus doses have a delayed onset, lower peak effect, and longer duration of action compared with intravenous boluses.

The transdermal route is available for fentanyl with patches at constant doses of 25, 50, 75, and 100 µg/hr. With initial application, plasma concentrations rise slowly, peak effect occurs after approximately 15 hours, and elimination half-life is over 20 hours. Therefore, fentanyl cannot be used to provide rapid analgesia, cannot be used to titrate doses, and is not the first choice for opioid-naive patients. The suggested equi-analgesic dose of transdermal fentanyl, 25 µg/hr, is oral morphine, 45–135 mg/day.

The intraspinal route (epidural and intrathecal) of opioid delivery is by intermittent injection through reservoir devices or by continuous infusion through implantable or external pumps. The advantage of spinal opioids is a long duration of analgesia (18–24 hr) with a small dose of opioid (MSO_4, 5–10 mg) compared to parenteral doses. Prolonged use of spinal administration, however, results in increased plasma drug levels, systemic delivery to the CNS, and rostral cerebrospinal fluid redistribution of the drug, thus obviating the initial advantages. Side effects such as nausea and vomiting, respiratory depression, sedation, and pruritus may not be avoided with the spinal route. Also, tolerance may develop rapidly with this route. Finally, this technique is invasive and carries risks for patients with bleeding disorders and infection. In carefully selected cases, however, it may provide excellent analgesia with few difficulties. The principle supporting the use of spinal opioids is the binding of the injected agent to spinal opioid receptors. Intraventricular morphine delivery has been used for patients with refractory head and neck pain and with advanced metastatic disease. The indications for this treatment have not been fully studied.

Additional but, as yet, investigational routes of opioid delivery are buccal, nasal, and sublingual. A nasal form of a mixed agonist–antagonist agent, butorphanol, is available, but, as previously mentioned, these medications are not recommended for cancer pain patients.

As with oral opioids, when a change from one drug to another is being made, only one half to two thirds of the new drug's equi-analgesic dose should be prescribed because of potential incomplete cross-tolerance between any two opioids. Equi-analgesic doses of the commonly used opioids are summarized in Appendix V. Attention should be paid to the enteral/parenteral equi-analgesic ratios of the different opioids. The ratio for morphine, for example, is 1:3 (morphine sulphate:10 mg IM = 30 mg PO); for hydromorphone it is 1:5. Thus, the equi-analgesic ratios of both the old versus the new drug and of the one route of administration versus the other should be taken into account when choosing the dose of a new drug. For example, a patient received 8 mg of levorphanol q4h around the clock and 4 mg of hydromorphone q3h prn. He also received two injections of meperidine, 100 mg each, since his pain was not manageable. Intravenous morphine infusion is now an optional alternative treatment. What should be the correct infusion dose? The patient received:

Levorphanol: 8 mg × 6 = 48 mg PO; equal to 360 mg of morphine PO (1:7.5).

Hydromorphone: 4 mg × 7 PO (he actually received only 7 of the 8 prn doses prescribed) = 28 mg; equal to 106 mg of morphine PO (1:4).

All previous oral medications equal 466 mg of morphine PO, which is equi-analgesic to 156 mg of morphine IM (3:1).

Meperidine: 100 mg × 2 = 200 mg IM; equal to 15 mg of morphine IM (7.5:1).

The total equivalent parenteral dose is 171 mg of morphine. For safety purposes, this should be cut by one third to one half so the baseline infusion rate could be 96 mg/24 hr or 4 mg/hr.

An exception to the rule is the use of intravenous methadone in patients tolerant to morphine or Dilaudid. Such patients should only receive 10–20% of the calculated equianalgesic dose since equianalgesic doses of methadone may produce severe respiratory depression and even death. The reason for intravenous methadone producing such analgesic effects in patients tolerant to or not responding to escalating doses of morphine or Dilaudid is unclear.

One should bear in mind that when changing from a long half-life to a short half-life opioid, the blood level of the short half-life drug increases much faster than the level of the long half-life drug drops; as a result, toxic effects may appear several hours after the change has been made. The reduction of the new drug dose by one third to one half should usually be sufficient to avoid the toxic effects, although careful monitoring of the patient is necessary. Alternatively, the change can be made gradually, e.g., substitute only 50% of the drug one day and the other 50% the next day.

Adverse Effects of Opioids

Side effects of opioids include constipation, nausea, vomiting, pruritus, sedation, confusion, and respiratory depression. Dry mouth, myoclonus, and urinary retention may also occur. These adverse effects are often readily treatable and should be anticipated in all patients on opioids.

Constipation is the most common adverse effect and does not diminish during the course of therapy. Morphine is known to increase sphincter tone, increase segmentation, increase electrolyte and water absorption, and impair the defecation reflex. Therefore, stool softeners and stimulating laxatives are concurrent treatments for patients on opioids. Patients with a rare case of refractory constipation, with intact bowel mucosa, may undergo a brief trial of oral naloxone—0.4–0.8 mg q4h until a favorable effect, no longer than 24 to 48 hours. This oral antagonist putatively acts selectively on opioid receptors in the bowel.

Opioids may produce nausea and vomiting by central effects on the chemoreceptive trigger zone and vestibular system and by peripheral effects on the gastrointestinal tract. These effects most frequently occur with the initiation of opioid therapy, and tolerance often develops within weeks. Treatment includes antiemetics, such as neuroleptics, antihistamines, and benzodiazepines, and antivertiginous drugs, such as prochlorperazine or scopolamine.

Sedation is usually related to a marked increase in opioid dose. Tolerance to this effect develops rapidly. Persistent sedation may be treated with stimulants, such as dextroamphetamine or methylphenidate.

Confusion, hallucinations, and dysphoria may also occur with opioid therapy, especially in elderly patients. Opioids may be decreased initially by 75% without precipitating withdrawal and may then be converted to an agent with a short half-life to use as needed. Concurrent assessment for other potential contributory factors, such as metabolic derangement, hypoxia, use of other medications, or cerebral metastases, is essential.

Urinary retention may require opioid discontinuation or a change to an alternative opioid. Pruritus is treated with antihistamines and, of the spinal opioids, low doses of intravenous naloxone.

Respiratory depression is the most feared and least common adverse effect of opioid therapy, especially with chronic treatment. The risk of this problem is increased by rapid dose escalation, high titration of long-acting opioids such as methadone and levorphanol, renal failure, and high-dose use in an opioid-naive patient. Pain is a potent respiratory stimulant. If respirations decrease to less than 6–8/min, physical stimulation is often sufficient, and, rarely, diluted intravenous naloxone (0.1-mg increments) may be used cautiously.

Tolerance and physical dependence are normal pharmacologic responses to the chronic use of opioids. Tolerance is characterized by decreasing efficacy with repeated administration and is treated with an increased dosage. Physical dependence is characterized by withdrawal symptoms if treatment is stopped abruptly. Neither of these factors should limit appropriate opioid use. Addiction is psychologic dependence—a behavioral pattern characterized by a craving for a drug and an overwhelming concern with obtaining it. Addiction is extremely rare in cancer patients.

Tolerance, Physical, and Psychologic Dependence

Tolerance is defined as the need for increased doses of an opioid for the maintenance of its original effect. Tolerance to both desired (analgesia) and undesired (sedation, respiratory depression) effects can develop. Cancer pain patients commonly build tolerance to the analgesic effect in the clinical setting, and the first clinical sign is usually a shortened duration of the analgesic effect. When tolerance occurs, the opioid dose should be titrated upward until analgesia is achieved again or intolerable side effects develop. If a rapid increase in opioid dose is needed, however, the patient should be re-evaluated for tumor progression.

Physical dependence is defined as the occurrence of an abstinence (withdrawal) syndrome after abrupt discontinuation of an opioid agonist. It is characterized by anxiety, irritability, insomnia, abdominal cramps, nausea and vomiting, lacrimation, rhinorrhea, salivation, and diaphoresis. The time of occurrence depends on the opioid half-life (6 to 12 hours for morphine). The development of the syndrome can be avoided by slowly reducing the opioid dose (not more than 25% every second day). In case of opioid-induced respiratory depression, careful titration of naloxone dose is necessary to avoid abstinence syndrome.

Psychologic dependence or addiction is defined as continued opioid-craving behavior and the use of opioids for purposes other than pain relief. The fear of psychologic dependence or addiction is believed to be one of the major barriers to cancer pain control. Clinical data, however, strongly suggest that there is virtually no risk of iatrogenic opioid addiction in cancer pain patients. Fear of psychologic dependence or addiction in patients with cancer is unjustified and should never be a barrier to early and aggressive use of opioids in these patients.

Adjuvant Analgesics

Adjuvant drugs are a heterogeneous group of agents that either enhance the effectiveness of opioids and nonopioids or have independent analgesic effects in specific pain states, such as neuropathic pain. They may be indicated at each step in the WHO ladder. They include tricyclic antidepressants, anticonvulsants, stimulants (as already described), and corticosteroids.

Tricyclic antidepressants are considered to provide a direct analgesic effect by blocking the reuptake of serotonin and norepinephrine at CNS synapses and are used in cancer patients with any neuropathic pain syndrome. Their analgesic effects are independent of their effects on mood. The most commonly used agent is amitriptyline, but imipramine, doxepin, nortriptyline, and desipramine are alternatives. Anticonvulsants are particularly useful in treating chronic neuralgias or in any neuropathy characterized by paroxysmal, electrical pain. The putative mechanism of analgesia is sodium-channel blockade in damaged axons. Carbamazepine and clonazepam are most commonly used; phenytoin or valproic acid may also be tried. Intravenous lidocaine or the oral lidocaine analog, mexiletine, may also be useful in neuropathic pain via sodium-channel blockade as well as a poorly described spinal effect.

Baclofen may be an adjuvant therapy for patients with facial pain, spasm, and neuropathic pain, putatively due to its GABA-b agonist effects.

Corticosteroids are useful in relieving pain from bony metastases, nerve compression, spinal cord compression, and headache due to raised intracranial pressure. They may also be used for mood enhancement and appetite stimulation.

ANESTHETIC PROCEDURES

Anesthetic procedures may be either nondestructive or destructive. The former includes epidural/intrathecal use of opioids, with or without local anesthetics, and local anesthetic blockade of peripheral nerves and sympathetic ganglia. Destructive procedures include injections of lytic agents, such as phenol or alcohol, near peripheral nerves and ganglia.

The most commonly used destructive procedure is the celiac plexus lytic block. Its efficacy is greater than 80% in visceral pain originating from both pancreatic and nonpancreatic intra-abdominal cancer. The duration of analgesia may last for months and significant complications are rare.

NEUROSURGICAL PROCEDURES

Neurosurgical procedures for pain relief are indicated in a select minority of patients. These procedures only provide temporary pain relief and are associated with the risk of subsequent neurologic dysfunction or persistent deafferentation pain, or both. These procedures include peripheral neurectomy, dorsal rhizotomy, anterolateral cordotomy, commissural myelotomy, and hypophysectomy. Unilateral cordotomy is indicated for persistent contralateral somatic pain below spinal level C5. Bilateral cordotomies can be effective for bilateral somatic and visceral pain. Complications include respiratory failure (high cervical cordotomy), sexual and sphincter dysfunction, ataxia, and paresis below the cordotomy level. Hypophysectomy is indicated for refractory, widespread metastatic cancer pain. It is usually performed stereotactically via a transsphenoidal approach, putatively creating a deafferentation lesion of the hypothalamus and activating descending analgesic systems. Complications include diabetes insipidus, cerebrospinal fluid leakage, and optic or oculomotor nerve damage. Chapter 10 discusses neurosurgical procedures for pain management in detail.

Conclusions

Pain control is but one part of a comprehensive approach to treat cancer patients. Continuing care and assessment are essential to ensure the best quality of life. This goal necessitates a comprehensive medical evaluation and accurate diagnosis, from initial therapy through to the final stages of disease. Currently available treatments, especially analgesic medications, can relieve pain in the majority of patients. Patients with intractable and severe pain would benefit from a referral to cancer pain and palliative care specialists.

Selected Readings

Amano K, et al. Bilateral versus unilateral percutaneous high cervical cordotomy as a surgical method of pain control. *Acta Neurochir (Wien)* 52(Suppl);143–145, 1991.

American Pain Society. *Principles of Analgesic Use in the Treatment of Acute and Cancer Pain.* Skokie, IL: American Pain Society, 1992.

Bates T, et al. Bone metastasis consensus statement. *Int J Radiat Oncol Biol Phys* 23;215–216, 1992.

Cherny NI and Foley KM. Current approaches to the management of cancer pain: A review. *Ann Acad Med Singapore.* 23: 139–159, 1994.

Coyle N, Adelhardt J, Foley KM, and Portenoy RK. Character of terminal illness in the advanced cancer patient: Pain and other symptoms during the last four weeks of life. *J Pain Symptom Manage* 5;83–93, 1990.

Du Pen SL, et al. Chronic epidural bupivacaine-opioid infusion in intractable cancer pain. *Pain* 49;293–300, 1992.

Ferrer-Brechner T. Anesthetic techniques for the management of cancer pain. *Cancer* 63;2343–2347, 1989.

Fitzgibbon DR and Galer BS. The efficacy of opioids in cancer pain syndromes. *Pain* 58:429–431, 1994.

Foley KM. Pain syndromes in patients with cancer. *Med Clin North Am* 71;169–184, 1987.

Gonzales GR, Eliott KJ, Portenoy RK, and Foley KM. The impact of a comprehensive evaluation in the management of cancer pain. *Pain* 47;141–144, 1991.

Hare BD. The opioid analgesics: Rational selection of agents for acute and chronic pain. *Hosp Formul* 22;64–83, 1987.

Kaiko RF, et al. Central nervous system excitatory effects of meperidine in cancer patients. *Ann Neurol* 13;180–185, 1983.

Leng G and Finnegan MJ. Successful use of methadone in nociceptive cancer pain unresponsive to morphine. *Palliative Med* 8:153–155, 1994.

Levine DN, Cleeland CS, and Dam R. Public attitudes toward cancer pain. *Cancer* 56;2337–2339, 1985.

Max MB, et al. Amitriptyline relieves diabetic neuropathy pain inpatients with normal or depressed mood. *Neurology* 37;589–596, 1987.

Melzack R. The tragedy of needless pain: A call for social action. *Sci Am* 262;27–33, 1990.

Payne R. Role of epidural and intrathecal narcotics and peptides in the management of cancer pain. *Med Clin North Am* 71; 313–328, 1987.

Portenoy RK. Constipation in the cancer patient: Causes and management. *Med Clin North Am* 71;303–312, 1987.

Portenoy RK. Management of common opioid side effects during long-term therapy of cancer pain. *Ann Acad Med Singapore.* 23:160–170, 1994.

Portenoy RK, and Hagan NA. Breakthrough pain: Definition, prevalence and characteristics. *Pain* 41;273–281, 1990.

Porter J, and Jick H. Addiction rare in patients treated with narcotics. *N Engl J Med* 302;123, 1980.

Schug SA, et al. A long-term survey of morphine in cancer pain patients. *J Pain Symptom Manage* 7;259–266, 1992.

Walsh TD. Opiates and respiratory function in advanced cancer. Recent results. *Cancer Res* 89;115–117, 1984.

World Health Organization Expert Committee. *Cancer Pain Relief and Palliative Care.* Geneva, Switzerland, World Health Organization, 1990.

19

Cancer Pain in Children

Alyssa A. LeBel

"Infants do not cry without some legitimate cause."

OMNIBONUS FENARIUS

Until recently the pain suffered by infants and children has been universally underestimated and therefore undertreated. Nowhere is the situation more unfortunate than in the management of pain associated with childhood cancer.

Most children with cancer experience pain. A prospective study assessing the prevalence and etiology of pain in children and young adults treated by the pediatric branch of the National Cancer Institute over a 6-month period demonstrated that pain was present in 54% of hospitalized patients and 25% of outpatients. The individual frequencies of the various causes of pain differed markedly from those reported in a similar adults series. Specifically, tumor-related pain accounted for 34% of the pain experienced by hospitalized children and only 18% of the pain experienced by outpatients. **Treatment-related pain** (mucositis, infection, postoperative state, neuropathic pain including vincristine-associated neuropathy and phantom limb pain, prolonged lumbar puncture headache, abdominal pain from intractable vomiting, and radiation dermatitis) **predominated in both inpatient and outpatient children**. Even in patients with active malignancy, tumor-associated pain accounted for only 46% of the pain experienced, and therapy-related pain accounted for 39%; pain of both etiologies was reported by 14% of the patients.

Several obvious differences between adult and pediatric malignancies contribute to these reported differences. First, the spectrum of malignancies seen in children is different from that in adults. Specifically, the most common malignancies seen in children—acute lymphoblastic leukemia, primary brain tumors, rhabdomyosarcoma, neuroblastoma, and other soft-tissue and bone sarcomas—are rarely seen in adults. Likewise, carcinoma, the most common adult malignancy, rarely occurs in children. Second, as a reflection of this pattern, most pediatric malignancies become widely metastatic and are rapidly fatal once they become refractory to standard therapy. An adult, however, may survive for many years with advanced disease. Third, most pediatric cancers are initially managed with aggressive multimodality treatment regimens that combine surgery, radiation therapy, and chemotherapy and are not only very effective in inducing tumor remission but also result in considerable morbidity. Fourth, when conventional therapy is no longer effective, many children continue to receive anticancer treatment which is often investigational, until shortly before their death. This approach is designed to test new treatment strategies; however, it inevitably leads to an increase in treatment-related morbidity and pain for children.

Assessment

Assessment of pain in children is similar to the assessment of pain in adults, since pain can never be seen primarily as a biologic event or a psychologic phenomenon, nor can it be separated from the social context in which it occurs. It is always a complex, multidimensional experience, including biologic, psychologic, and social interactions. Specifically in children, cognitive development and an understanding of pain influence the measurement of pain. Piagetian theory is often used to describe the developmental levels of understanding pain in school-age children; these levels are listed in Table 19-1. Speculations about younger children have been extrapolated from that framework. However, recent findings have shown that younger children have a more sophisticated understanding of pain than was previously thought. Children of 18 months of age can express and localize pain. In addition, they can recognize pain in another individual and will try to eliminate that pain. Although younger children may recover more frequently from surgery and report less pain after surgery, they typically have more pain from needle procedures than older children have. Young children's limited cognitive development may preclude an understanding of the context of the needle pain, the realization that the pain will be over quickly, and the use of effective cognitive coping strategies.

Developmental Issues and the Pain System

Until recently many clinicians have assumed that "neurologic immaturity" prevents children from experiencing pain. Cur-

Table 19-1. Development sequence of children's understanding of pain

Age	Expression of pain
6–18 mo	Fear of painful situations; use of simple words associated with pain; development of localization of pain
18–24 mo	"Hurt" used to describe pain
24–36 mo	Describes pain and external cause of pain
36–60 mo	Defines intensity of pain; use of descriptive adjectives and emotional terms
5–7 yr	Clear differentiation of levels of pain intensity
7–10 yr	Explanation of why pain hurts
> 11 yr	Explanation of the value of pain

Adapted from McGrath PJ, and Craig KD. Developmental and psychological factors of children's pain. *Ped Clin North Am* 36:823–836, 1989.

rent research disputes this contention. Pain transmission pathways develop during fetal life. Nerve tracts in the spinal cord and brainstem begin to myelinate around the gestational age of 22 weeks and are completely myelinated by 28 to 30 months after birth. More specifically, myelination is complete up to the thalamus by 30 weeks' gestation, and the thalamocortical pain connections to the cortex are myelinated by 37 weeks' gestation. Thus, pathways that can conduct noxious information from nociceptor to cortex are present in the newborn infant.

The majority of neurotransmitters and neuromodulators are present in the fetus. Calcitonin gene–related peptide and substance P are present at 8 to 10 weeks' gestation, while others such as enkephalin and vasoactive intestinal peptide appear 2 to 4 weeks later. Catecholamines are present in late gestation, and, in the human fetus, serotonin has been found at 6 weeks postnatally. Neurotransmitters that **enhance** the perception of pain are produced earlier in the fetus than are endogenous opioids.

The pain pathways of the nervous system in the mature fetus and newborn are therefore adequately developed so that the infant may exhibit a behavioral and physiologic response to noxious stimuli and may even have enhanced nociception. Because infants cannot communicate verbally, behavioral and physiologic responses can be used to assess pain in the very young, including facial expression, tachycardia, and stress related hormones. These may not be specific to pain, however

Recent research has demonstrated that pain control is very important in managing the newborn and young infant. Pain may result in a cascade of physiologic changes defined as a **stress response**.

In the past, opioid and other analgesics have been infrequently used in the treatment of the newborn and infant Although there are certain physiologic factors that force us to alter the method of providing opioid analgesia—for example, that morphine is slowly metabolized in infants under 3 to 6 months of age—our current understanding dictates that there are few contraindications to providing opioids for effective analgesia to the very young.

NEONATAL OPIOID ABSTINENCE SYNDROME

Newborn infants of mothers who are on chronic opioids may have manifestations of opioid abstinence syndrome similar to those seen in the adult, i.e., marked autonomic changes as well as encephalopathy (tremors, hyperreflexia, hypertonia, irritability). This abstinence syndrome is reportedly less prominent in preterm infants, which may relate to the stage of the developing nervous system and the ability to mount a stress response to the opioid withdrawal. Interestingly, in young animals (<8 to 10 days of age), a stress response is not seen to other non-noxious stressful stimuli.

COGNITIVE DEVELOPMENT

Coping strategies are also influenced by cognitive development. Children as young as 18 months indicate, through structured play sessions, the awareness of ways to eliminate their pain, generally by seeking hugs and kisses and asking for medicine. Children who are 3 to 4 years of age spontaneously use distraction and also report that play makes them feel better. Although they may use this technique spontaneously, children cannot deliberately distract themselves or use self-initiated cognitive strategies to decrease pain before the age of about 5 years. As a result, cognitive and behavioral strategies, such as relaxation, are generally beyond their capabilities.

Communicating pain is also influenced by cognitive development. Children as young as 18 months can indicate their pain and give a location, but it is not possible to obtain a self-report of intensity of pain before about 3 years of age. Children who are 3 years of age can give a gross indication, such as "no pain," "a little pain," and "a lot of pain." Similarly, many children at this age can use concrete measures such as "poker chips" of "pieces of hurt" to convey the intensity of their pain. The use of more abstract self-report instruments, such as the "smiling faces scale," are generally not valid for use in children under 5 years of age.

Simple self-report measures are recommended for children older than 6 years of age. Among the most useful scales for measuring intensity of pain are visual analog scales, either vertical or horizontal, and simple numeric scales—for example, "If 0 means no hurt or pain and 10 means the biggest hurt or pain you could ever have, tell me how much hurt or pain you have now." In contrast to measurement of adult pain, the use of adjectival categorical scales such as "mild," "moderate," "severe," and "excruciating" are not recommended for children younger than 13 years of age.

PAIN BEHAVIOR

Behavioral observations should not be used in lieu of self-report. However, behavioral observations are invaluable when self-report is not available—for example, in children younger than 2 years of age or in children without verbal ability due to disability or disease. In the presence of noxious stimuli, behavioral pain indicators may arouse suspicion and prompt investigations even in the absence of a verbal report of pain. Behavioral indicators of pain are listed in Table 19-2.

Neonates and infants feel pain, and neonates are no less sensitive to noxious stimulation than are older children and adults. Therefore, assessment of pain, though more complex than in older children, should be considered essential in the care of neonates and infants. In infants, reliance on facial expression, crying, posture, and physiologic variables such as heart rate, respiratory rate, blood pressure, and palmar sweating are important as potential indicators of pain.

Table 19-2. Behavioral indicators of pain

Crying
Fussing, irritability
Withdrawal from social interaction
Sleep disturbance
Facial grimacing
Guarding
Not easily consoled
Reduction in eating
Reduction in play
Reduction in attention span

Adapted from McGrath PJ. An assessment of children's pain: A review of behavioral, physiological, and direct scaling techniques. *Pain* 31:147–176 1987.

However, there are currently no physiologic measures that reliably indicate pain. Treatment of pain should never be withheld based on a lack of physiologic evidence alone.

Management

The administration of analgesics to children is according to the World Health Organization's ladder approach, as discussed in Chapter 18 for the adult cancer pain patient (see p. 314).

PHARMACOLOGIC TREATMENT

Table 19-3 lists the pediatric dosages for common pain medications.

Acetaminophen and Nonsteroidal Anti-inflammatory Drugs

Acetaminophen has been shown to be safe even for newborns in whom the immature hepatic metabolism system is protective, with decreased production of toxic metabolites. In children who are unable to take acetaminophen by mouth, the rectal route is the next option. However, in the child with cancer, bacterial seeding is a concern.

Aspirin salicylates, such as choline magnesium trisalicylate and several nonsteroidal anti-inflammatory drugs, including naproxen (Naprosyn) and tolmetin (Tolectin), are used, particularly for children with pain of inflammatory origin. The use of these medications, however, is limited in the child with thrombocytopenia, coagulopathy, or gastritis.

Opioids

As in adults, opioid analgesics are the drugs of choice for moderate to severe pain. For infants 3 to 6 months of age, clearance and analgesic effects of morphine, fentanyl, sufentanyl, and methadone resemble those for young adults. Six-

Table 19-3. Analgesic medications in children (see also Appendix V)

Drug	Dose	Route	Frequency
Acetaminophen	10–15(20) mg/kg	PO (PR)	q4h
Aspirin	10–15 mg/kg	PO	q4h
0.1% Bupivacaine	2–7 ml/hr	Epidural	continuous
Choline magnesium salicylate	10–15 mg/kg	PO	q4h
Codeine	0.5–1.0 mg/kg	PO	q4h
Fentanyl/0.1%	0.5–2.0 μg/kg	IV	q1–2h
3 μg Fentanyl/0.1% bupivacaine mix	2–7 ml/hr	Epidural	continuous
Ibuprofen	4–10 mg/kg	PO	q6–8h
Imipramine	0.2–3.0 mg/kg	PO	every night
Morphine	0.05–0.06 mg/kg per hr	IV, SQ	continuous
	0.08–0.10 mg/kg	IV	q2h
	0.10–0.15 mg/kg	IV, IM	q3–4hr
	0.2–0.4 mg/kg	PO	q4h
Morphine time release	0.3–0.6 mg/kg	PO, PR	q12h
Meperidine	0.8–1.3 mg/kg	IV	q2h
	0.8–1.0 mg/kg	IM, SQ	q3–4h
Methadone	0.1 mg/kg	IV, PO	q4h × 2, then q6–12 h
Naproxen	5–7 mg/kg	PO	q8–12h
Naloxone	0.5–1.0 μg/kg	IV	q10–15min

Adapted from Berde CB, et al. Report of the Subcommittee on Disease Related Pain in Childhood Cancer. *Pediatrics* 86:818–825, 1990.

month-old infants show no more respiratory depression from fentanyl than do adults. It is the general clinical impression that all opioids, including morphine, have a wide margin of safety and excellent efficacy for most children older than 6 months of age with cancer pain.

Premature and term infants show reductions in clearance of most opioids. The sensitivity of newborns to morphine is due, in part, to kinetic factors, including a smaller volume of distribution, diminished clearance, and, possibly, increased entry through the blood-brain barrier. An increased sensitivity on a pharmacodynamic basis, associated with immaturity of ventilatory responses to hypoxemia and hypercarbia, may be present.

For nonintubated infants younger than 3 to 6 months of age, the opioid must be used cautiously and only with close observation, and the dose is approximately one third to one fourth of that used for older children. In contrast to respiratory effects, hemodynamic effects of opioids in newborns receiving assisted ventilation are mild and may be beneficial.

For children with cancer, the oral route is most effective. However, this route may be limited by nausea, mucositis, and difficulty with swallowing pills or elixirs.

When parenteral administration is required, the intravenous or subcutaneous route can be used. Intramuscular injections should not be used, since they are painful and frightening, and children may accept pain rather than asking for a "shot."

In cases of severe pain in a patient whose dose requirement is unknown, 0.5 mg/kg of morphine can be given and reassessed every 15 minutes, with additional increments of 0.05 mg/kg administered until relief is obtained. Intermittent bolus injections of morphine or its equi-analgesic can then be provided around the clock. Continuous infusions of morphine may begin at a starting dose of 0.02–0.04 mg/kg per hour for children older than 6 months of age.

Patient-controlled analgesia (PCA) is effective for children and adolescents aged 7 years and older. However, some children and adolescents may not have the cognitive, emotional, or physical resources to use PCA.

The pharmacologic approach to the management of side effects is similar to that in adults. However, children may have difficulty communicating subjective symptoms which reflect difficulties with pruritus, nausea, and dysphoria. Therefore, if an infant or child becomes restless or irritable with increased opioid dose, treatment of side effects is suggested empirically, as is a change to an alternative opioid.

For acute respiratory depression, as dictated by professional judgment, children may receive naloxone titrated to the desired effect. The **initial dose of naloxone in a child is 0.5–1.0 mg/kg**.

Adjuvant Medications

Adjuvant medications such as tricyclic antidepressants and stimulants are beneficial as co-analgesics in children with cancer pain, with doses extrapolated from the adult dosage by weight. In general, the starting dose is low, approximately 0.3 mg/kg of amitriptyline with an increase to approximately, 1–2 mg/kg per day. A baseline ECG may be useful in patients who have received other cardiotoxic medications. The starting dose for stimulants such as dextroamphetamine and methylphenidate is 0.05 mg/kg. Corticosteroids are helpful owing to their anti-inflammatory, antiemetic, and mood-altering effects.

Analgesic Blockade

Regional blockade techniques have been developed for children of all ages, including newborns, and are generally performed with sedation or light general anesthesia because of patients' fear of needles. Regional, caudal epidural, or lumbar epidural blockade provides excellent analgesia with wide margins of safety. Hemodynamic and respiratory effects of epidural or subarachnoid blockade in infants are mild. The distribution and clearance of bupivacaine and lidocaine following regional blockade in children over 6 months of age resemble those in adults. Bupivacaine clearance is mildly delayed in newborns. Epidural and subarachnoid infusions of opioid and local anesthetics have been effectively used in infants and children who have refractory cancer pain. It is important to administer local anesthetic slowly in children, with constant assessment for clinical signs of intravascular effect.

Infants and children may also receive viscous lidocaine for mucosal analgesia. A single mucous dose of lidocaine should not exceed 4 mg/kg; a repeated oral administration of up to 2 mg/kg is generally safe. Infants and young children should receive dilute lidocaine sprays, such as 1% in neonates and 2% in children versus the 4% to 10% used in adults.

Transdermal Local Anesthetic Preparations

TAC (a mixture of tetracaine, epinephrine, and cocaine) and Emla (a eutectic mixture of 2.5% lidocaine and 2.5% prilocaine) are used in the pediatric population. TAC is administered in a maximum safe dose of 0.3–0.5 ml/kg for children. It is ineffective through intact skin but is rapidly absorbed from mucosal surfaces and is generally used during suturing of wounds. The use of Emla is risky in patients with a history of congenital methemoglobinemia. The maximum recommended application areas based on body weight are 100 cm for up to 10 kg, 600 cm for 10–20 kg, and 2000 cm for more than 200 kg. The application is applied with use of an occlusive dressing 1 hour before the procedure.

Other Techniques

Finally, children are also excellent subjects for **hypnosis, relaxation**, and **biofeedback training**, all of which are especially useful for recurrent pain such as headache and for brief painful medical procedures. Developmentally, children over the age of 7 years generally benefit from such programs, but some treatment strategies have been applied to children as young as 3 to 4 years.

Selected Readings

Anand KJS, and Hickey PR. Pain and its effects in the human neonate and fetus. *N Engl J Med* 317:1321–1329, 1987.

Berde CB, et al. Report of the Subcommittee on Disease Related Pain in Childhood Cancer. *Pediatrics* 86:818–825, 1990.

Berde CB. The Treatment of Pain in Children. In: MR Bond, JE Charldon, and CJ Woolf (eds), *Proceedings of the Seventh World Congress on Pain*. New York: Elsevier, 1991. Pp. 435–440.

Beyer JE, and Wells N. Assessment of cancer pain in children. In: RB Patt (ed), *Cancer Pain*. Philadelphia: Lippincott, 1993.

Burrows FA, and Berde CB. Optimal pain relief in infants and children. *Br Med J* 307:815–816, 1993.

Eliott K, and Foley KM. Neurologic pain syndromes in patients with cancer. *Neurol Clin* 7:333–360, 1989.

Ferrell BR, et al. The experience of pediatric cancer pain. Part I: Impact of pain on the family. *J Pediatr Nurs* 9:368–379, 1994.

Leahy S, Hockenberry-Eaton M, and Sigler-Price K. Clinical management of pain in children with cancer: Selected approaches and innovative strategies. *Cancer Practice* 2:37–45, 1994.

McCarthy PJ, et al. Report of the Subcommittee on Assessment and Methodologic Issues in the Management of Pain in Childhood Cancer. *Pediatrics* 36:814–817, 1990.

McGrath PJ, and Craig KD. Developmental and psychological factors in children's pain. *Ped Clin North Am* 36:823–836, 1989.

Zeltzer LK, et al. Report of the Subcommittee on the Management of Pain Associated with Procedures in Children with Cancer. *Pediatrics* 86:826–831, 1990.

Pain in AIDS

Ursula Wesselmann and David Borsook

> *"Oh, write of me, not 'Died in
> bitter pains,' But 'Emigrated to
> another star!'"*
>
> HELEN HUNT JACKSON

In 1983, Luc Montagnier of the Pasteur Institute published the first report on the virus that is now known to cause AIDS. The World Health Organization (WHO) estimates that, as of mid-1993, over 13 million young people and adults have become infected with the human immunodeficiency virus (HIV) since the start of the pandemic. Of the cumulative infections in adults, over 1.5 million have occurred in North America and western Europe and over 8 million have occurred in subsaharan Africa. In the United States 56% of all AIDS patients are homosexual or bisexual males and 19% are male and female drug abusers. Approximately 3% of patients at risk for HIV are hemophiliacs or other recipients of infected blood and blood products. The spread of HIV by heterosexual contact currently accounts for 5% of cases. Heterosexual transmission is the fastest growing group of AIDS cases in the United States.

Pain is the second most common reason for hospitalization of AIDS patients. The prevalence of pain is reported to be 50 to 60% in hospital and hospice inpatients, 68% in patients at home, and 97% in patients close to death. Despite the fact that pain is a relatively common symptom in HIV-infected patients, there are remarkably few studies on the management of pain syndromes in HIV disease. Although AIDS is a fatal disease, due to the lack of specific disease-oriented treatment, the life-span of HIV-infected patients can be prolonged by early antiviral therapy and prophylaxis for opportunistic infections. Quality of life becomes an increasingly important issue in these patients. However, pain in HIV-positive patients is often inadequately treated. Knowledge of the clinical presentation of pain syndromes in HIV-infected patients is essential to treat such pain appropriately.

This chapter reviews the etiology of pain manifestations in HIV-positive patients in different organ systems and discusses appropriate treatment strategies. Pain treatment is based on the underlying cause, when possible. Symptomatic measures, however, should not be delayed while the workup for the underlying etiology is in progress or if the underlying cause can not be treated effectively. Specific problems of pharmacologic and nonpharmacologic symptomatic pain relief in HIV-positive patients is also discussed subsequently. Figure

20-1 shows the most prevalent pain locations reported in HIV-positive patients. Figure 20-2 is an outline of the clinical approach to the treatment of pain in HIV-positive patients.

Gastrointestinal Pain Manifestations

ORAL CAVITY

Candidal infection (pseudomembranous, erythematous, hyperplastic, angular cheilosis) is the most common cause of oral cavity pain in HIV-positive patients. Treatment includes topical antibiotics such as nystatin, clotrimazole, topical amphotericin, and systemic antibiotics. If frequent relapses occur, topical antibiotics such as imidazoles and triazoles are used.

Perioral and intraoral painful and nonpainful ulcers are common early signs of symptomatic HIV infection. The differential diagnosis includes herpes simplex virus (HSV), varicella zoster virus (VZV), cytomegalovirus (CMV), Epstein-Barr virus (EBV), cryptococcal infection, histoplasmosis, and

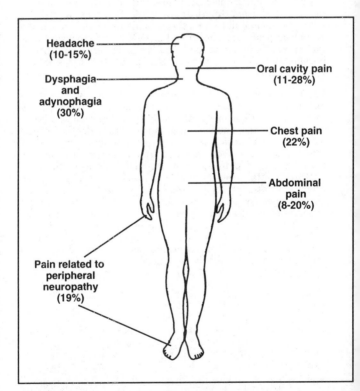

Fig. 20-1. Pain symptoms in AIDS patients.

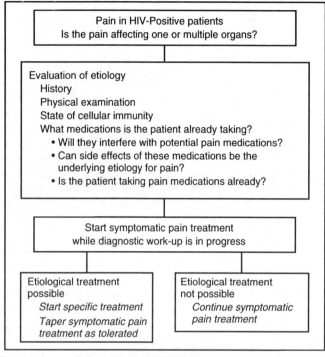

Fig. 20-2. Approach to patients with AIDS.

typical and atypical mycobacterial infections. Herpetic lesions are usually very painful, and sometimes debilitating. They should be treated with systemic acyclovir. Often the etiology of painful aphthous ulcers cannot be identified. If they are very painful and not responsive to topical therapy, a trial of steroids might be indicated, if not otherwise contraindicated in the immunocompromised host. A beneficial role of thalidomide in these patients has been reported in Great Britain; however, this drug is not available in the United States.

Kaposi's sarcoma is the most prevalent of oral neoplastic lesions in HIV-positive patients. The most common site is the palate. Oral Kaposi's sarcoma is seldom painful; however, opportunistic infections superimposed on the tumor may result in painful lesions, difficulty swallowing, and difficulty chewing.

Bacterial oral infections, necrotizing gingivitis, and dental abscesses are more common in the HIV-positive population and need to be treated with appropriate antibiotic therapy and debridement, if necessary. Regular dental hygiene is a necessity in these patients.

In addition to treatment directed at the etiology of the lesion, painful oral lesions can often be effectively treated with topically applied 2% lidocaine gel.

ESOPHAGUS

Approximately 30% of AIDS patients develop dysphagia and odynophagia. Candida infection is the most common cause and needs to be treated with systemic antifungal agents. The differential diagnosis of other infectious agents includes CMV, EBV, mycobacterium, cryptosporidium, *Pneumocystis carinii*, *Torulopsis glabrata*, and *Histoplasma capsulatum*. Endoscopy with biopsy is usually necessary to make the diagnosis, so the infectious agent can be treated appropriately. Neoplasms, such as Kaposi's sarcoma or non-Hodgkin's lymphoma of the esophagus, usually cause dysphagia but no pain. Esophageal ulcers secondary to zidovudine (AZT) therapy have been reported.

ABDOMEN

The prevalence of abdominal pain in AIDS patients ranges from 8% to 20%. Abdominal pain in HIV-positive patients includes a large differential diagnosis: infectious etiologies, neoplastic etiologies, side effects of drug therapy, and also common types of abdominal pathology such as peptic ulcer disease.

Intestinal infections usually present with abdominal cramps and diarrhea and require a thorough search for the infectious agent. Watery diarrhea is commonly caused by giardiasis, cryptococcal infection, *Mycobacterium avium-intracellulare* (MAI), or *Isospora belli*. Dysenteric symptoms are commonly associated with bacterial pathogens (*Shigella, Salmonella, Campylobacter, Yersinia*), CMV, or amebiasis. Venereal infections such as syphilis, gonorrhea, chlamydiosis, and HSV have to be included in the differential diagnosis. Large- and small-bowel perforations may be seen in CMV infections and secondary to tumor involvement (lymphoma, Kaposi's sarcoma), and *Campylobacter* infections may be associated with intussusception.

Visceromegaly can be the cause of abdominal pain related to tumor involvement or infection (CMV hepatitis, MAI, or perihepatitis associated with tubal gonococcal or chlamydial infection) in AIDS patients.

Pancreatitis in HIV-positive patients is often related to drug therapy (pentamidine, didanosine, dideoxycytidine) and may resolve with discontinuation of the drug. Acute pancreatitis can be caused by CMV infection. Acalculous cholecystitis and sclerosing cholangitis are most commonly associated with CMV and cryptosporidium infection. Extrahepatic biliary obstruction can be secondary to infections, especially MAI infection, or tumor.

HIV-positive patients are more likely to develop unusual malignancies, especially Kaposi's sarcoma and non-Hodgkin's lymphoma, which must be considered in the differential diagnosis of abdominal pain. Gastrointestinal bleeding, intestinal obstruction, and intestinal perforation due to tumor may require emergent laparotomy.

The treatment of abdominal pain includes alimentary rest, antibiotic therapy directed against the etiologic agent, if possible, antidiarrheal agents (caveat: in some abdominal infections such as *Salmonella* and *Shigella* antidiarrheal medications may prolong the illness), and antispasmodic agents. A laparotomy might be indicated if the patient presents with an acute abdomen. For patients with upper abdominal pain not responding to pharmacologic therapy, a celiac plexus block should be considered.

ANORECTAL

Thirty-four percent of homosexual or bisexual patients present with anorectal diseases. Perirectal abscesses, fissures, fistulas, and hemorrhoids are common presentations. CMV, HSV, *Neisseria gonorrhea*, *Chlamydia trachomatis*, and *Entamoeba histolytica* can cause proctitis. A slight increase in the number of anal carcinomas in HIV-positive homosexuals has been reported. Therapy is directed at the underlying etiology. Symptomatic therapy should include stool softeners to decrease pain during bowel movements.

Pulmonary Pain Manifestations

Of the few available studies that have evaluated the prevalence of pain in AIDS patients, one study found that the most prevalent pain location or syndrome was **chest pain secondary to *P. carinii* pneumonia**. Other infectious agents include opportunistic infections with CMV, MAI, *Cryptococcus neoformans*, *H. capsulatum*, *Toxoplasma gondii*, HSV, pyogenic bacteria (*Streptococcus pneumoniae*, *Haemophilus influenzae*), or mycobacteria. Therapy primarily consists of antibiotic treatment, but should also include symptomatic relief with nonsteroidal anti-inflammatory drugs (NSAIDs), if not otherwise contraindicated.

Rheumatologic Pain Manifestations

Musculoskeletal involvement has been reported in up to 72% of HIV-infected patients.

ARTHRITIS AND ARTHRALGIA

The most frequently reported type of arthritis with HIV infection is **Reiter's syndrome**. These patients predominantly present with a severe, persistent oligoarticular arthritis, primarily affecting the large joints of the lower extremities. Few patients also have a sacroiliitis. In addition many patients have other nonarticular clinical features of Reiter's syndrome such as urethritis, conjunctivitis, *Keratoderma blennorrhagicum*, balanitis, and painless oral ulcers. Patients who lack these nonarticular features are classified as having reactive arthritis. The response of articular pain in HIV-positive patients with Reiter's syndrome or reactive arthritis to NSAIDs is poor. Some patients improved with intra-articular steroids, azothioprine, methotrexate, or gold.

The prevalence of psoriasis and psoriatic arthritis is significantly higher in HIV-positive patients than in the general population. Septic arthritis caused by unusual organisms, such as *C. neoformans, Mycobacterium haemophilum,* and *Sporothrix schenckii* has been described in HIV-positive patients, but these cases are rare. HIV-related arthritis that usually affects the lower extremities and lasts about 1 month has been described. During acute HIV infections, arthralgias are often present. In addition, sudden-onset, intermittent, debilitating arthralgias lasting 2 to 24 hours have occurred in HIV-positive patients. In contrast to patients with Reiter's syndrome and reactive arthritis, the majority of HIV-positive patients with nonspecific arthralgias and HIV-related arthritides respond well to NSAIDs.

MYOPATHY

The most common type of myopathy seen in HIV-positive patients is an **inflammatory myopathy**, which is clinically identical to the idiopathic seronegative polymyositis. These patients present with proximal muscle weakness, myalgia, and muscle cramps. Creatine kinase is elevated and the EMG shows evidence of myopathy. The diagnosis can be confirmed by muscle biopsy. Treatment with corticosteroids and intravenous immunoglobulin has been advocated with variable response. The evidence of myositis as a primary manifestation of HIV infection is inconclusive.

A toxic myopathy, which is clinically indistinguishable from polymyositis, has been described after 6 to 12 months of AZT therapy with more than 500 mg/day. Symptoms frequently improve after discontinuation of AZT.

Other rare types of myopathies reported in AIDS patients have included necrotizing noninflammatory myopathy associated with and without AZT, pyomyositis, microsporidiosis of the muscle, nemaline rod myopathy, and myositis ossificans. Finally, nonspecific myalgias are common during acute HIV infection.

VASCULITIS

Seven cases of **necrotizing vasculitis** of the polyarteritis nodosa type have been reported in HIV-positive patients. In all cases the patients presented with a peripheral sensory or motor sensory neuropathy.

Hyperalgesic pseudothrombophlebitis has been described in AIDS patients, manifesting as painful calf swelling with erythema, cutaneous hyperalgesia, and fever. The treatment is elevation of the calf and NSAIDs. The differential diagnosis includes deep venous thrombosis, Baker's cyst, and cellulitis.

Neurologic Pain Manifestations

Approximately 40% of HIV-positive patients develop a neurologic symptom. Ten percent of patients experience neurologic symptoms as the initial manifestations of AIDS.

HEADACHE

Headache is a common complaint in HIV-positive patients and includes a broad differential diagnosis ranging from simple causes to life-threatening HIV-related infections or neoplasms. In AIDS patients with neurologic disease, headache has been reported to be a symptom in 55%. Knowledge of the stage of HIV disease and the immune status is necessary, because the likelihood of underlying etiologies differs with different stages of the disease. In most healthy HIV carriers with normal CD4 counts, no previous opportunistic infections, no clinical signs of immunosuppression, and no abnormal neurologic findings on clinical examination, serious neurologic complications are unlikely. Review of the headache characteristics in HIV-positive patients at the University of California, San Francisco, Headache Clinic showed that **headache that was not accompanied by intracranial pathology was usually not accompanied by nausea**. Common underlying causes for headache in healthy HIV carriers are stress, anxiety, migraine, and sinusitis.

In 1% to 2% of HIV-positive patients, acute HIV infection is associated with **aseptic meningitis**, manifesting as fever, headache, meningism, and occasionally cranial neuropathies and transient encephalopathy. The acute symptoms of HIV-related meningitis are usually self-limited and resolve within a few weeks. Treatment is symptomatic with NSAIDs; however, it should be kept in mind that NSAIDs can also be the cause of aseptic meningitis. Up to 30% of HIV carriers present with a more indolent variant of HIV-related meningitis with chronic headaches and pleocytosis. In addition to meningitis related to the HIV, the differential diagnosis of meningitis in AIDS includes other viruses, fungi, mycobacteria, or tumor cells (carcinomatous meningitis). Bacterial infections are rare.

Cryptococcal meningitis occurs in approximately 10% of patients with AIDS. The most common clinical symptoms are headache, meningism, fever, nausea, altered mental status, and cranial neuropathies. The diagnosis is made by cerebrospinal fluid (CSF) analysis (usually normal cell count, normal protein, positive cryptococcal antigen, and fungal cultures).

Amphotericin B is the treatment for cryptococcal meningitis; for severe infections a second antifungal medication—flucytosine—is sometimes added. Life-long maintenance therapy with fluconazole is necessary after recovery from the acute infection.

HIV-positive patients are at an increased risk of developing **encephalitis** due to opportunistic infections. Encephalitis may present with headache and is accompanied by alterations in the state of consciousness. HIV-related encephalitis and CMV encephalitis usually present without focal neurologic findings. Encephalitis due to cerebral toxoplasmosis, cryptococcosis, VZV, HSV, *Mycobacterium tuberculosis*, and neurosyphilis is generally associated with focal neurologic abnormalities. The diagnosis can usually be made by CT or MRI with/without contrast media and CSF analysis. Treatment is specifically directed against the infectious agent.

Cerebral toxoplasmosis occurs in 5% to 10% of HIV-positive patients who present clinically with persistent headache, changes in mental status, seizures, or other focal neurologic signs. Standard treatment includes pyrimethamine, folinic acid, and sulfadiazine. To reduce the mass effect of the intracranial focal lesion, a short course of dexamethasone is often recommended.

The differential diagnosis of headache in HIV-positive patients, in addition to infectious etiologies, includes **primary CNS lymphomas, metastatic systemic lymphomas, and very rarely cranial Kaposi's sarcoma**. Four percent of patients with AIDS develop a primary CNS lymphoma, usually of the B cell type. Stereotactic brain biopsy is often necessary to distinguish CNS lymphoma from toxoplasmosis in AIDS patients. The lymphoma is radiosensitive; however, survival time is often short (3 to 6 months after radiation). Whole-brain radiation and steroids often cause a significant improvement of symptoms, particularly headache, which is an important aspect of quality of life.

Progressive multifocal leukoencephalopathy occurs in up to 4% of AIDS patients and is caused by an opportunistic papovavirus. Clinical manifestations include headache, hemiplegia progressing to quadriplegia, sensory abnormalities, aphasia, ataxia, dementia, and confusion. Death occurs 3 to 6 months after the onset of neurologic symptoms.

Headache can also result from therapy of HIV disease. A recent study reported that 16% of patients have AZT-associated headache. Another study found that 8% of patients requiring a reduction in AZT due to myelosuppression experienced a self-limited acute meningoencephalitis.

AIDS patients who present with headache frequently undergo a diagnostic spinal tap, where 10–15 ml of spinal fluid is removed, in view of the wide differential diagnosis of HIV-related infectious etiologies of headache. The percentage of AIDS patients suffering from post–lumbar-puncture headache is lower than in the non–HIV-infected comparable age group. AIDS patients who developed post–lumbar-puncture headaches responded well to epidural blood patches.

CENTRAL PAIN

Central pain is defined as pain associated with a lesion of the somatosensory pathway at any level of the CNS. It is characterized by spontaneous pain with allodynia, hyperesthesia, hyperalgesia, and hyperpathia with evidence of damage to the thalamus or structures of the CNS that supply the affected region. Central pain usually involves one half of the whole body. Etiologies include infarcts, metastases, primary brain tumors, arteriovenous malformations, aneurysms, hemorrhages, multiple sclerosis, and traumatic lesions. Recently there have been reports of AIDS patients who developed central pain due to *Toxoplasma* abscesses in the thalamic region. Treatment with amitriptyline resulted in substantial pain relief, while treatment with hydromorphone and nortriptyline was ineffective.

NEUROPATHY

Painful peripheral neuropathies have been reported in 6% to 30% of AIDS patients. The incidence of painful peripheral neuropathies is significantly increased in the advanced stages of HIV disease. Peripheral neuropathies are probably underreported in HIV-positive patients, since they are often characterized by an insidious progression while the clinician is concentrating on more life-threatening complications of AIDS.

Primary HIV-related Distal Symmetrical Polyneuropathy

The most common type of peripheral neuropathy that occurs in HIV-positive patients is a distal, predominantly sensory polyneuropathy. It can be diagnosed clinically and electrophysiologically in over one third of patients with AIDS, and pathologically in almost all patients dying of AIDS. Most AIDS patients develop this neuropathy late in the course of HIV infection, and usually in association with systemic opportunistic infections. Patients complain about a burning pain on the soles of the feet, contact hypersensitivity, or numbness of the feet. On examination, ankle jerks are decreased or absent and thresholds to sensory stimuli are elevated in the feet and legs. The sensory complaints are typically symmetrical. Weakness of the intrinsic muscles of the feet is less common. Electrodiagnostic studies are indicative of a polyneuropathy with features of both axonal loss and demyelination. The CSF cell count is normal, and there is only minimal, if any, elevation of protein. Pathologic examination of the sural nerve shows axonal degeneration of myelinated and unmyelinated axons, demyelination, and mononuclear inflammation. Gracile tract degeneration has been documented at autopsy in AIDS patients with sensory neuropathy, implying that the distal axonal degeneration affects central as well as peripheral projections of dorsal root ganglion cells.

Treatment is aimed at symptomatic relief. There are isolated reports in the literature of improvement of distal sensory polyneuropathy with AZT; however, the majority of patients do not appear to benefit from this therapy. This neuropathy does not seem to respond to plasmapheresis. Tricyclic antidepressants (amitriptyline and nortriptyline), anticonvulsants (carbamazepine, phenytoin, and clonazepam), and topical capsaicin have been used successfully for symptomatic pain relief. Mexiletine and intravenous lidocaine, which have been found to result in considerable improvement in the symptomatic treatment of painful diabetic peripheral neuropathies, have recently also been used for symptomatic pain relief in HIV-related distal sensory neuropathies, with good results in our own experience and other groups. Also, locally applied lidocaine cream has been shown to provide transient relief of burning dysesthesias. Many patients have significant pain relief with the combination of an opioid and amitriptyline.

In patients not responding to medications, as described above, or in patients who respond to these medications but suffer from intolerable side effects, local anesthetic block techniques (lumbar sympathetic blocks or lumbar epidural blocks) should be considered.

Distal Symmetrical Polyneuropathy Related to Toxic and Nutritional Causes

Distal symmetrical polyneuropathy in HIV-positive patients can also be secondary to toxic and nutritional causes, and careful, thorough history taking is essential to differentiate these neuropathies from primary HIV-related distal symmetrical polyneuropathy. The clinical presentation is the same.

Vincristine (used for chemotherapeutic protocols for Kaposi's sarcoma or lymphoma), isoniazid (used to treat tuberculosis), and the antiretroviral agents didanosine and dideoxycytidine are known to cause distal painful peripheral neuropathies. Peripheral neuropathy occurred in 34% of patients treated with didanosine in phase 1 studies. Neuropathy occurred more frequently in patients with a history of neuropathy or neurotoxic drug therapy. In patients treated with dideoxycytidine who developed a distal painful polyneuropathy acutely, the symptoms resolved 3 to 5 weeks after dideoxycytidine was discontinued. Zidovudine is not known to cause a peripheral neuropathy.

Vitamin B_6 deficiency caused by nutritional deficits or associated with isoniazid treatment (isoniazid results in a marked excretion of pyridoxine) has been shown to result in painful distal neuropathies. Supplementation of vitamin B_6 results in improvement of neuropathy. Paradoxically, vitamin B_6, when consumed in large amounts for a prolonged time (overdosage of pyridoxine prescribed to be taken with isoniazide or megadoses of "over-the-counter" multivitamins) can also cause sensory neuropathy, which improves with discontinuation of the oral intake of vitamin B_6.

Pantothenic acid deficiency has been shown to result in a predominantly sensory neuropathy, reversed by the administration of pantothenic acid.

Paresthesias consisting of tingling and pins-and-needles sensations in the distal lower extremities are one of the early signs of vitamin B_{12} deficiency. In a recent study, the clinical characteristics of distal symmetrical polyneuropathy in HIV-positive patients were similar in patients with and without vitamin B_{12} abnormalities. The majority of patients in this study, with abnormalities of vitamin B_{12} metabolism, had significant improvement of pain in their feet when treated with parenteral vitamin B_{12}.

Other common etiologies for distal symmetrical painful neuropathies include alcohol abuse and diabetes. These common causes should also be kept in mind in the differential diagnosis of "painful feet" in HIV-positive patients, since correction of the underlying metabolic abnormalities can often result in significant reduction of pain.

Inflammatory Demyelinating Polyneuropathy

Inflammatory demyelinating polyneuropathy has been described in 30% of HIV-positive patients who were evaluated for peripheral neuropathy. Acute inflammatory demyelinating polyneuropathy has been associated with HIV seroconversion, but may occur at any stage of HIV infection. Typically, in both acute and chronic inflammatory demyelinating polyneuropathies there is profound motor weakness. Sensory symptoms may precede the onset of weakness and can present as painful paresthesias.

In general, HIV-associated inflammatory demyelinating polyneuropathy is similar to the presentation in patients not infected with HIV. However, HIV-positive patients frequently have up to 50 mononuclear leukocytes per cubic millimeter in the CSF, while patients without HIV infection rarely have more than 10 mononuclear leukocytes per cubic millimeter of CSF. Plasmapheresis is currently the treatment of choice. In patients not responding to plasmapheresis, or when plasmapheresis is impractical, intravenous immunoglobulin treatment or a short course of prednisone (caveat: this can trigger additional immunosuppression) might be indicated. Prospective studies comparing these different treatment modalities in HIV-positive patients are necessary. Painful paresthesias usually resolve with treatment directed at the presumed underlying autoimmune etiology. Janisse (1993) reported a patient with Guillain-Barré syndrome but without HIV infection who was ventilator dependent and who presented with paresthesias and dysesthesias not relieved by conventional treatment. He had complete pain relief with a continuous epidural infusion of 0.0625% bupivacaine. Such options should be considered for pain relief in HIV-positive patients with inflammatory demyelinating polyneuropathy, where therapy directed against the autoimmune response fails to relief paresthesias and conventional pain medications have failed or are contraindicated in view of decreased ventilatory function.

Multiple Mononeuropathy

Patients with multiple mononeuropathies present with multifocal sensory and motor complaints in the distribution of cutaneous nerves, mixed nerves, and nerve roots. There are at least two forms of multiple mononeuropathies in HIV-positive patients. Some HIV-positive patients present with mononeuropathies of only one or two peripheral nerves and are otherwise healthy (CD4 count usually greater than 200). In these patients the mononeuropathies usually improve spontaneously or with immunosuppressive therapy, including corticosteroids, plasmapheresis, or intravenous immunoglobulin therapy. Other patients present with more widespread mononeuropathies (three or more nerves involved) and usually have a CD4 count less than 50. In these patients CMV infection is often found on nerve biopsy. Other signs of systemic CMV infection (retinitis, gastroenteritis) are frequently present. CMV neuropathy has been shown to respond to ganciclovir therapy.

In addition to therapy directed at the underlying etiology, symptomatic therapy with tricyclic antidepressants or anticonvulsants for painful sensory disturbances is often helpful.

Polyradiculopathy

Progressive polyradiculopathy usually occurs in the later stages of HIV disease, when CD4 counts are low and opportunistic infections are present. Clinically, it is characterized by lower extremity and sacral paresthesias, radiating pain in the distribution of the cauda equina, and progression to ascending sensory loss, paraparesis, areflexia, and urinary retention, developing over 1 to 4 weeks. The CSF shows a polymorphonuclear pleocytosis, elevated protein, and decreased glucose. Often CMV can be isolated by culture. EMG and nerve conduction velocity studies are consistent with widespread proximal axonal pathology in lumbar and sacral nerve root segments. Ganciclovir usually reverses the radiculopathy if the treatment is initiated before paralysis is complete. Other etiologies of progressive polyradiculopathy that have been described in HIV-positive patients are lymphomatous meningitis and neurosyphilis. Syphilitic polyradiculopathy improved with intravenous penicillin therapy.

HERPES ZOSTER

Herpes Zoster Radiculitis

Five to ten percent of HIV-positive patients develop herpes zoster radiculitis. Herpes zoster (shingles) is an acute, topically limited illness caused by a recrudescence of VZV that has been latent in one or more sensory ganglia. While one attack of herpes zoster usually confers immunity (recurrence 2% or less) in the nonimmunocompromised patient, HIV-positive patients often have repeated attacks of herpes zoster. Herpes zoster outbreaks are uncommon before age 50, and young patients with herpes zoster infections should be evaluated for immunodeficiency status.

Clinically, patients present with sharp, burning, lancinating pain and often decreased sensibility in the affected dermatomal area. Pain may occur before the typical rash appears (characteristic crops of vesicles on an erythematous base). The treatment of herpes zoster is still controversial. For patients with disseminated herpes zoster IV acyclovir is the treatment of choice (5 mg/kg q8h for 5 days). If herpes zoster is only restricted to one dermatome, the decision whether to admit the patient for intravenous acyclovir treatment will depend on the overall immune status of the individual HIV-positive patient and the risk of dissemination of herpes zoster. How often dissemination occurs in HIV-positive patients is not well known. HIV-positive patients have a higher incidence of neurologic complications of herpes zoster, specifically stroke, cranial neuropathy, or myelitis. Some authors have therefore suggested that all such patients receive acyclovir therapy.

Symptomatic pain management during the acute attack of herpes zoster includes NSAIDs, amitriptyline, doxepin, trazodone, or fluoxetine. Severe pain not improved by these medications may require narcotic agents. Subcutaneous local anesthetic and steroid injections have been reported to reduce pain, shorten the course of the acute phase of shingles, and reduce the incidence of postherpetic neuralgia in patients with and without HIV infection. Somatic blocks (intercostal nerve blocks) prior to subcutaneous infiltration allow for analgesia in the affected dermatome. Little success has been reported with somatic nerve blocks alone. Epidural anesthetic blocks with bupivacaine have been shown to result in excellent pain control in HIV-positive patients with shingles, where conventional treatment resulted in little improvement. Sympathetic blockade early in the course of the disease has been reported by some authors to provide excellent analgesia in patients with acute herpes zoster and to reduce the incidence of postherpetic neuralgia, while others found no benefit. Prospective long-term studies are necessary in the HIV-positive population to clarify this issue.

Postherpetic Neuralgia

AIDS patients with acute herpes zoster outbreaks seem to have an increased risk of developing postherpetic neuralgia, which is defined as pain in the affected dermatome lasting longer than 3 months after crusting of the skin lesions. Reports on how to prevent postherpetic neuralgia are anecdotal, and adequately controlled prospective studies involving large groups of patients are necessary. Early pain control seems to be an important factor. Clinically, the patients present with three components of pain: a constant, deep, aching, burning sensation; a spontaneous shooting pain; and a superficial dysesthetic sensation evoked by light touch or wearing clothes. The only oral medications shown to be effective for postherpetic neuralgia in controlled clinical trials are amitriptyline and desipramine. In patients who do not tolerate tricyclic antidepressants due to altered cardiac conduction, hypotension, dry mouth, constipation, urinary retention, or CNS side effects (confusion, seizures), the use of opioid analgesics should be considered, since effective pain control without untoward effects has been reported. No long-term clinical prospective trials have been performed, however.

The topical agents are another option. They are especially useful in the HIV-positive population because they have no major systemic side effects. Topical lidocaine cream applied to the painful region has been shown to decrease the pain intensity significantly with minimal systemic drug absorption. Also, aspirin in chloroform applied to the painful area (King's formula: 700 mg of aspirin dissolved in 15–30 ml of chloroform) has been shown to result in substantial pain relief. Capsaicin preparations have been advocated for postherpetic neuralgia, but in our experience patients are not able to tolerate the burning sensation when applying the cream topically.

Neural blockade provides short-term relief of postherpetic neuralgia, but the long-term efficacy of repeated neural blockade is not clearly established. Repeated epidural blocks or continuous epidural infusions with local anesthetics with or without opioids have been helpful in patients who failed topical therapy and oral medications.

Finally, patients who failed pharmacologic and local anesthetic treatment and who suffer from intractable postherpetic neuralgia should be considered for dorsal root entry zone lesions or posterior rhizotomy.

A transcutaneous electrical nerve stimulation unit is associated with almost no side effects and is occasionally of major benefit in patients with postherpetic neuralgia. A trial of this modality is warranted in every HIV-positive patient with postherpetic neuralgia.

NERVE COMPRESSION INJURIES

The bed-bound, malnourished AIDS patient is susceptible to developing pain from nerve compression. The most common symptoms are ulnar nerve compression at the elbow, resulting in pain and paresthesias in the forearm and the fourth and fifth digits, and common peroneal nerve compression at the fibular head, resulting in paresthesias and numbness over the lateral lower extremity and dorsum of the foot. These sensory symptoms usually go along with weakness in the muscles supplied by the damaged nerve. Padding of the appropriate area and limb positioning help to avoid further trauma.

BACK PAIN

Back pain in HIV-positive patients includes a wide differential diagnosis. A thorough neurologic examination, including attention to bowel and bladder function, is essential. An MRI or CT scan of the spine with and without contrast media is usually necessary to further elucidate the cause of the pain. Common causes include disk disease, spinal stenosis, spondylolysis, spondylolisthesis, facet arthropathy, and scoliosis.

Epidural steroid injections often result in considerable pain relief. Oral pain medications include NSAIDs and muscle relaxants. Physical therapy should be offered to every patient with mechanically induced back pain. In addition, epidural abscesses (bacterial, tuberculous, fungal) need to be considered in the HIV-positive population. In cases of cauda equina epidural abscesses, pain may be severe with minimal other neurologic symptomatology, unless the infection extends upward. Treatment is directed against the infectious agent, and surgical decompression may be indicated. Other epidural lesions include metastases from lymphoma requiring radiation therapy. If the platelet count is extremely low, spontaneous epidural or retroperitoneal hematoma must be considered.

Back pain can also be caused by radiculopathy, as described in the previous section of this chapter. EMG and nerve conduction velocity studies are necessary to confirm the diagnosis, and a lumbar puncture is essential to evaluate for infectious (CMV, syphilis) or malignant (lymphoma) etiologies.

Up to 20% of patients with AIDS develop a noninflammatory vacuolar myelopathy; clinically, they present with sensory ataxia and spastic paraparesis. Localized back pain and a sensory level are unusual. Spasticity can cause significant muscle pain, which is often improved with antispastic agents such as baclofen.

Although therapy of back pain is focused primarily on the underlying etiology, if possible, symptomatic pain relief should not be forgotten.

TABETIC NEUROSYPHILIS

Tabes dorsalis is characterized by lancinating or lightning pains, most frequently in the legs, but the pain can roam over the body from face to feet. Pain attacks come in bouts lasting hours to days. Other symptoms are ataxia and urinary incontinence. Homosexual men are at an increased risk for both syphilis and HIV infection. Infection with HIV may modify the natural history of syphilis and decrease the latency period before the onset of neurosyphilis. Intravenous penicillin G is the treatment of choice for neurosyphilis. The lancinating pains can be ameliorated by anticonvulsants (phenytoin or carbamazepine). Cordotomy has been reported to be successful in non–HIV-positive patients in whom medications failed to relieve the pain.

Symptomatic Pharmacologic Pain Management

Pain treatment in HIV-positive patients consists of correcting the underlying cause of the painful syndrome and of symptomatic pain management. As in cancer pain management, it is useful to start with a nonopioid drug such as acetaminophen or an NSAID for mild to moderate pain (Fig. 20-3).

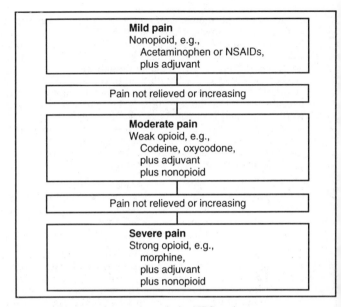

Fig. 20-3. Pharmacotherapy for pain in AIDS patients.

These medications are available for oral or rectal administration, and most recently, intramuscular or intravenous ketorolac has become available. However, we do not use ketorolac IV or IM for longer than 5 days because of its hematologic and renal side effects. If the pain is not adequately controlled by this regimen, a weak opioid such as codeine or oxycodone should be added. If the pain continues to persist, the weak opioid is replaced by a strong opioid. Different opioids can be delivered by the oral, rectal, subcutaneous, transdermal, intravenous, intramuscular, epidural, or intrathecal route. Pain medications should be given at regular intervals and additional medication should be available for breakthrough pain.

Neuropathic pain may not respond to opioid medication, but is frequently ameliorated with adjuvant analgesic drugs such as tricyclic antidepressants, anticonvulsants, and membrane-stabilizing agents. Topical applications are helpful in post-herpetic neuralgia, and viscous lidocaine has been used to reduce the pain of oropharyngeal ulcers.

Table 20-1 lists typical starting doses for commonly used pain medications (see also Chaps. 4 and 5 and Appendix 6 for a detailed discussion of these drugs).

Regional anesthetic techniques are indicated in patients who do not have adequate pain relief with analgesic medications or who cannot tolerate these medications due to severe side effects.

Table 20-1. Pain medications frequently used to treat pain in HIV-positive patients

Drug	Dose
Nonopioid analgesics	
Acetaminophen	650 mg q4h PO
Trisalicylate	750 mg tid PO
Opioid analgesics	
Codeine	30 mg q4h PO
Oxycodone	5 mg q4h PO
Morphine elixir	5–20 mg q3h PO
MS Contin	15 mg bid PO
Morphine	5–10 mg q3h IV or SQ
Fentanyl patch	25 µg/hr q3d transdermal
Levorphanol	2 mg q6h PO
Methadone	5 mg q8h PO
Antidepressants	
Amitriptyline	10–25 mg every night PO
Desipramine	25 mg qd PO
Nortriptyline	25 mg qd PO
Anticonvulsants	
Carbamazepine	100 mg bid PO
Phenytoin	100 mg tid PO
Membrane-stabilizing agent	
Mexiletine	150 mg every night PO

Other aspects of symptomatic pharmacologic pain treatment include careful wound management in this immunosuppressed group. Pain due to ileus can be difficult. Naloxone (0.4 mg q8h PO) can often improve bowel function in patients who need to continue opioids for pain control.

Pain Treatment in HIV-positive Patients with a History of Drug Abuse

Nineteen percent of AIDS patients are male and female intravenous drug abusers (IVDAs). Surprisingly, these patients have not been found to complain of more pain and did not require more analgesics than non-IVDAs in one study. In our own experience, some HIV-positive IVDAs require higher doses of opiates to control pain because they are tolerant to opioids, but their pain can be well controlled. Adequate pain control should not be withheld from this group, but specific treatment protocols that take the risk of physical and psychologic dependence into account need to be established (e.g., supervised opioid regimen by visiting nurse in outpatient setting).

Specific Problems in the Use of Drugs for HIV-positive Patients

In view of the multiple organs involved in HIV-related diseases requiring multiple drugs, careful attention to side effects, contraindications, and drug interactions is necessary when administering pain medications. Multidisciplinary consultations may be necessary to address these issues. Fear of the complexity of these issues should not prevent effective pain management, and early consultation with a multidisciplinary pain center is helpful.

HIV-positive patients often present with thrombocytopenia in the later stages of their disease, and these patients are at increased risk for bleeding when NSAIDs or aspirin is used for pain relief.

Zidovudine is metabolized by glucuronidation and is then renally excreted. Other drugs may competitively inhibit glucuronidation, such as acetaminophen, aspirin, NSAIDs, and morphine, leading to drug toxicity. Phenytoin levels have been reported to be low or very high in patients receiving AZT concomitantly, and they need to be monitored carefully. The use of acetaminophen and AZT may lead to an increased incidence of granulocytopenia.

Carbamazepine can cause neutropenia, aplastic anemia, and agranulocytosis, requiring careful monitoring of hematologic parameters in HIV-positive patients. Steroids have to be used carefully in these patients, who are already immunosuppressed. Central-acting analgesics might lead to further sedation in an already fatigued HIV-patient. We and other investigators have successfully used dexedrine (2.5–10 mg every morning) to counteract opioid-induced sedation in patients with no cardiac contraindications.

Specific Problems in the Use of Regional Anesthesia Techniques in HIV-positive Patients

Nerve blocks and regional anesthetic techniques can be very useful in treating pain in HIV-positive patients in whom analgesic medications have failed or who cannot tolerate these drugs because of severe side effects. However, the immunocompromised host is more susceptible to an infection from invasive procedures.

Contraindications for invasive procedures for pain relief in HIV-positive patients are: (1) coagulation problems and thrombocytopenia, (2) signs of bacteremia, fungemia, or other types of blood-borne opportunistic infections, (3) leukopenia, and (4) infection at the site of needle puncture. Keeping these contraindications in mind, we have had excellent pain relief with regional anesthetic techniques without significant complications in HIV-positive patients in our pain center.

Nonpharmacologic Interventions

The majority of HIV-positive patients are young and faced with a fatal disease. Psychologic and social factors contribute to the pain experience, and a comprehensive approach to the pain problem, including psychologic interventions such as relaxation therapy, hypnosis, and group therapy, in addition to pharmacological therapy, is important. Physical therapy can decrease musculoskeletal pain and helps to maintain mobility. Good nursing care and appropriate beds and mattresses will prevent or ameliorate pain from pressure sores in the terminally ill cachectic patient.

Conclusions

Pain syndromes are underreported in the HIV-positive population, often because the effort of the clinician is usually focused mainly on the diagnosis and treatment of life-threatening complications of AIDS.

Accurate assessment of pain in HIV-positive patients is important to improve the quality of life in these patients facing a fatal disease.

Knowledge of the differential diagnosis of the various manifestations of pain in HIV-positive patients is essential to treat the underlying etiology.

Symptomatic pain treatment should be started as soon as the pain problem is identified.

A comprehensive multidisciplinary approach to pain management in HIV-positive patients, similar to the approach used in cancer pain, is desirable.

Selected Readings

Cornblath DR, et al. Peripheral Neuropathies in Human Immunodeficiency Virus Infection. In: PJ Dyck et al. (eds), *Peripheral Neuropathy*. Philadelphia: Saunders, 1993. Pp. 1343–1353.

Janisse T. Pain Management of AIDS Patients. In: PP Raj (ed), *Practical Management of Pain* (2nd ed). St. Louis: Mosby, 1992. Pp. 546–578.

O'Neill, WM, Sherrard JS. Pain in human immunodeficiency virus disease: A review. *Pain* 54:3–14, 1993.

Simpson DM, and Olney RK. Peripheral neuropathies associated with human immunodeficiency virus infection. *Neurol Clin* 10:685–711, 1992.

Palliative Care of Cancer Pain

Seth A. Waldman and David Borsook

> "... there's one thing I must tell
> you: there's no question of heroism
> in all this. It's a matter of common
> decency. That's an idea which may
> make some people smile, but the
> only means of fighting a plague is
> common decency."
>
> DR. BERNARD RIEUX IN *THE PLAGUE*,
> BY ALBERT CAMUS

Pain is, unfortunately, the final common pathway of many patients who suffer from advanced cancer; up to 80% of patients will have moderate to severe pain. In addition to the incidence of chronic, nonmalignant pain syndromes, these patients may also experience pain due to primary or metastatic progression of their cancer (e.g., pathologic fracture, tumor invasion, gastrointestinal obstruction, spinal cord compression) or side effects of its treatment (e.g., deafferentation, neuropathic, or ischemic pain).

Pain control has been poor, largely due to undertreatment by physicians. Many are inexperienced with prescribing strong analgesic drugs or are unfamiliar with ancillary procedures. Others are concerned with addiction or with beginning the "slippery slope" leading to euthanasia. As a result, fear of unrelieved pain is a major concern of patients and has partly fueled the recent debate in the United States regarding euthanasia and physician-assisted suicide. The fear and hopelessness resulting from unrelieved chronic pain, coupled with the depression that is associated with terminal illness, put cancer patients at a high risk for suicidal ideation. Addressing the issue of requests for physician-assisted suicide and euthanasia is premature when adequate social and analgesic palliation is not yet widely available.

Part of the difficulty some care givers have in recognizing the importance of palliative treatment of cancer pain is that it is regarded as mutually exclusive of curative treatment. As a result, it is thought of as the final step following the failure of curative treatment rather than as a goal in itself.

The advent of hospice care in the United States in the mid-1970s is a part of the trend in "social palliation," which describes modern care of the terminally ill. Just as the application of medical and surgical attempts to cure cancer must accommodate the psychologic and social needs of patients and their families, pain control must also be integrated into their care. Terminal palliation—symptom relief without the intent to cure—can greatly improve the quality of a patient's life;

however, to die at home pain free among family and familiar surroundings should be the ultimate goal.

The mainstays of treatment for cancer pain are the potent long-acting opiates and nonsteroidal anti-inflammatory agents (NSAIDs); when used properly, they are capable of controlling pain in more than 90% of patients in this population. Inasmuch as cancer can contribute to other general pain syndromes (e.g., neuropathic pain, ischemic pain), the treatment of these syndromes is not substantively different when cancer is the inciting cause. Because opiate and NSAID use, adjunctive procedures (e.g., anesthetic and neurolytic blockade), and treatment of associated pain syndromes are described in detail elsewhere, this chapter focuses on palliative radiotherapy, chemotherapy, and surgery.

Radiation Therapy

GENERAL PRINCIPLES

Palliative radiation therapy has been a mainstay of nonsurgical cancer treatment since early in this century. In principle, it is the delivery of ionizing radiation to tissue to reduce the number of cancer cells while maintaining normal tissue integrity. This can be delivered internally (by implantation of radioactive isotopes) or, more commonly, by external beam irradiation using megavoltage photons or electrons (via a linear accelerator) or gamma rays (via a cobalt unit).

External beam irradiation is prescribed in absorbed radiation dose (the SI unit is called the gray—1 Gy is equal to 100 rads) per unit volume of tissue in a selected field. The total dose is usually delivered in fractions, the dose and field of which are determined by the volume of tissue treated and the goals of treatment.

INDICATIONS FOR PALLIATIVE RADIATION THERAPY

The primary indications for radiotherapy in the treatment of cancer pain are bone pain due to metastases (with or without pathologic fracture), spinal cord compression, blockade of hollow viscera, and reduction of space-occupying lesions (particularly cerebral metastases). It is also valuable in reducing certain tumors that are producing symptoms other than pain. Table 21-1 lists indications for palliative radiotherapy.

RADIATION THERAPY AND PAIN CONTROL

Although the etiology of bone pain secondary to tumor metastasis is unclear, radiotherapy is an extremely effective means of treatment. Overall, the response rates are as high as 70% to 80%. Osseous metastases (most commonly associated with primary tumors of the prostate, breast, and lung) tend to regress more slowly than their painful symptoms, which can resolve within 24 hours of a single fraction of ir-

Table 21-1. Indications for palliative radiotherapy

Pain relief
Bone pain
Nerve root and soft-tissue infiltration

Control of bleeding
Hemoptysis
Vaginal bleeding
Hematuria
Rectal bleeding

Control of fungation and ulceration

Dyspnea

Oncologic emergencies
Superior vena cava obstruction
Spinal cord compression
Cerebral metastases causing raised intracranial pressure

Relief of blockage of hollow viscera

Shrinkage of tumor masses
Causing symptoms by virtue of site or space occupancy

Reprinted by permission of Elsevier Science Inc. from The Role of Radiotherapy in Palliative Care, by M. Ashby. *J Pain Symptom Manage* 6(6) 383, 1991. Copyright 1991 by the U.S. Cancer Pain Relief Committee.

radiation. This dissociation between the decrease in tumor bulk and pain relief suggests that the mechanism of bone pain is not entirely secondary to mechanical effect.

Pain due to tumor invasion of nervous and soft tissue can also be treated with radiotherapy; however, treatment frequently requires higher doses of radiation, and pain relief tends to correlate with regression of the tumor. This is usually prescribed for tumors invading the brachial plexus (e.g. Pancoast's tumor of the lung) and in tumors of the head and neck.

Pain due to vertebral metastasis can be the result of bone pain, spinal cord compression, or radicular compression.

SIDE EFFECTS

Effects of tissue irradiation are both localized and systemic. Acute skin reactions (often incorrectly called burns) are due to transient damage to the basal layer of the epidermis and are severe only in radical therapy. Alopecia can occur due to irradiation of the head, and patients should be made aware that treatment not involving the scalp is unlikely to produce this effect. Late radiation effects (damage to slowly dividing cells) are not usually of consequence in terminally ill patients due to their limited life expectancy.

Hormone Therapy and Chemotherapy

Drugs used primarily to effect a cure in the cancer patient are often given to relieve painful symptoms in patients in whom a cure is no longer a realistic goal. Reduction in tumor mass with cytotoxic drugs can relieve symptoms even in cancers not usually treated primarily with drug therapy. Similarly, patients with tumors that respond to suppression of endogenous hormones or whose tumor growth is decreased by the administration of exogenous hormone therapy may experience a decrease in painful symptoms with treatment despite our inability to cure the cancer with these treatments. Examples of this are breast cancer, which may be sensitive to estrogen or progesterone receptors and can be treated with oophorectomy, androgens, estrogens, and antiestrogens in addition to cytotoxic drugs; and prostate cancer, which may respond to orchiectomy, estrogens, luteinizing hormone–releasing hormone analogs, and antiandrogens.

Palliative Surgery

GENERAL PRINCIPLES

Surgical procedures intended to reduce the painful and otherwise uncomfortable symptoms of cancer are a part of the curative and palliative treatment of cancer. These involve reducing tumor mass, interrupting pathways of pain innervation, removing tissues whose endocrine products potentiate growth of the primary tumor, and removing or stabilizing osseous metastases and pathologic fractures. Table 21-2 lists indications for palliative surgery.

NEUROSURGICAL AND ANESTHETIC PROCEDURES

Chapters 9 and 10 offer information on neurosurgical and anesthetic palliative procedures.

ORTHOPEDIC PROCEDURES

Osseous invasion by primary or metastatic tumors is a frequent cause of pain in the cancer patient. The vast majority of osseous metastases are the result of primary prostate, breast, and lung carcinomas. Symptoms may manifest as a direct result of periosteal/endosteal irritation, compression of adjacent (central or peripheral) nervous tissue, or pathologic fracture.

Metastases to the calvarium and base of the skull can produce localized pain as well as symptoms related to their location. For example, metastases to the clivus can produce severe pain referred to the calvarium, which is exacerbated by movement, and can be associated with ipsilateral cranial nerve deficits. A similar referral pattern is associated with the jugular foramen syndrome; however, arm or shoulder re-

Table 21-2. Indications for palliative surgery

Urgent
Conspicuous bleeding
Closed stenosis of a hollow viscera
Intestinal perforation
Cardiac compromise
Spinal cord compression

Tumor debulking
Hepatic and pulmonary metastases
Ulcerated and necrotic tumors with distant metastases

Surgery of metastases
Osteolytic metastases (with or without pathologic fracture) due
   to slowly progressing primary tumors

Ablative surgery
Ovariectomy
Orchiectomy
Hypophysectomy

Adapted from Bonica JJ and Ventafridda V. Pain Control with Anticancer
Modalities. In: JJ Bonica (ed), *The Management of Pain* (2nd ed). Philadelphia: Lea and Febiger, 1992. Pp. 419–420.

ferral can also occur, as can cranial nerve involvement. These
lesions are often treated with radiotherapy rather than
surgery.

Pain due to metastasis to a vertebral body is associated with
varying degrees and patterns of spinal cord and radicular
compression depending on the vertebral level. These lesions
may progress to pathologic fracture if untreated. While osseous metastases respond well overall to external beam or
systemic intravenous irradiation, lesions that develop into
fractures may require surgical stabilization or decompressive
laminectomy, or both, to alleviate the patient's symptoms. Because of their proximity to the CNS, osseous lesions are often
associated with a greater degree of plexus infiltration.

GENERAL SURGICAL PROCEDURES

Visceral obstruction is common in patients with intra-abdominal and pelvic tumors—affecting approximately one third of
all patients with colon and ovarian cancer. Postlaparotomy
adhesions or fibrosis resulting from radiation therapy may
contribute to the high incidence of visceral obstruction in
these patients. Obstruction can result not only in pain but
also in dehydration, septicemia, and primary organ failure.

While pain secondary to obstruction can often be ameliorated
by intravenous hydration, nasogastric suction, opiates, and
antiemetics, venting procedures are often very beneficial. Obstruction of the gastrointestinal tract may be treated by percutaneous gastrostomy/jejunostomy or by laparotomy with di-
verting colostomy. Obstructions of the biliary tree, as occurs

in pancreatic and hepatic carcinoma, may require endoscopic stent placement or laparotomy for biliary bypass. Similarly, obstructions of the urinary tract may often be stented with cystoscopic guidance as an alternative to open surgical bypass.

Hospice and Home Care

The variety and quality of services available to patients outside of the hospital has expanded significantly over the past two decades. This has allowed a professionally supervised care plan developed in the hospital or clinic to be continued at home. Inpatient hospice care may be the first contact that a patient's family has with medical and social palliation, and is, in many ways, a transition phase between aggressive inpatient medical treatment and home care. Since the goal of palliative care is the subjective maintenance or improvement in quality of life, as perceived by patients and their family, it is ideally accomplished at home. Coordinating these services would not be possible without a well-organized team of health professionals including nurses, social workers, clergy, home-care suppliers, and pharmacists, all of whom remain in contact with the patient's physician. Working in concert, the home palliative care team can provide patients with most of the same modalities of pain control that are available in an institutional setting (e.g., intraspinal narcotics, epidural anesthesia, patient-controlled analgesia).

Conclusions

The widening scope of palliative care of the cancer patient reflects an understanding that palliative care and pain relief must coexist with attempts to cure, rather than be regarded as the unfortunate end of failed treatment. Because length of survival is the common gauge of successful treatment, factors such as emotional and physical comfort (so-called quality of life) are often ignored in clinical trials of cancer therapy. Effective pain relief can be achieved in most patients and should be a goal of treatment in both the early and terminal stages of cancer.

Selected Readings

Ashburn M, and Lipman A. Management of pain in the cancer patient. *Anesth Analg* 76:402–416, 1993.

Ashby M. The role of radiotherapy in palliative care. *J Pain Symptom Manage* 6:380–388, 1991.

Grossman SA. United States: Status of cancer pain and palliative care. *J Pain Symptom Manage* 8:437–439, 1993.

Mercadante S, Armata M, and Salvaggio L. Pain characteristics of advanced lung cancer patients referred to a palliative care service. *Pain* 59:141–145, 1994.

Rubens R, et al. Appropriate chemotherapy for palliating advanced cancer. *Br Med J* 304:35–40, 1992.

IV

Special Considerations

Opioid Management of Chronic Nonmalignant Pain

John F. DiCapua and Alyssa A. LeBel

> *"You are outside life, you are above life, you are afflicted with ills the ordinary person does not know, you transcend the normal level and that is what people hold against you, you poison their quietude, you corrode their stability. You feel repeated and fugitive pain, insoluble pain, pain outside thought, pain which is neither in the body, nor the mind, but which partakes of both. And I share your ills, I am asking: who should dare to restrict the means that bring us relief?"* (Plea for free use of opium for sufferers including lucid madmen, tabetics, cancer patients, and those afflicted with chronic meningitis.)
>
> ANTONIN ARTAUD

Managing patients with chronic nonmalignant pain may be one of the pain specialist's more difficult tasks. Most patients do best with multidisciplinary treatment based on psychologic interventions and physical therapy. In some pain programs, however, patients may improve function without increasing pain control. For these carefully monitored patients, chronic opioid therapy may complement a multidisciplinary approach. This chapter outlines factors that need to be considered when treating chronic pain patients with opioids. These factors include effectiveness of opioids for neuropathic pain; adverse effects of opioids; and opioid tolerance, dependence, and addiction. Figure 22-1 is a flowchart of issues that should be considered in the treatment of chronic pain (noncancer) patients with opioids.

Effectiveness

Opioid responsiveness, or effectiveness, is difficult to assess clinically owing to confounding patient issues such as psychologic distress, individual sensitivity to side effects, prior exposure to opioids, and, possibly, genetic factors. The temporal nature of the pain and its putative pathophysiology also influence opioid effectiveness. Finally, there is disagreement regarding the goal of treatment. Is analgesia enough, or is

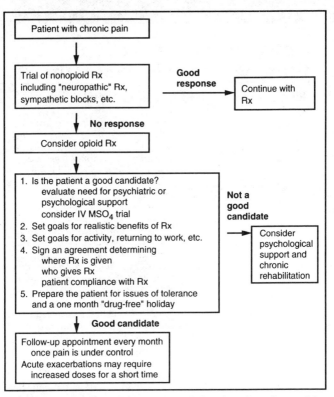

Fig. 22-1. Approach to the treatment of chronic pain patients with opioids.

improved function necessary? Overall, studies that adequately address either of these issues are scarce.

One such study by Robowtham and colleagues (1991) supports the use of opioids in neuropathic pain in humans. In this double-blind, placebo-controlled study of 19 patients with postherpetic neuralgia, both intravenous lidocaine and morphine reduced the pain of postherpetic neuralgia compared to saline control. In some survey studies, the usefulness of opioids is also supported. In one such study involving chronic pain patients managed with opioids, one third of the patients achieved adequate pain relief and one third achieved partial pain relief. Few patients had dramatic improvement in employment status or family relationships attributable to the treatment program. In another study of five patients with postamputation pain, opioids produced a 50% reduction in phantom pain for more than 22 months. In a study by Bouckoms and associates (1992) of 59 chronic pain patients referred for psychiatric evaluation, 20 (34%) were pain free on opioids by the end of 36 months of regular followup. Surveys by Taub (1982) and Tennant and colleagues (1988) also suggest that opioids can be used to decrease chronic pain; however, data from these surveys lack clinical detail of specific pain etiologies and can not be used to generalize.

Clinically, select patients with all types of chronic pain respond to opioid analgesia. Initially it was thought that neuropathic pain was unresponsive to opioids. However, more recently, evidence suggests that neuropathic pain may be resistant, but by no means always unresponsive, to opioids. "Opioid resistance" may be a matter of an inadequate dosage rather than an inappropriate drug. The dose-response curve for opioid therapy may be "shifted to the right" for patients with neuropathic pain.

Controlled and survey data that negate the effectiveness of opioid therapy in chronic nonmalignant pain are also limited. Tasker and Dostrovsky retrospectively reviewed 168 patients with neuropathic pain and reported that opioid analgesics are most effective against evoked pain, less effective against lancinating pain, and rarely effective against steady pain. Arner and Meyerson administered single doses of opioids to patients with neuropathic pain without benefit, possibly a dose-related effect. Max compared single doses of clonidine, codeine, ibuprofen, and placebo in patients with postherpetic neuralgia. He found that reported pain relief following 120 mg of codeine did not differ from placebo, again, possibly a dose-related phenomenon.

Overall, it is clear that there is a select group of chronic pain patients of all types that derives pain relief from opioids. However, evidence does not support that chronic pain patients on opioids frequently improve functionally. This factor should not necessarily limit treatment options. Conversely, pain treatment should not be withheld if a patient functions despite the pain.

Adverse Effects

The side effects of opioids have been discussed elsewhere in this handbook. An appropriate concern is that long-term opiate use can produce prolonged unwanted side effects or irreversible tissue damage. Most studies on this topic were done on cancer patients and methadone-maintenance patients. The following summarizes the findings:

1. Ten to twenty percent of patients report persistent constipation, increased sweating, insomnia, mental clouding, and decreased sexual function.
2. There is a tendency toward elevated serum albumin and disturbances in hypothalamic/pituitary regulation, particularly abnormalities in prolactin fluctuation.
3. Progressive hepatic dysfunction does not occur in methadone-maintenance patients in the absence of viral hepa-

titis or ethanol abuse. Other serious organ toxicity has not been found.

4. It is unclear whether chronic opioids produce subtle neuropsychologic abnormalities. Surveys that suggest the presence of mild neuropsychologic changes often do not control for the concurrent use of sedative/hypnotic drugs, history of head trauma, or premorbid neuropsychologic disturbances. In one study of methadone-maintenance patients these changes were not found, and a study of cancer patients indicates that tolerance to the cognitive impairment produced by opioids develops rapidly.

Overall, it appears that long-term side effects, tissue damage, or subtle neuropsychologic abnormalities do not appear to be a prohibitory problem of chronic opioid use.

Tolerance, Physical Dependence, and Addiction

The terminology relating to narcotic analgesic consumption is confusing. For example, drug addiction is defined differently by the World Health Organization, the DSM-IV, the American Medical Association, and multiple individual researchers, making it difficult to compare studies. The following definitions are adapted from Rinaldi and colleagues (1988).

Drug addiction is a disorder characterized by compulsive use of a substance resulting in physical, psychologic, or social harm to the user and continued use despite that harm.

Drug dependence is a generic term that relates to physical or psychologic dependence, or both. It is characteristic for each pharmacologic class of psychoactive drugs. Impaired control over drug-taking behavior is implied.

Drug abuse is any use of drugs that causes physical, psychologic, economic, legal, or social harm to the individual user or to others affected by the drug user's behavior.

Physical dependence is a physiologic state of adaptation to a drug or alcohol, usually characterized by the development of tolerance to drug effects and the emergence of a withdrawal syndrome during prolonged abstinence.

Psychologic dependence is the emotional state of craving a drug either for its positive effect or to avoid negative effects associated with its absence.

Tolerance is physiologic adaptation to the effect of drugs, so as to diminish effects with constant dosages or to maintain the intensity and duration of effects through increased dosage.

Neither tolerance nor physical dependence has been shown to be a limiting factor in the use of opiates for chronic pain or cancer pain. Many chronic pain patients have been managed with stable, constant doses of opiates as long as the disease does not progress. As seen with cancer patients, the need for progressive dose escalation is usually observed only in those with an obviously advancing painful lesion. On occasion, patients have an increase in opiate requirement to match a temporary increase in pain. Once the acute exacerbation in pain subsides, patients can often go back to their basal chronic opiate requirements. Physical dependence can be handled by tapering drug doses and the use of adjuvant drugs such as clonidine.

Drug addiction is far more complicated. Older surveys of addicted individuals suggested that a significant number of addicts became addicted following the therapeutic use of opiates. More recently, large prospective surveys of patients have found an extremely small risk of addiction following the short-term administration of opioids for pain. However, to date, no studies have directly assessed the risk of addiction among chronic nonmalignant pain patients administered opioids for prolonged periods.

In a recent review, Fishbain and associates (1992) found the prevalence of drug addiction among chronic pain patients to range from 3.2% to 16%. This means that of the patients attending chronic pain clinics, 3.2% to 16% display addictive behavior. It does not mean that 3.2% to 16% of patients in chronic pain clinics become addicts because they are given chronic opiates for management of their pain. Studies to address the latter statement have simply not been done.

Conclusions

The decision to use opioids for the management of chronic pain is not an easy one. Research tends to indicate the following:

1. There is a select group of chronic pain patients that derive pain relief from opioids.
2. Increased function has not been shown with chronic opioid pain management.
3. Even patients with neuropathic pain can respond to opioids.
4. Overall, it appears that long-term side effects, tissue damage, or subtle neuropsychologic abnormalities do not appear to be a prohibitory problem of chronic opioid use.
5. Neither tolerance nor physical dependence is a limiting factor in the use of opioids for chronic pain.
6. Addiction is a problem among chronic pain patients. However, the risk of becoming a drug addict from chronic opioid use is not known but is probably very low.

Although most clinicians will agree with the above statements, there is still a strong controversy about whether chronic pain patients should be managed with opiates. Portenoy (1990) believes that chronic pain patients should be given a therapeutic trial of opioids, and that the decision to continue opioids should depend on individual patient response. Chabal and colleagues (1992) present a biopsychosocial model of chronic pain management in which the emphasis is on behavioral therapy and self-reliance. The use of opioids is viewed as a distraction from the more useful therapeutic options. Opioids are used as an adjunctive component of therapy—that is, not to alleviate all pain but to provide a bridge until the patient no longer feels the compelling need to rely on them.

Clearly, patients must be individualized. Careful consideration of the potential risks and benefits is needed in every case. If opioids are offered for the management of chronic pain, strict guidelines should be followed. Portenoy suggests the following guidelines for the use of opioid maintenance therapy for chronic nonmalignant pain.

1. Opioids should be considered only after reasonable attempts at analgesia have failed.
2. A history of substance abuse should be viewed as a relative contraindication.
3. A single practitioner should take primary responsibility for treatment.
4. Patients should give informed consent before the start of therapy; points to be covered include recognition of the low risk of psychologic dependence as an outcome, the potential for cognitive impairment with the drug alone and in combination with sedative/hypnotics, and an understanding by female patients that children born when the mother is on opioid maintenance therapy will likely be physically dependent at birth.
5. After drug selection, doses should be given on an around-the-clock basis; several weeks should be agreed upon as the period of initial dose titration, and although improvement in function should be continually stressed, all should agree to at least partial analgesia as the appropriate goal of therapy.
6. Failure to achieve at least partial analgesia at relatively low initial doses in the nontolerant patient raises questions about the potential treatability of the pain syndrome with opioids.
7. Emphasis should be given to attempts to capitalize on improved analgesia by gains in physical and social function.
8. In addition to the daily dose determined initially, patients should be permitted to escalate dose transiently on days of increased pain. Two methods are acceptable: (1) prescription of an additional 4 to 6 "rescue doses" to be taken as needed during the month, and (2) instruction that 1 or 2 extra doses may be taken on any day, but must be followed by an equal reduction of dose on subsequent days.
9. Most patients should be seen and drugs prescribed at least monthly. Patients should be assessed for the efficacy of treatment, adverse drug effects, and the appearance of either misuse or abuse of the drugs during each visit. The results of the assessment should be clearly documented in the medical record.
10. Exacerbations of pain not effectively treated by transient, small dose increases are best managed in the hospital,

where dose escalation, if appropriate, can be observed closely and return to baseline doses can be accomplished in a controlled environment.
11. Evidence of drug hoarding, acquisition of drugs from other physicians, uncontrolled dose escalation, or other aberrant behaviors should be followed by tapering and discontinuation of opioid maintenance therapy.

Selected Readings

Bouckoms AJ, et al. Chronic nonmalignant pain treated with long-term oral narcotic analgesics. *Ann Clin Psychiatry* 4:185–192, 1992.

Chabal C, Jacobson L, Chaney EF, and Mariano AJ. The psychosocial impact of opioid treatment. *Am Pain Soc J* 1:289–291, 1992.

Fishbain DA, Rosomoff HL, and Rosomoff RS. Drug abuse, dependence, and addiction in chronic pain patients. *Clin J Pain* 8:77–85, 1992.

Jadad AR, et al. Morphine responsiveness of chronic pain: Double-blind randomized crossover study with patient-controlled analgesia. *Lancet* 339:1367–1371, 1992.

Portenoy RK. Chronic opioid therapy in nonmalignant pain. *J Pain Symptom Manage* 5(Suppl):S46–S62, 1990.

Portenoy RK, Foley KM, and Inturrisi DE. The nature of opioid responsiveness and its implications for neuropathic pain: New hypotheses derived from studies of opioid infusions. *Pain* 43:273–286, 1990.

Portenoy RK, and Foley KM. Chronic use of opioid analgesics in non-malignant pain: Report of 38 cases. *Pain* 25:171–186, 1986.

Porter J, and Jick H. Addiction rare in patients treated with narcotics. *N Engl J Med* 302:123, 1980.

Rinaldi RC, Steindler EM, Wilford BB, and Goodwin D. Clarification and standardization of substance abuse terminology. *JAMA* 259:555–557, 1988.

Rowobtham MC, Resiner Keller LA, and Fields HL. Both intravenous lidocaine and morphine reduce the pain of postherpetic neuralgia. *Neurology* 41:1024–1028, 1991.

Taub A. Opioid analgesics in the treatment of chronic intractable pain of non-neoplastic origin. In: LM Kitahata, and D. Collins (eds), *Narcotic Analgesics in Anesthesiology*. Baltimore: Williams & Wilkins, 1982. Pp. 199–208.

Tennant FS, et al. Chronic opioid treatment of intractable nonmalignant pain. *Pain Manage* Jan/Feb:18–36, 1988.

Tennant FS, Uleman GF. Narcotic maintenance for chronic pain: Medical and legal guidelines. *Postgrad Med* 73:81–94, 1983.

Special Problems in the Treatment of Pain

Scott M. Fishman and Donna B. Greenberg

> *"We all must die. But that I can save him from days of torture, that is what I feel as my great and ever new privilege. Pain is a more terrible lord of man than even death."*
>
> ALBERT SCHWEITZER

The patient with severe pain presents special problems that often make diagnosis and treatment difficult for either the clinician or the patient. While descriptions of pain and its location, time course, intensity, and behavioral effects are important factors in guiding diagnosis and evaluating therapy, pain is a subjective experience that varies greatly. Clinicians have few reliable objective measures of pain. Complaints of pain are impossible to verify. As a result, opioid-based pain management is often fraught with special problems, since opioids are often the only source of relief but are associated with a high abuse potential and side effects.

This chapter discusses the special set of potential drug-related complications. Most commonly, opioids produce constipation, nausea, vomiting, sedation, and respiratory depression. Any adverse effects from opioids may significantly limit therapy and some present serious consequences. Unfortunately, there are few predictors of which patients will experience which side effects and which opioids will produce them. It is prudent to expect side effects and to take preventive action. Because not all opioid-related toxicity can be prevented, patients should be closely monitored with a high level of suspicion. Effective management includes anticipation of adverse effects and preventive measures, choosing the best medication with careful administration, and clear communication with the patient, family, or nurse to ensure prompt recognition and response to adverse effects.

Side Effects of Opioids

CONSTIPATION

Constipation is the most common dose-dependent side effect of opioids. Tolerance does not develop. Constipation should be expected throughout the duration of opioid administration. Preventive therapy with cathartics and adequate fluid intake should be offered at the time opioids are started and continued throughout opioid treatment. Because opioid-related constipation results from increased tone and decreased gut motility, stool softeners and bulking agents such as bran or psyllium derivatives alone will be inadequate. Severe constipation may respond to oral naloxone (0.8–1.2 mg q6h PO until the first bowel movement).

To prevent and/or counteract constipation:

1. Start cathartic therapy and encourage fluids at the time of initiating opioid therapy.
2. Do not solely use a stool softener or bulking agent.
3. Continue bowel prophylaxis throughout the course of opioid therapy.
4. Suggested cathartic prophylaxis regimens include:
   Senna: 1 tablet of extract qd or bid PO
   Cascara: 4–12 ml at bedtime
   Bisacodyl: either 5 mg tablet qhs PO or 10 mg rectal suppository every night

NAUSEA AND VOMITING

Severe nausea and vomiting due solely to opioids are rare. Usually these symptoms are mild and may be managed with antiemetics or a reduction in the opioid dose to the minimal acceptable level of analgesia. A change in the route of administration may also alleviate symptoms. Fortunately, tolerance often occurs within several days of administering opioids, at which time antiemetic therapy should be discontinued. If nausea and vomiting persist, changing to a different equianalgesic opioid may reduce emetic side effects. If patients report a history of severe nausea with previous opioid treatment, antiemetic therapy may be started in advance. There is usually no need to discontinue the opioid in combination with the antiemetic. Why one opioid should produce nausea and vomiting while another does not is unclear.

Opioids produce nausea and vomiting by stimulating the medullary chemoreceptor trigger zone (CTZ), a potent sensory center responsible for afferent input to the emetic center. The importance of these anatomic centers relates to their rich endowment of neurotransmitter receptors, which correspond to antiemetic agents used clinically. These include histamine (H_1) blockers such as hydroxyzine; serotonin (5-HT$_3$) blockers such as ondansetron; dopamine (DA$_2$) blockers such as droperidol or haloperidol; anticholinergic agents such as scopolamine. Benzodiazepine agonists such as lorazepam may also possess antiemetic properties, although it is unclear whether this is due to direct action on benzodiazepine receptors found in the CTZ or indirect action on anxiety and conditioning. The single best agent is not always predictable, so choose the agent that offers secondary benefits such as promotility, sedative, antipruritic, anxiolytic, or antipsychotic properties.

Management of opioid-induced nausea and vomiting:

1. Severe nausea and vomiting due solely to opioids are rare.
2. Opioid-related nausea and vomiting are usually transient, with tolerance in 2 to 3 days.
3. Opioid-related nausea and vomiting vary with drug and patient; there are no clear patterns.
4. First-line adjustment in response to opioid-related nausea and vomiting:
   a. Reduce the opioid dose to the minimal acceptable level of analgesia.
   b. Change from one opioid agent to another equi-analgesic agent.
   c. Change the route of administration (IV to PR, etc.).
   d. Antiemetic therapy.
5. Increased risk of opioid-related nausea if the patient is ambulatory.
6. Remember other causes of nausea and vomiting:

   Chemotherapy
   Radiation therapy
   Metastases: brain and gastrointestinal
   Increased intracranial pressure
   Ulcer disease
   Gastroparesis
   Intestinal obstruction
   Esophagitis
   Gastritis
   Uremia
   Liver disease
   Infection: bacterial, viral, etc
   Pregnancy
   Fear/anxiety

SEDATION

Opioid-related sedation is common but temporary, resolving over time as patients accommodate to a new opioid drug. In those patients with persistent sedation, the opioid dose should be reduced to the minimal level required for adequate analgesia. Consider whether the medication may be accumulating and, if so, either increase the dose interval or change to a shorter-acting agent. For unremitting sedation, stimulants such as dextroamphetamine or caffeine can reduce sedation until accommodation occurs.

Management of opioid-related sedation:

1. Opioid-related sedation is common but usually temporary.
2. Severe or prolonged sedation may be treated by:
   a. Reducing the opioid dose to the minimal acceptable level of analgesia
   b. Increasing the dose interval or changing to a shorter-acting opioid to avoid accumulation
   c. Therapy with stimulants

PRURITUS

Pruritus is a common side effect of parenterally administered opioids. It is uncommon with oral opioids. Its frequency also varies with dose. Pruritus is found in the large majority of patients treated with intrathecal and epidural opioids and frequently in those treated with intravenous or intramuscular opioids. Usually parenteral opioids produce mild pruritus, but moderate to severe pruritus does occur in some patients. Fortunately, tolerance occurs and the severity of pruritus decreases with duration of opioid therapy. Opioid-related pruritus is usually localized to the face or, less often, the perineum and can also become generalized. The mechanism of opioid-induced pruritus is not well understood. Suggested hypotheses include mu-receptor stimulation, H_1 release, local excitation of posterior horn neurons, and central migration of spinal opioids to "itch centers" in the brain.

As with other opioid-related side effects, changing opioids may effectively relieve pruritus. Naloxone is currently the most effective therapy and is useful for opioid-related pruritus from any route of administration (5 µg/kg IVP q10min prn; hold for decreased analgesia). Antihistamines may be effective for opioid-related pruritus except when pruritus is due to spinal opioids. Antihistamines potentiate opioid analgesia, often allowing for a small reduction of opioid dose that might further reduce pruritus. Because nonsedating antihistamines are less effective than sedating antihistamines, the antipruritic efficacy of antihistamine therapy may, in part, be related to sedation. Recently, small amounts of propofol (10 mg IVP) have been found to effectively control pruritus due to spinal opioids. Propofol has no effect on analgesia and is effective for pruritus from spinal opioids. At this very low dose, adverse effects from propofol should be minimal.

When choosing an antipruritic treatment, consider that antihistamine poorly controls pruritus from spinal opioids, that sedative effects of antihistamines and opioids will be additive, and that naloxone may decrease analgesia.

Management of opioid-related pruritus:

1. Opioid-related pruritus is common.
2. Tolerance to this effect occurs over time.
3. Treatment involves either:
   a. Change in opioid agent
   b. Naloxone (5 µg/kg IVPq10min prn; hold for decreased analgesia)
   c. Antihistamine (hydroxyzine 25–50 mg IV or IM or 25–100 mg PO q6h prn)
   d. Propofol (10 mg IVP q10min, in 2–3 doses)

RESPIRATORY DEPRESSION

Respiratory depression is a potentially serious complication of opioid administration. Fortunately, tolerance occurs early in chronic therapy. Combining oral or intravenous opioids with epidural or intrathecal opioids may quickly depress respiration and should be avoided. Significant acute respiratory depression can be managed with the opiate receptor antagonist naloxone. Dosages of naloxone for treating respiratory depression are given below. While naloxone may provide a brisk response, its duration of action is short. Pay close attention to the patient after naloxone administration; more than one dose of naloxone may be required. Continuous intravenous administration of naloxone can be considered. Special care must be given to the patient taking prolonged opioids, since rapid administration of naloxone can precipitate withdrawal.

In special cases, reversal of opioid actions can promote pulmonary edema. This effect is likely the result in reversal of opioid-induced pulmonary vascular smooth muscle relaxation. However, this is usually of minimal concern, unless the patient is predisposed to pulmonary edema (congestive heart failure, adult respiratory distress syndrome, etc).

Issues of opioid-related respiratory depression:

1. Respiratory depression is a serious and reversible complication of opioid therapy.
2. Tolerance to this effect occurs early in chronic therapy.
3. Reverse opioid effects with naloxone at 0.1 mg IVP repeated q10–15 min as needed (one fourth of the usual 0.4-mg ampule of naloxone).
4. Duration of action of naloxone is shorter than most opioids; repeat doses may be necessary.

TOLERANCE

Tolerance occurs when a fixed dose of opioid provides decreasing analgesia. Tolerance may also occur with opioid side effects, developing at different rates for different side effects. Pain in the tolerant patient can usually be treated by either changing the opioid or increasing the dose. A patient who has become tolerant to one opioid drug may respond with ample analgesia to another opioid. Tolerance occurs at different rates with different opioids, illustrating that cross-tolerance between these drugs may be incomplete. Equi-analgesic doses are not appropriate in the opioid-tolerant patient. When starting a new opioid agent in a tolerant patient, the recommended starting dose is 50% greater than the equi-analgesic dose and is titrated to effective analgesia.

Issues of opioid tolerance:

1. Pain in the tolerant patient may resolve by either:
   a. Changing the opioid agent
   b. Increasing the dose of opioid
2. Incomplete opioid cross-tolerance: a tolerant patient may respond with ample analgesia to a second opioid.
3. Equi-analgesic doses are not appropriate in the opioid-tolerant patient:
   a. Starting dose in a tolerant patient is 50% greater than the equi-analgesic dose
   b. Titrate to effective analgesia

OPIOID DEPENDENCE AND WITHDRAWAL

Physical Dependence

Physical dependence implies that continuous exposure to a drug is necessary to avoid the withdrawal syndrome. Attempts to avoid dependency may lead to inadequate opioid doses and undertreatment of pain. Dependence reflects a biochemical adaptation from chronic exposure to opioids. Opioids inhibit cyclic adenosine monophosphate (cAMP). Sudden discontinuation of opioids or administration of an opioid antagonist can induce a rebound disinhibition of cAMP associated with symptoms of withdrawal.

Withdrawal

The least severe withdrawal symptoms typically appear earlier than the most severe. Withdrawal begins with increased irritability or restlessness and later progresses to agitation, tremors, insomnia, frequent yawning or sneezing, lacrimation, fever, tachycardia, and other features of heightened sympathetic activity. Sudden discontinuation of shorter-acting opioids such as morphine or hydromorphone are more likely to produce withdrawal symptoms than longer-acting agents such as methadone or transdermally administered fentanyl. However, the syndrome may be seen with discontinuation or antagonism of any opioid.

The withdrawal state can be avoided by slow, systematic tapering of the opioid dose at a daily rate of 15% to 20%. Withdrawal can usually be reversed by reintroducing the opioid at dosages of 25% to 40% of the previous daily dose. To avoid sleep disturbance, bedtime doses should be the last to be weaned. Treatment of sympathetic hyperactivity may halt further development of withdrawal symptoms. Effective sympatholytics include clonidine and beta-blockers. These agents can produce hypotension. Clonidine may produce sedation, and its antiwithdrawal effects may be antagonized by tricyclic antidepressants. However, when abrupt discontinuation of a chronic opioid is mandatory, clonidine detoxification can effectively blunt objective findings of sympathetic hyperactivity. It remains controversial whether clonidine may increase or mask subjective symptoms of withdrawal such as anxiety, insomnia, and restlessness.

Issues of opioid withdrawal:

1. Attempts to avoid dependency may lead to inadequate opioid doses and undertreatment of pain.
2. The withdrawal state can be avoided by slow, systematic tapering of the opioid dose at a daily rate of 15% to 20%.
3. Reversal of withdrawal can usually be seen upon reintroducing the opioid at doses that are 25% to 40% of the previous daily dose.
4. When abrupt discontinuation of a chronic opioid is mandatory, clonidine may be used instead of or in addition to other opioids.

      a. Clonidine detoxification can effectively blunt objective findings of withdrawal.

      b. It is usually started at doses of 10–20 μg/kg per day in 3 divided doses and adjustments are made to reduce signs of withdrawal while limiting hypotension.

      c. Clonidine can be maintained for between 4 days for short-acting opioids and 14 days for long-acting opioids.

      d. After that period, clonidine can be tapered over 4 to 6 days.

5. Clinical manifestations of withdrawal:

      a. Early: anxiety, insomnia, yawning, sweating, rhinorrhea, lacrimation

      b. Later: dilated pupils, gooseflesh, tremor, chills, anorexia, muscle cramps (18 to 24 hours after the last dose: hypertension, tachycardia, tachypnea, fever, nausea and vomiting)

      c. Laboratory findings: leukocytosis, ketosis, electrolyte imbalance

THE OPIOID-ADDICTED PATIENT

Patients with a history of substance abuse and severe pain present a particularly challenging dilemma because prior substance abuse is a relative contraindication to opioid administration. If possible, nonopioid analgesics remain the first line of therapy in these cases. For those with a history of substance abuse and pain that is acute, resistant to all other therapeutic options, or associated with terminal illness, the relative nature of this contraindication must yield to compassionate use of opioids. With an informed, cautious, and limited approach, opioids can be safe and effective for treating severe pain in the patient with opioid addiction or a history of drug abuse.

The high prevalence of illicit drug use and drug-seeking activities mandate that physicians maintain an extremely high level of caution when releasing opioids, particularly to the addicted patient. The opioid-addicted patient is often viewed by caregivers as already having had too much opioid, with any more opioid serving only to support their habit. In these patients, severe pain is often undertreated. In these cases, it is important to take a rational and dispassionate approach. Initially, determine whether the patient requires opioid analgesia and then determine the appropriate dose for a potentially opioid-tolerant patient.

Acute pain with a clear origin (postoperative, posttraumatic, etc) always warrants adequate analgesia with opioids, if necessary, based on a plan for short-term administration. When pain becomes chronic, the use of opioids in the drug-addicted or drug-abusing patient may be problematic. Addiction is often not acknowledged. These patients may present with dramatic complaints of pain and even offer serious reservations about taking "addictive" medicines. The clinician may feel consoled that the patient respects the potency and risks of using opioids. However, frequent or forceful protests over taking addictive drugs despite brisk or escalating use may suggest addiction. Once the addicted patient finds a preferred agent, further manipulations may be predicated on securing a steady opioid supply. Too often the clinician may foresee escalating complications and continue maintenance opioids as a compromise.

Ample analgesia in an opioid-abusing patient who is likely to be opioid tolerant may require a higher than normal opioid dose. However, this patient should not require analgesics for a longer than normal period. The clinician should watch for behavior reflecting craving for opioids. Attention should be paid to around-the-clock doses, since individual doses may mislead the clinician who is treating a patient who has requested every possible prn dose. Inquire as to whether the patient uses opioids to treat symptoms other than pain, such as sleep disturbance or anxiety. Limiting prn doses may suppress drug-seeking behaviors. Because opioids have a street value as illegal recreational drugs, limiting brand names or "do not substitute" orders will make it less likely that the drug will be resold illicitly. A patient's request for brand names or no-substitution order should raise the concern of resale.

When patients are undergoing methadone maintenance therapy and circumstances mandate opioid analgesia for severe pain, it is often best to view the need for methadone and the new pain problem as two separate entities. While methadone therapy will induce tolerance, requiring greater than normal analgesic doses of opioid, a different opioid can be added to specifically treat the pain. The new opioid, rather than starting at approximately 50% higher than the usual dose, would be administered, followed, and tapered as if the patient were on a single opioid agent.

Issues with opioid-addicted patients:

1. A history of substance abuse is a relative contraindication to opioid administration for nonmalignant pain.
2. The relative nature of this contraindication must yield to compassionate use of opioids, particularly in the setting of acute pain.
3. Dependent patients may be undertreated due to the common view by care givers that these patients have already had too much opioid, with any more opioid only serving to support their habit.
4. Methadone therapy will induce tolerance, requiring greater than normal analgesic doses of opioid for acute pain.

Selected Readings

American Pain Society. *Principles of Analgesic Use in the Treatment of Acute Pain and Chronic Cancer Pain* (2nd ed). Clinical Pharmacy. 9:601–611, 1990.

Foley KM. Controversies in cancer pain. *Cancer* 63:2257–2265, 1989.

Foley KM. Opioids. *Neurol Clin* 11:503–522, 1993.

Hyman SH and Cassem NH. Pain. In: E Rubenstein and DD Federman, (eds). *Scientific American Medicine: Current Topics in Medicine,* Subsection II. New York: Scientific American, 1989. Pp. 1–17.

NIH Consensus Development Conference. The integrated approach to the management of pain. *J Pain Symptom Manage* 2:35–41, 1987.

Portenoy RK. Chronic opioid therapy in nonmalignant pain. *J Pain Symptom Manage* 5:S46–S62, 1990.

Wall PD, and Melzack R, eds. *Textbook of Pain* (2nd ed). New York, Churchill-Livingstone, 1988.

Psychosocial Issues in the Treatment of Pain

Scott M. Fishman and Donna B. Greenberg

> *"It was a most repugnant undertaking to have to treat a group of complaints which, as all authors are agreed, are typified by instability, irregularity, fantasy, unpredictability—complaints which are governed by no law or rule, and whose diverse manifestations are connected to no serious theoretical formulation."*
>
> PAUL BRIQUET: TRAITE CLINIQUE ET THERAPEUTIQUE DE L'HYSTERIE

All pain has a psychological component. Psychological stress makes any pain more intense and less tolerable. Rather than dissecting the psychogenic from the somatic components of pain, it is more effective to assume that the complaint of pain always indicates subjective distress. Besides nociception, complaints of pain can express fear, dependency, or even a way of ensuring other benefits that come with illness.

Persistent pain can change behavior. Anxiety and depression are common in patients with pain, and more likely if the pain is persistent. It is often difficult to tell which came first— pain or psychologic dysfunction. Analgesia is always the first strategy and may relieve acute pain as well as its associated psychologic symptoms.

Disability compensation and litigation complicate pain management. Sternbach (1974) has said that the patient receiving financial reward for illness loses his or her amateur standing. Compensation for illness, whether deserved, fraudulent, financial, or social, sets the patient apart from others. This patient has a large counter-incentive to relinquish pain. Despite what seems to be adequate intervention, the litigious patient may report no analgesia until a pending law suit is settled. The patient interested in workers' compensation will seem eager to work, especially if it is clearly not possible to perform the previous job. The same patient may be unwilling to pursue other job options. Short-term disability must be offered in a prescribed time frame. After that, alternative employment will be expected.

Chronic Pain

Acute pain is often related to a discernible injury or focus of disease. It is usually self-limited and associated with autonomic changes such as tachycardia, hypertension, diaphoresis, mydriasis, and pallor. Pain that persists beyond the normal time of healing or for longer than 6 months is considered to be chronic pain. It is critical to appreciate that the sequelae of chronic pain may reflect a separate mechanism from that of the original insult that began the syndrome. The patient with chronic pain may have symptoms unlike those of an inciting injury and may develop new medical and psychiatric symptoms that defy diagnostic classification.

The transition from acute to chronic pain often reveals symptoms dissimilar from and less traceable to the original symptoms. A patient with chronic pain may be unable to give a clear description of pain despite strong, but often vague, complaints. Unlike acute pain, chronic pain presents without signs of heightened sympathetic activity due to chronic adaptation of the autonomic nervous system. Instead, the patient may be able to associate his or her pain with depression, bedrest, insomnia, hostility, or anxiety. Timing and localization are rarely offered. It is not hard to understand how the validity of a patient's complaints may be questioned by a physician faced with vague findings, the lack of evidence of focal disease, and the appearance of an individual who seems excessively preoccupied with his or her pain.

Chronic pain states are typically more complex than acute pain, often interwoven with medical, psychologic, and social facets. Cause and effect are difficult to establish because loss of function, either physical or psychologic, may reflect a predisposition to or consequence of the pain syndrome. Chronic pain conditions represent a challenge that usually requires a search for the initial cause of pain and, if possible, treatment of the cause.

Chronic pain patients may have seen multiple physicians and have received a broad spectrum of therapeutic interventions without relief of symptoms. Substance abuse is frequently associated with chronic pain patients, including alcoholism. Family or employment structures that reinforce pain require investigation and planning of alternatives. Chronic pain patients benefit from behavioral and insight-oriented treatments that improve coping and function, relieve anxiety, and decrease pain intensity. These techniques include biofeedback and relaxation training, hypnosis, desensitization, and behavioral modification (see Chaps. 6, 8, and 11). These techniques, however, require a capable, compliant, and supportive patient. Patients with severe psychopathology require specialized consultation from psychiatrists. Clinical suspicion of psychopathology is critical to the evaluation of the chronic pain patient.

Anxiety and Depression

Anxiety and depression may make patients less able to cope with ongoing pain. These conditions tend to result in varying degrees of hopelessness or vigilance, diminishing either the ability or the incentive to cast focus away from pain. Whether causative or reactive, anxiety and depression must be recognized in evaluating patients with pain, because analgesia may not be fully adequate without treatment of the underlying psychopathology.

DEPRESSION

Although it is often difficult to distinguish the causal relationship of depression to pain, recognizing and treating depression may enhance analgesia. Sadness and hopelessness are the symptoms that clinicians commonly associate with depression. However, these symptoms are among many and may not always be most prominent. Anxiety, irritability, and obsessive thoughts are less well-known features of depression. The signs and symptoms of clinical depression appear in Table 24-1. Chronic pain is commonly associated with complaints of diminished sleep, loss of appetite, decreased activity, lack of energy, loss of concentration, and decreased interest in experiencing pleasure—symptoms that overlap with neurovegetative signs of depression. In patients using opioids, it is important to avoid being misled by vegetative signs that seem solely due to opioid side effects such as psychomotor retardation, severe fatigue, anorexia, constipation, and hypersomnia, as these are also symptoms of major depression.

Assessment of depression will often require a complete history, including investigation of suicidal thinking. Direct questions about sadness, hope, and what the future holds for the patient may stimulate clear and clinically useful responses. Cognitive testing will clarify cognitive impairment. Major depressive disorders should be treated with antidepressant medications (Table 24-2). Tricyclic antidepressant therapy may potentiate analgesic efficacy, particularly if pain is neuropathic.

Table 24-1. Signs and symptoms of clinical depression

Chronic Pain is commonly associated with these features.

1. Depressed mood, subjective or observed
2. Markedly diminished interest or pleasure in all, or almost all, activities most of the day
3. Significant (more than 5% of body weight per month) weight loss or gain
4. Insomnia or hypersomnia
5. Psychomotor agitation or retardation
6. Fatigue or loss of energy
7. Feelings of worthlessness or excessive or inappropriate guilt
8. Diminished ability to think or concentrate, or indecisiveness
9. Recurrent thoughts of death or suicide

Reproduced with permission from Cassem NH. *Massachusetts General Hospital Handbook of General Hospital Psychiatry* (3rd ed). St Louis: Mosby–Year Book, 1991.

Table 24-2. Available preparations

Drug	Dosage forms (mg)	Usual daily dose (mg/day)	Extreme dose (mg/day)	Therapeutic plasma levels (ng/ml)
Cyclic compounds				
Imipramine (Tofranil and generics)	T: 10, 25, 50 C: 75, 100, 125, 150 INJ: 25 mg/2 ml	150–200	50–300	> 225[a]
Desipramine (Norpramin and generics)	T: 10, 25, 50, 75, 100, 150 C: 25, 50	150–200	50–300	> 125
Amitriptyline (Elavil and generics)	T: 10, 25, 50, 75, 100, 150 INJ: 10 mg/ml	150–200	50–300	> 120 (?)[b]
Nortriptyline (Pamelor and generics)	C: 10, 25, 50, 75 LC: 10 mg/5 ml	75–100	25–150	50–150
Doxepin (Adapin, Sinequan, and generics)	C: 10, 25, 50, 75, 100, 150 LC: 10 mg/ml	150–200	25–300	100–250 (?)
Trimipramine (Surmontil)	C: 25, 50, 100	150–200	50–300	
Protriptyline (Vivactil)	T: 5, 10	15–40	10–60	
Maprotiline (Ludiomil)	T: 25, 50, 75	100–150	50–200	
Amoxapine (Asendin)	T: 25, 50, 100, 150	200–300	50–300	
Clomipramine (Anafranil)	C: 25, 50, 75	150–200	50–250	

Atypical compounds			
Bupropion (Wellbutrin)	T: 75, 100	200–300	100–450
Trazodone (Desyrel and generics)	T: 50, 100, 150, 300	200–300	100–600
Fluoxetine (Prozac)	T: 20	20–60	5–100
Monoamine oxidase inhibitors			
Phenelzine (Nardil)	T: 15	45–90	15–90
Tranylcypromine (Parnate)	T: 10	30–50	10–90
Isocarboxazid (Marplan)	T: 10	20–50	10–90

C = capsules; INJ = injectable form; LC = liquid concentrate or solution; T = tablets.

aSum of imipramine plus desipramine.

bSum of amitriptyline plus nortriptyline.

Reproduced with permission from Arana GW, and Hyman SE. *Handook of Psychiatric Drug Therapy* (2nd ed). Boston: Little, Brown, 1991.

The selective serotonin reuptake inhibitors (SSRIs) and tricyclic antidepressants (TCAs) remain the first-line agents of pharmacotherapy. The SSRI antidepressants, such as fluoxetine, paroxetine, fluvoxamine, and sertraline, can produce anxiety as a side effect in some patients, have delayed onset of antidepressant effect, and have no known analgesic properties. The limitations of TCA therapy include delayed onset of antidepressant effect (analgesic effects may be immediate). Many of the TCAs have side effects such as confusion, urinary retention, erectile dysfunction, dry mucous membranes, sedation, and orthostatic hypotension.

ANXIETY

Both anxiety and pain are major sources of suffering, only to be compounded when occurring simultaneously. Thus, recognizing and treating anxiety in the patient with pain will likely improve the chance of successful analgesia.

Pain and anxiety have similar psychologic and somatic features. For instance, in the acute phase, each elicits a heightened state of autonomic arousal. When anxiety and pain become chronic, each tends to be maladaptive and marked by suffering. In other words, just as chronic anxiety often leads to phobic avoidance, chronic pain usually leads to pain behaviors, often with avoidance as a prominent feature. It is likely that when anxiety and pain occur simultaneously, their potential for any of these effects is increased.

The psychologic component of anxiety is characterized by apprehension, fear, or a sense of impending doom, or all of these. Patients do not always know why they are anxious. The somatic component of anxiety (Table 24-3) is characterized by autonomic hyperactivity and, as such, can imitate other organic disease processes like heart disease, acute anemia, pulmonary dysfunction, and seizure. Episodes of spontaneous and rapidly escalating anxiety may represent panic attacks, characterized by discrete periods of anxiety, ranging in intensity from mild to extreme, and associated with several of the usual physical symptoms listed in Table 24-4—the DSM-IV diagnostic criteria for panic attacks.

Recognition of stressors and reassurance may go a long way in reducing fear. Because opioids may be requested for the treatment of nonpainful symptoms, such as anxiety or insomnia, identifying and appropriately treating these problems with antianxiety agents may limit opioid exposure. Benzodiazepines are the first-line agents of drug therapy for all forms of anxiety including panic attacks. Clonazepam and alprazolam are well suited for the treatment of anxiety. Lorazepam and oxazepam are useful when treating anxiety in patients with diminished hepatic or renal function because neither has active long acting metabolites. Other antipanic agents include TCAs and SSRIs which are not useful for acute intervention because they will take several weeks to work. They require close follow-up for management of potential side

Table 24-3. Physical signs and symptoms of anxiety

Anorexia
"Butterflies" in stomach
Chest pain or tightness
Diaphoresis
Diarrhea
Dizziness
Dry mouth
Dyspnea
Faintness
Flushing
Headache
Hyperventilation
Light-headedness
Muscle tension
Nausea
Pallor
Palpitations
Paresthesias
Sexual dysfunction
Shortness of breath
Stomach pain
Tachycardia
Tremulousness
Urinary frequency
Vomiting

Reproduced from Cassem NH. *Massachusetts General Hospital Handbook of General Hospital Psychiatry* (3rd ed). St. Louis: Mosby–Year Book, 1991.

Table 24-4. Criteria for panic attack

A discrete period of intense fear or discomfort, in which four (or more) of the following symptoms develop abruptly and reach a peak within 10 minutes.
1. Palpitations, pounding heart, or accelerated heart rate
2. Sweating
3. Trembling or shaking
4. Sensations of shortness of breath or smothering
5. Feeling of choking
6. Chest pain or discomfort
7. Nausea or abdominal distress
8. Feeling dizzy, unsteady, lightheaded, or faint
9. Derealization (feelings of unreality) or depersonalization (being detached from oneself)
10. Fear of losing control or going crazy
11. Fear of dying
12. Paresthesias (numbness or tingling sensations)
13. Chills or hot flashes

Source: *Diagnostic and Statistical Manual of Mental Disorders* (4th ed). Washington, DC: American Psychiatric Association, 1995.

effects (see above). Persistent anxiety may lead to avoidance behaviors, requiring behavioral counseling.

Somatoform Disorders

Although the first order of managing pain is to identify an organic or metabolic cause, too often a cause is not found. Next, a possible psychiatric condition associated with the pain should be considered. The somatoform disorders are diagnosed when physical symptomatology does not correlate with demonstrable pathology or a reasonable mechanism that explains the symptom. For instance, somatoform disorders may occur in patients with known physical disease whose distress appears to be out of proportion to the physical evidence. These patients are not intentionally faking illness, as in malingering or factitious disorders.

The DSM-IV criteria for psychologic factors affecting physical conditions are listed in Table 24-5. The spectrum of psychosomatic diseases includes the somatoform disorders, which represent a group of six entities listed below. The DSM-IV diagnostic classification is given in Table 24-6 for Somatization Disorder; Table 24-7 for Somatoform Pain Disorder; Table 24-8 for Conversion Disorder; Table 24-9 for Hypochondriasis; Table 24-10 for Body Dysmorphic Disorder; and Table 24-11 for Undifferentiated Somatoform Disorder.

Once a physical etiology for the symptom is ruled out, it is common for these patients to resist a psychological explanation. Resistance may represent an inability to relinquish the symptom as a psychologic defense against emotional conflicts. For instance, some patients may prefer pain to acknowledgment of emotional conflict; others may find a psychiatric explanation a shameful sign of weakness. Factors sustaining pain may include interpersonal, religious, cultural, economic, or even medical issues, often requiring investigation before treatment can be successful.

The different somatoform disorders, while having clear diagnostic criteria in the DSM-IV, tend to overlap in clinical presentation. Strict adherence to diagnostic criteria may not be possible. Thus, it is important to consider patterns of behavior and to question whether a patient's pain is psychologically maintained. For purposes here, somatization disorder and somatoform pain disorder will be further discussed. Although the entities mentioned above are important, they are beyond the scope of this chapter and can be fully reviewed in most general psychiatric textbooks.

SOMATIZATION DISORDER

Patients with multiple somatic complaints without a discernible physical origin or mechanism may have somatization disorder, formerly known as hysteria or Briquet's syndrome. The DSM-IV diagnostic criteria for this disorder are outlined in

Table 24-5. The diagnostic and statistical manual (DSM-IV) criteria for psychological factors affecting physical conditions

A. A general medical condition is present.

B. Psychological factors adversely affect the general medical condition in one of the following ways.

   1. The factors have influenced the course of the general medical condition as shown by a close temporal association between the psychological factors and the development or exacerbation of, or delayed recovery from, the general medical condition.
   2. The factors interfere with the treatment of the general medical condition.
   3. The factors constitute additional health risks for the individual.
   4. Stress related physiologic responses precipitate or exacerbate symptoms of the general medical condition.

Choose name based on the nature of the psychological factors (if more than one factor is present, indicate the most prominent):

   Mental disorder affecting . . . [indicate the general medical condition] (e.g., an Axis I disorder such as major depressive disorder delaying recovery from a myocardial infarction)

   Psychological symptoms affecting . . . [indicate the general medical condition] (e.g., depressive symptoms delaying recovery from surgery, anxiety exacerbating asthma)

   Personality traits or coping style affecting . . . [indicate the general medical condition] (e.g., pathologic denial of the need for surgery in a patient with cancer; hostile, pressured behavior contributing to cardiovascular disease)

   Maladaptive health behaviors affecting . . . [indicate the general medical condition] (e.g., overeating, lack of exercise, unsafe sex)

   Stress-related physiologic response affecting . . . [indicate the general medical condition] (e.g., stress-related exacerbations of ulcer, hypertension, arrhythmia, or tension headache)

   Other or unspecified psychological factors affecting . . . [indicate the general medical condition] (e.g., interpersonal, cultural, or religious factors)

Source: *Diagnostic and Statistical Manual of Mental Disorders* (4th ed). Washington, DC: American Psychiatric Association, 1995.

Table 24-6. Somatization disorder

A. A history of many physical complaints beginning before age 30 years that occur over a period of several years and result in treatment being sought or significant impairment in social, occupational, or other important areas of functioning.

B. Each of the following criteria must have been met, with individual symptoms occurring at any time during the course of the disturbance.
   1. Four pain symptoms: A history of pain related to at least four different sites or functions (e.g., head, abdomen, back, joints, extremities, chest, rectum, during menstruation, during sexual intercourse, or during urination).
   2. Two gastrointestinal symptoms: A history of at least two gastrointestinal symptoms other than pain (e.g., nausea, bloating, vomiting other than during pregnancy, diarrhea, or intolerance of several different foods).
   3. One sexual symptom: A history of at least one sexual or reproductive symptom other than pain (e.g., sexual indifference, erectile or ejaculatory dysfunction, irregular menses, excessive menstrual bleeding, vomiting throughout pregnancy).
   4. One pseudoneurologic symptom: A history of at least one symptom or deficit suggesting a neurologic condition not limited to pain (conversion symptoms such as impaired coordination or balance, paralysis or localized weakness, difficulty swallowing or lump in throat, aphonia, urinary retention, hallucinations, loss of touch or pain sensation, double vision, blindness, deafness, seizures; dissociative symptoms such as amnesia; or loss of consciousness other than fainting).

C. Either 1 or 2:
   1. After appropriate investigation, each of the symptoms in criterion B cannot be fully explained by a known general medical condition or the direct effects of a substance (e.g., a drug of abuse, a medication).
   2. When there is a related general medical condition, the physical complaints or resulting social or occupational impairment are in excess of what would be expected from the history, physical examination, or laboratory findings.

D. The symptoms are not intentionally produced or feigned (as in factitious disorder or malingering).

Source: *Diagnostic and Statistical Manual of Mental Disorders* (4th ed). Washington, DC: American Psychiatric Association, 1995.

Table 24-7. Pain disorder

A. Pain in one or more anatomic sites is the predominant focus of the clinical presentation and is of sufficient severity to warrant clinical attention.

B. The pain causes clinically significant distress or impairment in social, occupational, or other important areas of functioning.

C. Psychological factors are judged to have an important role in the onset, severity, exacerbation, or maintenance of the pain.

D. The symptom or deficit is not intentionally produced or feigned (as in factitious disorder or malingering).

E. The pain is not better accounted for by a mood, anxiety, or psychotic disorder and does not meet criteria for dyspareunia.

Code as follows:

307.80   Pain disorder associated with psychological factors. Psychological factors are judged to have the major role in the onset, severity, exacerbation, or maintenance of the pain. (If a general medical condition is present, it does not have a major role in the onset, severity, exacerbation, or maintenance of the pain.) This type of pain disorder is not diagnosed if criteria are also met for somatization disorder.

Specify if:

Acute: duration of less than six months.

Chronic: duration of six months or longer

307.89   Pain disorder associated with both psychological factors and a general medical condition. Both psychological factors and a general medical condition are judged to have important roles in the onset, severity, exacerbation, or maintenance of the pain. The associated general medical condition or anatomic site of the pain is coded on Axis III.

Specify if:

Acute: duration of less than six months

Chronic: duration of six months or longer

Note: The following is not considered to be mental disorder and is included here to facilitate differential diagnosis.

Pain disorder associated with a general medical condition. A general medical condition has a major role in the onset, severity, exacerbation, or maintenance of the pain. (If psychological factors are present, they are not judged to have a major role in the onset, severity, exacerbation, or maintenance of the pain.) The diagnostic code for the pain is selected based on the associated general medical condition if one has been established or on the anatomic location of the pain if the underlying general medical condition is not yet clearly established—for example, low back (724.2), sciatic (724.3), pelvic (625.9), headache (784.0), facial (784.0), chest (786.50), joint (719.4), bone (733.90), abdominal (789.0), breast (611.71), renal (788.0), ear (388.70), eye (379.91), throat (784.1), tooth (525.9), and urinary (788.0).

Source: *Diagnostic and Statistical Manual of Mental Disorders* (4th ed). Washington, DC: American Psychiatric Association, 1995.

Table 24-8. Conversion disorder

A. One or more symptoms or deficits affecting voluntary motor or sensory function that suggest a neurologic or other general medical condition.

B. Psychological factors are judged to be associated with the symptom or deficit because the initiation or exacerbation of the symptom or deficit is preceded by conflicts or other stressors.

C. The symptom or deficit is not intentionally produced or feigned (as in factitious disorder or malingering).

D. The symptom or deficit cannot, after appropriate investigation, be fully explained by a general medical condition, or by the direct effects of a substance, or as a culturally sanctioned behavior or experience.

E. The symptom or deficit causes clinically significant distress or impairment in social, occupational, or other important areas of functioning or warrants medical evaluation.

F. The symptom or deficit is not limited to pain or sexual dysfunction, does not occur exclusively during the course of somatization disorder, and is not better accounted for by another mental disorder.

Specify type of symptom or deficit:
  With motor symptom or deficit
  With sensory symptom or deficit
  With seizures or convulsions
  With mixed presentation

Source: *Diagnostic and Statistical Manual of Mental Disorders* (4th ed). Washington, DC: American Psychiatric Association, 1995.

Table 24-6. These patients tend to present symptoms prior to the age of 30 years and their symptoms are associated with multiple organ systems. Symptoms are often offered in vague or dramatic terms. These individuals are often narcissistic, dependent, or manipulative, or all of these. They usually have seen numerous physicians ("doctor shopping") and have received numerous tests and therapies. Most complications result from medical intervention.

The course of the somatization disorder is chronic and often marked by a fluctuating pattern. Management requires ruling out organic disease with minimal hospitalization, invasive testing, and pharmacotherapeutic interventions. Once recognized, treatment requires an empathic clinician who can provide a medical environment where the patient can feel comfortable bringing forth frequent medical complaints. This medical environment must be reassuring while setting clear limits on time and workup and not alienating a patient who may be resistant to psychological explanations. Professional psychiatric consultation may be required.

SOMATOFORM PAIN DISORDER

Patients who have a severe preoccupation with their pain may have somatoform pain (psychogenic pain), which is often

Table 24-9. Hypochondriasis

A. Preoccupation with fears of having, or the idea that one has, a serious disease based on the person's misinterpretation of bodily symptoms.

B. The preoccupation persists despite appropriate medical evaluation and reassurance.

C. The belief in criterion A is not a delusional intensity (as in delusional disorder, somatic type) and is not restricted to a circumscribed concern about appearance (as in body dysmorphic disorder).

D. The preoccupation causes clinically significant distress or impairment in social, occupational, or other important areas of functioning.

E. The duration of the disturbance is at least six months.

F. The preoccupation is not better accounted for by generalized anxiety disorder, obsessive-compulsive disorder, panic disorder, a major depressive episode, separation anxiety, or another somatoform disorder.

Specify if:

With poor insight. If for most of the time during the current episode, the person does not recognize that the concern about having a serious illness is excessive or unreasonable.

Source: *Diagnostic and Statistical Manual of Mental Disorders* (4th ed). Washington, DC: American Psychiatric Association, 1995.

associated with a particular psychological focus such as avoiding work, social stressors, or a need for attention. Somatoform pain disorder is classified by DSM-IV as a preoccupation with pain for longer than 6 months (see Table 24-7). Usually a complete workup fails to reach an organic pathophysiologic explanation, or the pain and its associated symptoms and behaviors are grossly out of proportion to the physical findings or known lesion. Frequently, patients complain of pain in a nonanatomic distribution, with or without sensory and motor changes. Disuse atrophy may even be present. Such patients may be extremely difficult to treat and may require multi-

Table 24-10. Body dysmorphic disorder

A. Preoccupation with an imagined defect in appearance. If a slight physical anomaly is present, the person's concern is markedly excessive.

B. The preoccupation causes clinically significant distress or impairment in social, occupational, or other important areas of functioning.

C. The preoccupation is not better accounted for by another mental disorder (e.g., dissatisfaction with body shape and size in anorexia nervosa).

Source: *Diagnostic and Statistical Manual of Mental Disorders* (4th ed). Washington, DC: American Psychiatric Association, 1995.

Table 24-11. Undifferentiated somatoform disorder

A. One or more physical complaints (e.g., fatigue, loss of appetite, gastrointestinal or urinary complaints).
B. Either 1 or 2:
  1. After appropriate investigation, the symptoms cannot be fully explained by a known general medical condition or the direct effects of a substance (e.g., a drug abuse, a medication).
  2. When there is a related general medical condition, the physical complaints or resulting social or occupational impairment is in excess of what would be expected from the history, physical examination, or laboratory findings.
C. The symptoms cause clinically significant distress or impairment in social, occupational, or other important areas of functioning.
D. The duration of the disturbance is at least six months.
E. The disturbance is not better accounted for by another mental disorder (e.g., another somatoform disorder, sexual dysfunction, mood disorder, anxiety disorder, sleep disorder, or psychotic disorder).
F. The symptom is not intentionally produced or feigned (as in factitious disorder or malingering).

Source: *Diagnostic and Statistical Manual of Mental Disorders* (4th ed). Washington, DC: American Psychiatric Association, 1995.

disciplinary intervention. Use of opioids in this group is not recommended. Treatment involves the following: (1) opioid detoxification, if necessary; (2) cognitive and behavioral therapy to enhance coping and insight; (3) physical and occupational therapy to increase movement and general functionality; (4) recognition and treatment of depression; and (5) inpatient chronic pain rehabilitation—an aggressive consolidated approach for all of the above.

Malingering

Presentation of false or greatly exaggerated symptoms constitutes malingering and should raise suspicions of secondary gain. Hyman (1988) and Cassem (1991) describe four factors that should prompt suspicion of malingering: (1) presentation in the medicolegal context; (2) marked discrepancy between claimed distress and objective findings; (3) a lack of cooperation with the diagnostic and treatment regimen; and (4) the presence of antisocial personality disorder or polysubstance abuse.

The distinction between somatoform disorder and malingering is often less than clear; the difference rests on the degree to which the patient is conscious of producing a symptom. Malingering reflects psychopathology but does not respond to psychologic interpretation, suggestion, or pharmacotherapy. If the patient does not have pain, do not treat it. All findings should be clearly and directly discussed without distortion and documented in writing, particularly when patients display manipulative behavior.

Main Points

1. Pain is frequently associated with social and psychologic disturbances, particularly when it becomes chronic.
2. Anxiety and depression are particularly common correlates of pain.
3. Anxiety and depression should be diagnosed and treated.
4. Persistent psychopathology should not prevent thoughtful consideration of diagnosis and treatment of specific pain problems.
5. Willing patients with chronic pain can benefit from behavioral interventions including biofeedback and relaxation training, hypnosis, desensitization, and behavioral modification.
6. Chronic pain is commonly associated with indicators of major depression including diminished sleep, loss of appetite, decreased activity, lack of energy, loss of concentration, decreased interest in experiencing pleasure, and suicidal ideation.
7. Conscious presentation of false or greatly exaggerated symptoms constitutes malingering.

Selected Readings

Breitbart W. Psychiatric management of cancer pain. *Cancer* 63: 2336–2342, 1989.

Cassem NH. *Massachusetts General Hospital Handbook of General Hospital Psychiatry* (3rd ed). St. Louis: Mosby–Year Book 1991.

Hyman S. *Manual of Psychiatric Emergencies.* Boston: Little, Brown, 1988.

Sternbach R. *Pain Patients: Traits and Treatments.* New York: Academic Press, 1974.

Obstacles in the Treatment of Pain

Robert O. Ong

> *"Divinum est sedare dolorem — It is divine to allay pain."*
>
> GALEN

Over the past decade a great effort has been made to identify problems in the management of pain. Many of the problems were linked to misconceptions and myths perpetuated not only by physicians and health professionals but by patients as well.

In this chapter, we provide a brief survey of various myths that individuals may harbor toward receiving pain treatment. We also discuss issues such as the process of maintaining a high standard of care and the difficulties in providing this due to state laws, issues with local pharmacists, and patient and family attitudes.

The Roots of Inadequate Pain Control in the General Population

THE ROLE OF HEALTH CARE PROFESSIONALS

Health care professionals may harbor **misconceptions** and myths about the use of analgesics, most notably opioids. Furthermore, health professionals do not always adequately assess pain. Some of these issues are outlined below.

Misconception: Use of Potent Opioid Analgesics Will Always Result in Drug Addiction.

In reality, less than 0.1% of patients develop drug abuse when these drugs are used legitimately. Tolerance and dependence are easily managed medically. Patients at risk for dependence may be recognized by the following observations:

1. Usage out of control
2. Obsession with obtaining supply
3. Usage causes personal and legal difficulties
4. Usage continues despite problems
5. User denies taking the substance
6. Quality of life is not improved

Misconception: Physical Dependence and Drug Tolerance Are Often Equated with Drug Abuse.

Physical dependence is defined as the altered physiologic state produced by the repeated administration of a drug, which necessitates its continuation to prevent appearance of a withdrawal reaction or abstinence syndrome. **Drug tolerance** exists when increasingly larger doses are needed to provide the same effect as the original dose. In contrast, drug abuse or addiction is characterized by a behavior pattern of compulsive drug use and procurement of its supply with a high tendency for relapse after withdrawal. It is therefore possible to be physically dependent on drugs without being addicted (babies of addicted mothers will show signs of withdrawal and physical dependence at birth) and to be addicted without being physically dependent (as in patients taking cocaine) (Rogers 1989).

Misconception: Patients Who Show Signs of Withdrawal Are Often Considered to be Addicted.

Patients will often exhibit signs of withdrawal and are not necessarily addicted. A withdrawal syndrome is often the result of stopping opioid analgesics abruptly in patients who have received an opioid for more than 1 week, or inappropriate equi-analgesic conversions from one opioid to another. Opioids may be safely tapered by decreasing the previous day's dose by 75% and then further decreasing it by 25% every 2 or 3 days.

Misconception: Drug Addiction Can Be Prevented By Withholding Opioid Analgesics.

This erroneous concept reflects the lack of knowledge about the pharmacokinetics of opioid analgesics. In fact, the longer the patient waits for pain relief, the more medications are required to achieve an adequate plasma concentration. This is the very basis of providing patient-controlled analgesia.

Misconception: Patients Who Respond to Placebo Are Considered Not To Have Real Pain.

A positive response to placebo does not indicate that the patient's pain is not real or existent because several factors vary considerably from one patient to another and also at different times even in the same patient. Placebo is not considered a reliable tool in assessment of pain. Studies have shown that its effect results from physician–patient relationship, the significance of therapeutic effort, and the frame of mind imparted by the physician as well as the therapeutic setting.

The descending analgesic system may account for placebo-induced analgesia and the apparent analgesic effects of acupuncture and hypnosis.

Misconception: Patients' Pain Behavior Is Often Regarded as a Dependable Index in the Assessment of Pain.

Responses to noxious stimuli can generally be classified into two distinct categories—one is a subjective experience of pain and the other is a complex set of observable behaviors. We rely on the patient's verbal and nonverbal communication of pain.

Unfortunately, health professionals pay little attention to nonverbal pain behaviors. Their own attitudes and conceptions about pain may obscure their assessment of pain. Patients who have a flat affect may not be regarded as credible as someone who moans, groans, grimaces, and exhibits other pain behaviors. The problem of assessment may also be compounded by the fact that patients' reaction to pain may also vary greatly depending on other factors such as culture, religious beliefs, intensity, location and quality of pain, and psychologic makeup.

Misconception: Presence of Visitors and Family Members May Make a Patient's Pain Worse.

Patients' reluctance to request opioid analgesics often leads to family members demanding the medications for them. Some patients are also noted to exhibit increased pain behavior in an effort to seek more attention from family members and visiting friends. It is therefore important to determine what is considered adequate analgesia for the patient.

Misconception: Sleep Is a Reliable Indicator of Pain Relief.

Patients commonly complain that persistent pain interferes with their sleep. This problem leads to chronic fatigue and sleepless nights. On the other hand, patients are sometimes awakened to assess their pain and pain relief. When awakened, some may report severe pain; others manage to sleep despite having severe pain. This may be due to the sedative effects of different medications.

Misconception: Patients Who Time the Duration of Their Pain Medications and "Watch the Clock" Are Said To Be "Addicted."

When patients find that the time interval between medications are getting longer, they may actually be developing tolerance, since the first sign of tolerance is a shortening of the duration of analgesic effect. It is thus important to recognize this and to increase either the dosage or the frequency of analgesics to provide adequate pain relief.

Another factor in the failure of pain management, commonly ascribed to health professionals, is the observation that some doctors are said to underprescribe analgesics while nurses underdose them. In some instances, drugs are not given regularly at scheduled intervals. In general, this reflects the lack of education in pain therapy and knowledge about certain chronic pain syndromes, such as cancer pain, among health professionals.

Attitudes expressed verbally or nonverbally by health professionals certainly affect the willingness of patients to verbalize their legitimate needs for pain medications. Questions such as "What do you need?" strongly reinforce a sense of dependency on the part of the patient. A patient might feel less awkward and helpless if he or she were to be greeted by the health care provider with a friendly pat on the shoulder and the question "What can I do to help you feel more comfortable?"

THE PHARMACIST

The problem of poor pain management can originate in the pharmacies. Statistics show that 38% of hospitalized patients with cancer have pain that necessitates use of analgesics, and this percentage rises to over 60% in the terminal phase. However, one hospital survey revealed that less than half of the hospital pharmacies stock class II analgesics which are useful for treating severe cancer pain. Medications such as morphine and methadone represented less than 2% of the analgesics actually prescribed. The dearth of such drugs is even greater in outpatient neighborhood pharmacies for fear of robbery.

There is an insufficient supply of drugs for many reasons. National regulation and legislation, such as stringent Drug Enforcement Administration requirements for triplicate forms in some states, non-refills, and maximum 30-day supply prescriptions (see Appendix III), as well as rising health costs contribute to the limited availability of analgesics for patients in pain. Some physicians argue that they do not prescribe narcotic analgesics because the pharmacies do not stock them. In turn, pharmacists insist that they do not stock them because of a lack of demand.

For those pharmacies that do stock narcotic analgesics, there have been reports of their reluctance to fill pain prescriptions in "exceptionally large doses or in unusual combinations." It is unfortunate that there is often a strict adherence to the concept of prescribing a "standard dosage" for pain medications. Such a standard dosage may, of course, be quite different from the truly therapeutic dosage, as shown in clinical studies. Hence any attempts to alter this concept should start in medical school and pharmacy education programs.

The Patient's Role

The responsibility for inadequate pain relief may well rest with the patient.

PATIENTS' RELUCTANCE TO TAKE OPIOID ANALGESICS

Studies found that the majority of patients in moderate pain wait to ask for pain relief until it becomes severe and unbearable.

PATIENTS' RELUCTANCE TO COMMUNICATE THEIR PAIN

There are several reasons why patients undercomplain or underreport their pain. Foremost is the fear of addiction. They dread loss of control and becoming dependent on pain medications. Other patients fear the stigma attached to taking narcotics and therefore the loss of self-esteem. They feel that when they frequently ask for pain medications, this places an unfair burden on relatives and nurses. Finally, some patients equate continued or increasing pain with a worsening of their condition and thus are hesitant to admit any such increase in their pain level either to themselves or to health care providers.

PATIENTS' DESIRE TO CONTINUE THEIR SUFFERING

There are patients whose religious traditions lead them to believe that pain has an associated redemptive meaning—i.e., suffering is regarded as a means of purification. However it is important to draw the fine line between religious fanaticism and sadomasochism. Here, the expertise of a chaplain or pastoral counselor is key to the successful management of pain.

PATIENTS' MEANS OF VERBALIZING THEIR PAIN

One patient may relate all of his or her pain to a family member who, in turn, reports this problem to the nurse. But when interrogated by the nurse, the patient will then deny having any pain. In other instances, one may complain of pain to a nurse only to deny it later when questioned by a physician. Such contradictions in patient communication quickly become a source of disbelief by medical staff that pain exists when in fact it is very real to the patient.

PATIENTS' POOR COMPLIANCE WITH PAIN MEDICATIONS

This problem stems from a lack of understanding of proper pain therapy and the pharmacokinetics of the drugs used. For example, antidepressants used to treat neuropathic pain are frequently discontinued by patients before allowing an adequate time (a few weeks) for the drug to build up sufficient in the blood level to take its effect on the body. Proper patient education is essential to a successful therapeutic outcome.

PATIENTS' FEAR OF OVERMEDICATION AND SIDE EFFECTS

In dealing with patients who express such fears and concern about the side effects of pain medications, one should exercise extreme caution.

Some factors that are responsible for inadequate pain relief in adults apply also to children. However, some of these factors are exaggerated in children.

Causes of Undertreatment of Pain in Children

DIFFICULTIES IN PAIN ASSESSMENT AND MEASUREMENT

The task of assessing the severity of pain in children is considerably more difficult than in adults. Because children, especially preschool age, cannot express their pain verbally, they may become withdrawn and sullen when in pain, and this may be mistaken for good pain control. Alternatively, crying may not necessarily connote pain but may be associated with other emotions such as fear, anxiety, or loneliness.

Young children are not able to express their pain level in terms of the standard visual analog scales used for adults. Instead, simpler self-report tools have been developed for children over age of 4, including the Oucher, poker chip tool, and face scales. For children older than 7, pain intensity can be assessed through the use of a horizontal word-graphic rating scale, numeric rating scale, or visual analog scale.

PARENTAL STRESS

Parental stress or reluctance to cooperate with health care providers may greatly interfere with the child's response to pain control. Pain can be effectively managed when there is harmonious interaction between the child, his or her parent(s), nurses, physicians, and other health care providers. Although the preferences of the child and family deserve respect and careful consideration, the primary responsibility of health professionals is to ensure safe and competent care. If the child were to undergo painful procedures in a hospital setting, allowing the parents to be with their child during the procedure as well as preparing the child and the parents on what to expect for pain medications will help allay their anxiety and distress.

LACK OF INFORMATION

Lack of information regarding the safety and efficacy of analgesics in young children has prevented health professionals from using analgesics effectively to control pain. The risk of opioid-induced respiratory depression is also a limiting concern.

SOCIETAL PREJUDICES

As in adults, societal prejudices exist regarding opioid addiction. Even within the medical community, there exists a serious misconception that children do not experience as much pain postoperatively, and so most surgeons try to avoid the use of opioid analgesics. Many children who receive continuous caudal infusions of narcotic and local anesthetic mixture are not provided with adequate analgesic supplements by the primary service once their caudal catheters are discontinued prematurely.

FEAR OF INJECTIONS

Children may deny the presence of pain for fear of injections. This is especially true in postoperative situations, where oral analgesics are poorly absorbed because of delayed gastric emptying during the recovery period. To compound the problem, nurses and doctors are more reluctant to give injections to children who may fear injections. It is therefore best to administer pharmacologic agents whenever possible by a route that is not painful (e.g., oral, transmucosal, intravenous).

Causes of Undertreatment of Pain in the Elderly

LACK OF FOCUS IN TREATMENT

Each year over 4000 publications can be found on Medline on the topic of pain, but only less than 1% of these deal with the pain experience or pain syndromes of the elderly. Epidemiologic data on pain in the elderly are lacking and studies that exist are often inconclusive. For instance, it has been shown that with increasing age, the age-specific morbidity rate also increases and that the prevalence of pain complaints in the elderly is 73% to 80%. In contrast, the large Nuprin epidemiologic survey showed an age-related reduction in the prevalence of chronic pain at all sites other than the joints. This latter survey reflects the existing misconception among clinicians, lay public, and patients that aging results in an increased pain threshold and that acute and chronic pain may be a part of normal aging. Perhaps it is not the sensation of pain itself that declines with aging but that the elderly are less inclined to complain about pain.

DELIBERATE UNDERREPORTING OF PAIN

Elderly patients may deliberately underreport their pain for a number of reasons. For instance, they are afraid that an analgesic will make them confused and drowsy, which may lead to more severe injuries from falls and accidents. Some patients may simply believe that pain is a physiologic part of aging and that a certain amount of it must be tolerated. Elderly patients tend to be passive recipients of health care—

partly from being uninformed about the availability of pain relief and partly from being afraid to complain about pain.

PHARMACOKINETIC STUDIES

A lack of adequate pharmacokinetic studies to determine adequate analgesic dosage requirements in the elderly has prevented health professionals from administering analgesics effectively. Gastrointestinal side effects, renal toxicities, respiratory depression, and unusual drug reactions in the elderly are always a concern for the clinician. Careful monitoring of the side effects of analgesics is even more important in treating pain of nursing home patients who may have moderate to severe cognitive impairment.

Process of Maintaining Standards of Care

To ensure that pain treatment is providing patients adequate relief, interventions that directly influence the routine behaviors of clinicians and patients need to be enforced, in addition to traditional educational approaches.

ROLE OF NATIONAL QUALITY ASSURANCE COMMITTEES

On a national scale, the Joint Commission on Accreditation of Healthcare Organizations (JCAHO) is an example of one such "quality assurance committee" that makes regular inspections of facilities including pain clinics to assess how well they are monitoring care. Because successful accreditation of the facility means economic viability, administrators provide strong incentives for health professionals to comply.

THE ROLE OF SPECIALTY SOCIETIES

The American Pain Society has developed quality assurance standards for the relief of acute pain and cancer pain. These draft standards were based on recommendations by a recent National Institutes of Health consensus conference in 1986, and is aimed at supporting individual clinicians in achieving their targeted outcome of pain relief in their facilities.

The standards focus on the treatment of acute pain and chronic pain, because there is already a scientific consensus regarding treatment methods, particularly the use of analgesic drugs. Areas that are still understudied include treatment of chronic pain not due to cancer and the outcomes of nonpharmacologic treatments (see Appendix II).

More recently, a clinical practice guideline on acute pain management of operative or medical procedures and trauma was developed under the sponsorship of the Agency for Health Care Policy and Research (AHCPR), Public Health Service, U.S. Department of Health and Human Services.

ACCREDITATION AND CREDENTIALING OF PHYSICIANS IN PAIN MANAGEMENT

To date, there is little consensus regarding the credentialing of health professionals considered qualified to provide pain treatment. There are numerous organizations that provide their own criteria for accreditation based on examinations, licensures, fellowship training, references, and clinical experience. Examples of these organizations are the American Academy of Pain Management, American Academy of Pain Medicine, American Board of Anesthesiology, and American Academy of Orofacial Pain. In addition, the International Association for the Study of Pain (IASP) has published a curriculum for pain fellowship training.

STANDARDS OF CARE FOR THE DIFFICULT PATIENT

Aside from following the general guidelines for prescription of narcotics set by Drug Enforcement Administration (see Appendix III), careful steps should also be taken to avoid turning a practice into a chronic pain drug practice.

Requests for "no substitution—brand medically necessary" should be perceived with extra caution, because police and pharmacists believe that brand name prescriptions, if specifically requested by the patient, suggest that the drug is sought for resale to other addicts or narcotic traffickers. Percocet, Percodan, Demerol, and Dilaudid are said to have high street value, because in their brand name formulations they can be readily identified by prospective purchasers.

Also, patients' stories about repeated accidents to their opioid prescription or drugs may indicate either abuse or some other problem such as diversion. Disappearing medicine is rare among the general public, but most pharmacists have heard these stories repeatedly from known drug abusers.

The medical condition causing pain that requires the prescription of controlled substances should be documented. Also, the following items must be clear or attained: that the diagnosis comes from a careful history and physical examination; that a written treatment plan with recorded measurable objectives has been obtained; that the need for controlled substances is clearly laid out; and the reason other treatment options are not chosen is explicitly stated.

At least every 3 months, patients who are receiving chronic narcotic prescriptions should be brought to the attention of the pain unit as a whole and carefully discussed in the light of the patients' response to treatment and progress toward treatment goals.

Use of a multidisciplinary approach to the treatment of pain is highly encouraged, and consultations by physicians outside of the pain unit are sought as appropriate. The team consists of physical therapists, behavioral therapists, a chaplain, pharmacists, and a social worker. At Massachusetts General Hospital, we also conduct weekly cancer pain meetings chronic pain conferences, acute and postsurgical pain rounds, and journal discussions with the pain team.

Selected Readings

Acute Pain Management Guideline Panel. Acute pain management: Operative or medical procedures and trauma. *Clinical Practice Guideline*. Rockville, MD: Agency for Health Care Policy and Research, Public Health Service, U.S. Department of Health and Human Services, 1992. AHCPR Pub. No. 92-0032.

Commission of the Provision of Surgical Services. Why is pain relief a particular problem in children? *Report of the Working Party on Pain After Surgery*. London, 1990.

Committee on Quality Assurance Standards. American Pain Society quality assurance standards for relief of acute pain and cancer pain. M Bond, J Charlton, and C Woolf (eds), *Proceedings of the VIth World Congress on Pain*. New York: Elsevier, 1991.

Crook J, Weir R, and Tunks E. An epidemiologic follow-up survey of persistent pain sufferers in a group family practice and specialty pain clinic. *Pain* 36:45–61, 1989.

Ferrell B. Pain management in elderly people. *J Am Geriatr Soc* 39:64–73, 1991.

Foley KM. The practical use of narcotic analgesics. *Med Clin North Am* 66:1091–1104, 1983.

Grossman SA. Undertreatment of cancer pain: Barriers and remedies. *Supportive Care in Cancer* 1:74–78, 1993.

Hodes RL. Cancer patients' needs and concerns when using narcotic analgesis. In CS Hill, Jr, and WS Fields (eds), *Drug Treatment of Cancer Pain in a Drug-Oriented Society*. New York: Raven, 1989.

Kanner RM. Are the people who need analgesics getting them? *Am J Nurs* 86:589, 1986.

Lisson E. Ethical issues related to pain control. *Nurs Clin North Am* 22:655, 1987.

Marks RM, and Schar EJ. Undertreatment of medical patients with narcotic analgesics. *Ann Intern Med* 78:173–181, 1973.

Morgan JP. American opiophobia: customary underutilization of opioid analgesics. In B Stimmel (ed), *Controversies in Alcoholism and Substance Abuse*. New York: Haworth, 1986.

O'Leary DS. The joint commission looks to the future. *JAMA* 238:951–952, 1987.

Porter J, and Jick H. Addiction rare in patients treated with narcotics. *N Engl J Med* 302:123, 1980.

Rogers AG. Analgesics: The physician's partner in effective pain management. *Virginia Med* 116:164–170, 1989.

Sternbach RA. Survey of pain in the United States: The Nuprin Pain Report. *J Clin Pain* 2:49–54, 1986.

Stjernsward J, and Teoh N. The scope of the cancer pain problem. KM Foley, et al (eds), *Advances in Pain Research and Therapy.* New York: Raven, 1990.

Weis OF, et al. Attitudes of patients, housestaff and nurses toward postoperative analgesia care. *Anesth Analg* 62:70–74, 1983.

Emergencies in Pain Management

Asteghik Hacobian, Milan Stojanovic, Cassandra L. Tribble, Paolo L. Manfredi, Jacqueline A. Tejeda, Juliet M. Cowin, and Ervant Nishanian

> *"In medicine, rules may be absolute, but consequences are variable."*
>
> CELSUS

Procedure-Related Emergencies

VASOVAGAL SYNCOPE

Vasovagal syncope is a common reaction that may occur even during a minor procedure. In patients with a history of vasovagal syncope, it can usually be prevented by a supine posture and sedation before the procedure. It is always associated with bradycardia.

Symptoms and Signs

Presyncopal symptoms and signs include nausea, epigastric distress, perspiration, lightheadedness, confusion, tachypnea, and pupillary dilatation.

Syncopal signs include loss of consciousness, generalized muscle weakness and loss of postural tone, pallor or cyanosis, brief tonic-clonic seizure–like activity, and hypotension.

Treatment

1. Stop the procedure.
2. Place the patient in the Trendelenburg position.
3. Administer oxygen, evaluate and protect the airway, and support ventilation depending on the severity of the case. Monitor oxygenation ventilation and vital signs.
4. Establish intravenous access if not present. Administer atropine 0.4–1.0 mg IV for a heart rate of less than 45 beats per minute, or for a progressively decreasing heart rate. Apply standard monitoring and evaluate ECG tracing for other possible causes of bradycardia (e.g., junctional rhythm).
5. Keep the patient supine until fully alert and recovered from bradycardia and weakness.
6. Always place the patient supine for procedures (e.g., intravenous line placement).

PNEUMOTHORAX

Pneumothorax is the presence of air within the intrapleural space. It may occur as a complication of intercostal nerve blocks, stellate ganglion blocks, celiac plexus blocks, intrascalene nerve blocks, and supraclavicular nerve blocks. Despite the frequent concern about the incidence of pneumothorax with intercostal blocks, it is rare in experienced hands.

Symptoms and Signs

A small pneumothorax usually causes no symptoms, although chest pain or dyspnea may occur. Tension pneumothorax manifests as decreased breath sounds, wheezing, hypotension, and circulatory collapse. Depending on the severity of the pneumothorax, signs on physical examination include tachypnea, asymmetrical expansion of the chest on the affected side, deviation of the trachea away from the pneumothorax, hyperresonance to percussion, and diminished breath sound on the affected side. A chest x ray should be taken in the upright position and at the end of maximal expiration to confirm the diagnosis.

Treatment

1. In life-threatening situations, when cardiovascular collapse is imminent, large-bore (14-gauge) catheter should be inserted at the midclavicular line in the second intercostal space just above the rib. To prevent air from entering the interpleural space, a syringe should be placed over the catheter before insertion. It should be followed by insertion of a chest tube with placement on water seal and suction.
2. Airway, breathing, and circulation should be supported and standard monitoring applied. Oxygen should be administered.
3. Small pneumothoraces occupying less than 25% of the hemithorax in asymptomatic individuals can be treated on an outpatient basis without removing the air. Serial chest radiographs to confirm nonexpansion should be obtained. The pneumothoraces should spontaneously resolve in 7 to 10 days.

SYSTEMIC LOCAL ANESTHETIC TOXICITY

Toxicity may result from an intra-arterial small-volume injection (e.g., during stellate ganglion block); drug overdose with a single injection; and administration at high infusion rates or frequent bolus intervals with resultant drug accumulation. Toxicity may manifest as either CNS or cardiovascular toxicity.

CNS Toxicity

Toxic effects are concentration dependent. Low concentrations of local anesthetics produce sedation, whereas high concentrations produce seizures. CNS toxicity parallels anesthetic potency.

Symptoms and Signs

These include metallic taste, tinnitus, visual disturbances, numbness of the tongue and lip, and lightheadedness. It may progress to loss of consciousness, generalized seizure activity, or coma.

Treatment

1. Oxygen should be administered by mask and/or bag on the first sign of toxicity; in mild cases it may be sufficient treatment. Airway, breathing, and circulation are assessed and standard monitoring is applied.
2. If seizure activity interferes with ventilation or it is prolonged, midazolam 1–2 mg IV or diazepam 5–10 mg IV should be administered. Alternatively thiopental 50–200 mg IV should be given with endotracheal intubation if the patient's airway is compromised. Succinylcholine 1.5 mg/kg IV may be given to facilitate intubation. It should be kept in mind that muscle relaxation abolishes muscle activity, but that neuronal seizure activity continues with elevated cerebral metabolic requirements for oxygen.

Cardiovascular Toxicity

Local anesthetics at low doses produce beneficial myocardial effects such as the prevention and treatment of arrhythmias. However, higher concentrations produce a dose-dependent decrease in myocardial contractility and can produce refractory arrhythmias and cardiovascular collapse.

The cardiovascular system is more resistant than the CNS to toxic effects, but when it occurs it may be difficult to treat.

Bupivacaine and etidocaine may be more cardiotoxic than the other local anesthetics.

Symptoms and Signs

Toxicity manifests as a decrease in cardiac contractility, a decrease in conduction with subsequent hypotension, and/or cardiac arrhythmias and cardiovascular collapse.

Treatment

1. Airway, breathing, and circulation should be supported according to Acute Cardiac Life Support (ACLS) protocol. Oxygen should be administered. Call for assistance.
2. Ventricular tachycardias are difficult to treat but will subside over time secondary to drug redistribution. Adequate circulatory support should be attempted in the meanwhile.
3. Ventricular arrhythmias induced with bupivacaine may be more responsive to treatment with bretylium 5–10 mg/kg IV q15–20min to a maximum of 30 mg/kg, than lidocaine.
4. Prolonged CPR or cardiopulmonary bypass may be required until the cardiotoxic effects subside.

EPIDURAL HEMATOMA

This is extremely rare if coagulation parameters are normal.

Symptoms and Signs

These include rapid onset of neurologic deficit and severe back pain.

Treatment

The immediate courses of action are MRI, steroids, and surgical decompression/laminectomy.

EPIDURAL ABSCESS

Symptoms and Signs

These include severe back pain, local back tenderness, fever, leukocytosis, and neurologic deficit.

Treatment

The immediate courses of action are MRI, surgical decompression/laminectomy, and intravenous antibiotics.

HIGH SPINAL ANESTHETIC

This may occur as a result of an unintentional subarachnoid injection of local anesthetics during an epidural, celiac plexus block, lumbar sympathetic block, stellate ganglion, and occipital nerve block.

Symptoms and Signs

These include dyspnea, nausea, vomiting, hypotension, and bradycardia. High sensory level which can progress to apnea and unresponsiveness.

Treatment

1. Establish adequate airway, administer oxygen, assess sensory and motor level.
2. Support ventilation; if the muscles of respiration are affected and the airway cannot be protected, endotracheal intubation may be necessary.
3. Support blood pressure and heart rate until the local anesthetic wears off.

HYPOTENSION

Iatrogenic Etiology

1. Intrathecal or subdural injection of local anesthetic
2. Excessive epidural block with local anesthetic
3. Celiac plexus neurolytic block or with local anesthetic
4. Tension pneumothorax
5. Drugs such as labetalol, guanethidine, bretylium and intravenous phentolamine are associated with hypotension if there is a rapid release of tourniquet during Bier blocks.

Preexisting Causes

1. Hypothyroidism
2. Dysrhymthmia
3. Thyroid storm
4. Sepsis
5. Left ventricular dysfunction
6. Cardiomyopathy

Acute Systemic Causes

1. Vasovagal
2. Allergic reaction
3. Myocardial ischemia
4. Adrenal insufficiency
5. Pulmonary embolism

Symptoms and Signs

These include lightheadedness, pallor, nausea, tachycardia, tachypnea, pupillary dilatation, confusion, and decreased muscle tone.

Treatment

1. Give supplemental oxygen.
2. Immediately establish intravenous access if not already in situ. Give intravenous fluids, e.g., 250–500 ml bolus of lactated Ringer's Solution.
3. Monitor the patient's vital signs, ECG tracing, oxygen saturation, and verbal communication.
4. Put the patient in the Trendelenburg position or elevate lower extremities
5. Administer vasopressors, if necessary, ephedrine 5–10 mg q5–10min IV; phenylephrine 50–100 µg IV bolus; or start infusion at 100 µg/min and maintain at 40–60 µg/min.

HYPERTENSION

Pain Etiology

1. Acute versus exacerbation of chronic pain
2. Anxiety
3. Essential hypertension
4. Preexisting disease
5. Rebound hypertension (sudden discontinuation of alpha-blockers such as clonidine or beta-blockers such as propranolol)

Drug Interactions

(e.g., meperidine/monoamine oxidase inhibitor, tricyclic antidepressants, and ephedrine/monoamine oxidase inhibitor)

1. Hypoxia
2. Hypercarbia
3. Intravascular injection

4. Systemic absorption of epinephrine, topical cocaine, or phenylephrine

Treatment

1. Supplemental oxygen
2. Ensure adequate ventilation
3. Treat underlying cause
4. Cancel procedure for diastolic blood pressure greater than 110 mm Hg
5. Treat with nifedipine 10 mg sublingual or labetalol 2.5–5.0 mg IV q5–10min.

Medication-Related Emergencies

ANAPHYLAXIS

Symptoms and Signs

Cardiovascular

1. Hypotension
2. Tachycardia
3. Dysrhymthmias

Pulmonary

1. Bronchospasm
2. Dyspnea
3. Pulmonary edema
4. Laryngeal edema
5. Hypoxemia
6. Cough

Dermatologic

1. Urticaria
2. Facial edema
3. Pruritus

Treatment

1. Stop administration of the drug.
2. Administer oxygen.
3. Assess the airway and ventilation; use endotracheal intubation if necessary.
4. Epinephrine 50–100 μg IV, or for persistent bronchospasm epinephrine 0.5 μg/min IV, then titrate against the patient's response.
5. Administer IV fluids (LR).
6. H_1 Blocker (benadryl 50–100 mg IV), H_2 blocker (cimetidine 150–300 mg IV).
7. Steroids (hydrocortisone 5 mg/kg IV, or dexamethasone 1–5 mg/kg IV)
8. In the event of circulatory collapse:

a. endotracheal intubation
b. epinephrine 1–5 mg IV or via endotracheal tube if no IV access. Titrate to response.
c. For cardiac arrest follow ACLS protocol.

OPIOID OVERDOSE

Symptoms and Signs

1. Sedation
2. Coma
3. Hypoventilation
4. Apnea
5. Miosis

Treatment

1. Support ventilation (Ambu bag, intubation), supplemental oxygen.
2. Naloxone 0.4 mg IV—maximal dose.

If the patient has been on chronic opioid therapy it is wise to administer naloxone 0.02–0.04 mg q2min, which will avoid precipitation of profound withdrawal. Due to naloxone's half-life of 1 hour, close monitoring and repeated injections might be needed in the event of opioid overdose. Close monitoring and naloxone infusion (0.5–1.2 mg/hr) might be required when overdose is caused by opioids with a longer half-life, such as methadone, propoxyphene, and levorphanol. Because vomiting is associated with naloxone administration, it is useful to keep the patient in the lateral decubitus position to prevent aspiration (endotracheal intubation should be also considered). When treating a patient on chronic opioid therapy, and an opioid overdose is causing sedation but not significant hypoventilation, observation for a few hours is the best therapeutic approach.

Opioid Withdrawal

Opioid withdrawal very rarely causes life-threatening symptoms. An exception is a patient on chronic opioids who receives naloxone: The withdrawal syndrome precipitated by opioid antagonists is much more severe than the one that occurs upon discontinuation of the drug.

Symptoms and Signs

1. Hypertension
2. Nausea
3. Vomiting (aspiration pneumonia might be a complication)
4. Fever
5. Shivering
6. Diarrhea
7. Muscle aches

Treatment

Resumption of opioid treatment is, in general, the best way to stop the withdrawal syndrome: 25% of the previous dose will usually abort all symptoms. When the withdrawal symptoms are less dramatic, clonidine 0.1–0.2 mg PO 3 tid can be added for the symptomatic treatment of nausea (prochlorperazine, metoclopramide, droperidol), muscle aches, (nonsteroidal anti-inflammatory drugs) and diarrhea (loperamide).

STEROIDS (EPIDURAL)

When used inappropriately in a cyclical weekly fashion for 1 month, epidural triamcinolone (150–300 mg) has been shown to suppress adrenal production of cortisol and the pituitary synthesis of endogenous corticotropin.

Symptoms and Signs

Adrenal insufficiency can present as weakness, fatigue, hypotension, weight loss, and anorexia. In its ultimate form— adrenal crisis—nausea, vomiting, and abdominal pain may become persistent. Lethargy may deepen to somnolence. Hypovolemic shock may be precipitated with a poor hemodynamic performance, although such poor hemodynamic performance is usually not evident when exogenous hormone is available, because mineralocorticoid activity of the adrenal medulla is still maintained. Long-term survival of adrenal-insufficient patients is dependent on the avoidance of stress that occurs with infection, trauma, surgery, gastrointestinal upsets, or hypoglycemia in insulin-dependent diabetics.

Treatment

It would be wise to supplement patients with stress dose steroids prior to any surgical stress or infection if patients have had a course of epidural steroids in the last 1 to 3 months. Should acute adrenal insufficiency occur, immediate treatment is necessary. The minimal therapy includes fluid and electrolyte resuscitation and steroid replacement.

Other Emergencies

THE SUICIDAL PATIENT

Symptoms and Signs

Pain patients may become suicidal. Suicidal ideation may represent a spectrum of intents, from self-harm to manipulation to reach a secondary gain. At times, patients will offer direct statements that raise the suspicion of suicide. Otherwise, some patients may only offer behavior that raises concerns about possible suicidal tendencies. Any signs or symptoms of suicidal tendency require prompt and direct inquiry about the suicidal thinking.

Treatment

1. Prepare for the acutely suicidal patient: Know how to (1) activate security personnel for emergent assistance should a suicidal patient require safety precautions prior to obtaining psychiatric evaluation and (2) access acute psychiatric intervention for rapid evaluation and containment of suicidality with the institution of appropriate safety measures.
2. Take all evidence of suicidal thinking or behavior seriously and always obtain acute psychiatric evaluation when acute suicidality is in question.
3. Be direct and do not be afraid to raise the issue of suicidality.

References

1. Barash PG, Cullen BF, and Stoelting RK. *Clinical Anesthesia.* Philadelphia: Lippincott, 1989.

2. Cousins M, and Bridenbaugh P. *Neuronal Blockade in Clinical Anesthesia and Management of Pain* (2nd ed). Philadelphia: Lippincott, 1988.

3. Isselbacher K, Braunwald E and Wilson JD. *Harrison's Principles of Internal Medicine* (13th ed). New York: McGraw-Hill, 1994.

4. Kay J, Findling JW, and Ralf H. Epidural triamcinolone suppresses the pituitary-adrenal axis in human subjects. *Anesth Anal* 79:501-505, 1994.

5. Levy JH Allergic reactions during anesthesia. *J Clin Anesth* 1:44, 1988.

6. Moore DC. *Regional Block: A Handbook for Use in the Clinical Practice of Medicine and Surgery* (4th ed). Springfield, IL: Thomas, 1981.

7. Orkin FK, and Cooperman LH (eds). *Complications in Anesthesiology.* Philadelphia: Lippincott, 1988.

8. Wingarden J, Smith J, and Lloyd H. *Cecil's Textbook of Medicine.* WB Saunders, 1992.

Appendixes

IASP Classification of Chronic Pain

To facilitate differential diagnoses for the reader, the International Association for the Study of Pain (IASP) Classification of Chronic Pain is summarized below.

I. Relatively Generalized Syndromes
   1. Peripheral neuropathy
   2. Stump pain
   3. Phantom pain
   4. Causalgia
   5. Reflex sympathetic dystrophy
   6. Central pain (including thalamic and pseudo-thalamic pain)
   7. Syndrome of syringomyelia (when affecting the head or limb)
   8. Polymyalgia rheumatica
   9. Fibrositis or diffuse myofascial pain syndrome
   10. Rheumatoid arthritis
   11. Osteoarthritis
   12. Calcium pyrophosphate deposition disease (CPPD)
   13. Gout
   14. Hemophilic arthropathy
   15. Burns
   16. Pain of psychologic origin
       a. Muscle tension
       b. Delusional or hallucinatory
       c. Hysterical or hypochondriacal
   17. Factitious illness and malingering

II. Neuralgias of the Head and Face
   1. Trigeminal neuralgia (tic douloureux)
   2. Secondary neuralgia (trigeminal) from CNS lesions
   3. Secondary trigeminal neuralgia from facial trauma
   4. Acute herpes zoster (trigeminal)
   5. Postherpetic neuralgia (trigeminal)
   6. Geniculate neuralgia (cranial nerve VII): Ramsay Hunt syndrome
   7. Glossopharyngeal neuralgia (cranial nerve IX)
   8. Neuralgia of the superior laryngeal nerve (vagus nerve neuralgia)
   9. Occipital neuralgia

III. Craniofacial Pain of Musculoskeletal Origin
   1. Acute tension headache
   2. Tension headache: chronic form (scalp muscle contraction headache)
   3. Temporomandibular pain and dysfunction syndrome

4. Osteoarthritis of the temporomandibular joint
5. Rheumatoid arthritis of the temporomandibular joint

IV. Lesions of the Ear, Nose, and Oral Cavity
1. Maxillary sinusitis
2. Odontalgia: toothache 1: due to dentino-enamel defects
3. Odontalgia: toothache 2: pulpitis
4. Odontalgia: toothache 3: periapical periodontitis and abscess
5. Odontalgia: toothache 4: tooth pain not associated with lesions (atypical odontalgia)
6. Glossodynia and sore mouth (also known as burning tongue or oral dysesthesia)
7. Cracked tooth syndrome
8. Dry socket

V. Primary Headache Syndromes
1. Classic migraine
2. Common migraine
3. Migraine variants
4. Carotidynia
5. Mixed headache
6. Cluster headache
7. Chronic paroxysmal hemicrania (chronic stage)
8. Chronic cluster headache
9. Cluster-tic syndrome
10. Posttraumatic headache

VI. Pain of Psychologic Origin in the Head and Face
1. Delusional or hallucinatory pain
2. Hysterical or hypochondriacal

VII. Suboccipital and Cervical Musculoskeletal Disorders
1. Myofascial syndrome: cervical sprain or cervical hyperextension injury (whiplash)
2. Myofascial syndrome: sternocleidomastoid muscle
3. Myofascial syndrome: trapezius muscle
4. Stylohyoid process syndrome (Eagle's syndrome)

VIII. Visceral Pain in the Neck
1. Carcinoma of thyroid
2. Carcinoma of larynx
3. Tuberculosis of larynx

IX. Pain of Neurologic Origin in the Neck, Shoulder, and Upper Extremity
1. Prolapsed disc
2. Osteophyte: cervical spondylosis
3. Intraspinal tumor
4. Fracture or collapse of cervical vertebrae
5. Epidural abscess
6. Vertebral tumor
7. Herpes zoster: acute

8. Postherpetic neuralgia
9. Syphilis: tabes dorsalis and hypertrophic pachymeningitis
10. Meningitis and arachnoiditis
11. Traumatic avulsion of nerve roots
12. Superior pulmonary sulcus syndrome (Pancoast's tumor)
13. Thoracic outlet syndrome
14. Cervical rib or malformed first rib
15. Pain of skeletal metastatic disease of the arm or shoulder girdle

X. Lesions of the Brachial Plexus
1. Tumors of the brachial plexus
2. Chemical irritation of the brachial plexus
3. Traumatic avulsion of the brachial plexus
4. Postradiation
5. Painful arms and moving fingers

XI. Pain in the Shoulder, Arm, and Hand
1. Bicipital tendinitis
2. Subacromial bursitis (subdeltoid bursitis, supraspinatus tendinitis)
3. Rotator cuff tear: partial or complete
4. Lateral epicondylitis (tennis elbow)
5. Medial epicondylitis (golfer's elbow)
6. DeQuervain's tenosynovitis
7. Osteoarthritis of the hands
8. Carpal tunnel syndrome
9. Pain of psychologic origin in the shoulder and arm
   a. Tension
   b. Delusional or hallucinatory
   c. Hysterical or hypochondriacal

XII. Vascular Disease of the Limbs
1. Raynaud's disease
2. Raynaud's phenomenon
3. Frostbite and cold injury
4. Erythema Pernio (chilblain)
5. Acrocyanosis
6. Livedo reticularis

XIII. Collagen Disease of the Limbs
1. Scleroderma
2. Ergotism

XIV. Vasodilating Functional Disease of the Limbs
1. Erythromelalgia
2. Thromboangiitis obliterans
3. Chronic venous insufficiency

XV. Arterial Insufficiency in the Limbs
1. Intermittent claudication
2. Rest pain

XVI. Pain in the Limbs of Psychological Origin
1. Tension

2. Delusional
3. Conversion

XVII. Chest Pain
1. Acute herpes zoster
2. Postherpetic neuralgia
3. Postinfectious and segmental peripheral neuralgia
4. Angina pectoris
5. Myocardial infarction
6. Pericarditis
7. Aneurysm of the aorta
8. Disease of the diaphragm
   a. Infection: chest or pulmonary source
   b. Neoplasm: chest or pulmonary source
   c. Musculoskeletal
   d. Infection: gastrointestinal source
   e. Neoplasm: gastrointestinal source
   f. Cholelithiasis
9. Fracture or collapse of thoracic vertebrae
10. Slipping rib syndrome
11. Postmastectomy pain: acute and subacute
12. Postmastectomy pain: chronic nonmalignant
13. Last postmastectomy pain or regional carcinoma
14. Postthoracotomy pain syndrome

XVIII. Chest Pain of Psychologic Origin
1. Muscle tension
2. Delusional
3. Conversion

XIX. Chest Pain: Referred from Abdominal or Gastrointestinal Tract
1. Subphrenic abscess
2. Herniated abdominal organs
3. Esophageal motility disorders
4. Esophagitis
5. Reflux esophagitis with peptic ulceration
6. Carcinoma of esophagus
7. Gastric ulcer with chest pain
8. Duodenal ulcer with chest pain
9. Thoracic visceral disease with pain
   a. Referred to abdomen
   b. Pericarditis
   c. Diaphragmatic hernia

XX. Abdominal Pain of Neurologic Origin
1. Acute herpes zoster
2. Postherpetic neuralgia
3. Segmental or intercostal neuralgia
4. Twelfth rib syndrome
5. Abdominal cutaneous nerve entrapment syndrome

XXI. Abdominal Pain of Visceral Origin
1. Cardiac failure
2. Gallbladder disease

3. Postcholecystectomy syndrome
4. Chronic gastric ulcer
5. Chronic duodenal ulcer
6. Carcinoma of the stomach
7. Carcinoma of the pancreas
8. Chronic mesenteric ischemia
9. Crohn's disease
10. Chronic constipation
11. Irritable bowel syndrome
12. Diverticular disease of the colon
13. Carcinoma of the colon

XXII. Abdominal Pain Syndromes of Generalized Diseases
1. Familial Mediterranean fever (FMF)
2. Abdominal migraine
3. Intermittent acute porphyria
4. Hereditary coproporphyria
5. Variegate porphyria

XXIII. Abdominal Pain of Psychological Origin
1. Muscle tension
2. Delusional or hallucinatory
3. Conversion

XXIV. Diseases of the Uterus, Ovaries, and Adnexa
1. Mittelschmerz
2. Secondary dysmenorrhea
   a. With endometriosis
   b. With adenomyosis or fibrosis
   c. With congenital obstruction
   d. With acquired obstruction
   e. Psychologic causes
3. Primary dysmenorrhea
4. Endometriosis
5. Posterior parametritis
6. Tuberculous salpingitis
7. Retroversion of the uterus
8. Ovarian pain
9. Chronic pelvic pain without obvious pathology (CPPWOP)

XXV. Pain in the Rectum, Perineum, and External Genitalia
1. Neuralgia of iliohypogastric, ilioinguinal or genitofemoral nerves
2. Tumor infiltration of the sacrum and sacral nerves
3. Rectal, perineal, and genital pain of psychologic origin

XXVI. Backache and Pain of Neurologic Origin in the Trunk and Back
1. Prolapsed intervertebral disc
2. Acute herpes zoster
3. Postherpetic neuralgia
4. Intraspinal tumor
5. Fracture of lumbar vertebrae

6. Collapse of lumbar vertebrae
7. Epidural abscess
8. Vertebral tumor
   a. Nerve involvement: thorax
   b. Musculoskeletal involvement: thorax
   c. Nerve involvement: abdomen
   d. Musculoskeletal involvement: abdomen
   e. Nerve involvement: low back
   f. Musculoskeletal metastasis: low back
9. Retroperitoneal tumor
10. Syphilis
11. Meningitis and arachnoiditis
12. Meningeal carcinomatosis
13. Tumor infiltration of the lumbosacral plexus

XXVII. Back Pain of Musculoskeletal Origin
   1. Osteophyte
   2. Lumbar spondylolysis
   3. Spinal stenosis
   4. Sacralization or lumbarization (transitional vertebra)
   5. Abnormal articular facets (facet tropism)
   6. Acute low back strain
   7. Recurrent low back strain
   8. Trauma: acute
   9. Chronic mechanical low back pain
   10. Prolapsed disc lesion
   11. Cauda equina lesion
   12. Ankylosing spondylitis
   13. Quadratus lumborum syndrome
   14. Gluteal syndromes

XXVIII. Back Pain of Visceral Origin
   1. Carcinoma of the rectum

XXIX. Low Back Pain of Psychologic Origin
   1. Tension
   2. Delusional
   3. Conversion

XXX. Local Syndromes in the Leg or Foot—Pain of Neurologic Origin
   1. Lateral femoral cutaneous neuropathy (meralgia paresthetica)
   2. Obturator neuralgia
   3. Femoral neuralgia
   4. Sciatical neuralgia
   5. Interdigital neuralgia of the foot (Morton's metatarsalgia)
   6. Injection neuropathy
   7. Painful legs and moving toes
   8. Metastatic disease

XXXI. Pain Syndromes of the Hip and Thigh of Musculoskeletal Origin
   1. Ischial bursitis
   2. Trochanteric bursitis
   3. Osteoarthritis of the hip

XXXII. Musculoskeletal Syndromes of the Leg
1. Spinal stenosis
2. Osteoarthritis of the knee
3. Night cramps
4. Plantar fasciitis

Source: With permission from the International Association for the Study of Pain (IASP).

Useful Contacts

Table AII-1. National and international pain societies

American Pain Society	5700 Old Orchard Rd. Skokie, IL 60076	(708) 966-5595
International Association for the Study of Pain	909 NE 43rd St., Suite 306 Seattle, WA 98105-6020	(206) 547-6409

Table AII-2. Listing of selected U.S. pain clinics

Alabama

University of Alabama Pain Center	1813 6th Ave. Birmingham, AL 35294	(205) 801-8250

Arizona

University Medical Center Pain Clinic	1501 N. Campbell Ave. Tucson, AZ 85724	(602) 626-6793

Arkansas

University of Arkansas Medical Sciences Pain Clinic	4301 W. Markum Little Rock, AR 72205	(501) 686-5270

California

Loma Linda University Medical Center	P.O. Box 933 Loma Linda, CA 92354	(909) 824-4475
Scripps Clinic Medical Institutions Pain Treatment Center	10666 N. Torrey Pines Rd. LaJolla, CA 92037	(619) 554-8898
Stanford University Hospital	S268-A Grant Bldg. 300 Pasteur Dr. Stanford, CA 94305	(415) 725-5852
University of California, Irvine	P.O. Box 14091 Orange, CA 92613-1491	(714) 456-6437
University of California, Los Angeles Pain Management Center	10833 Le Conte Ave. Los Angeles, CA 90024-6909	(213) 825-4291
University of California, San Diego	9500 Gilman Dr. La Jolla, CA 92093	(619) 543-3162
University of California, San Francisco Pain Management Center	3350 Parnassus, Suite 307 San Francisco, CA 94117	(415) 476-4276

Colorado

| University of Colorado Medical Center Pain Clinic | 4200 E. 9th Ave., B113 Denver, CO   80262 | (303) 372-1650 |

Connecticut

| Hartford Hospital | 80 Seymour St. Hartford, CT   06102-5037 | (203) 545-2117 |

District of Columbia

| Georgetown University Medical Center | 3800 Reservoir Rd., NW Washington, DC   20007 | (202) 784-2090 |

Florida

| Mayo Clinic, Jacksonville | 4500 San Pablo Rd. Jacksonville, FL   32224 | (904) 296-5288 |

| University of Florida College of Medicine
• Shands Hospital at the University of Florida
• Veterans Affairs Medical Center, Gainesville | JHMHSC, P.O. Box 100254 Gainesville, FL   32610-0254 | (904) 395-0077 |

| University of Miami Jackson Memorial Medical Center | P.O. Box 016370 Miami, FL   33101 | (305) 585-6283 |

| University of South Florida College of Medicine
• James A. Haley Veterans Hospital
• H. Lee Moffit Cancer Center and Research Institute | Department of Anesthesiology, MDC-59 12901 Bruce B. Downs Blvd. Tampa, FL   33612 | (813) 251-7438 |

Georgia

| Emory University Hospital Crawford Long Hospital of Emory University | 550 Peachtree St., NE Atlanta, GA   30365 | (404) 686-2320 |

Illinois

| McGaw Medical Center of Northwestern University Northwestern Memorial Hospital | 303 E. Superior St., Rm. 360 Chicago, IL   60611 | (312) 908-2500 |

| Northwestern University Department of Anesthesia Pain Control Service | 303 E. Superior St., Rm. 360 Chicago, IL   60611 | (312) 908-8254 |

Rush Pain Center	1725 W. Harrison St., Suite 262 Chicago, IL 60090	(312) 356-2320
University of Illinois College of Medicine at Chicago Michael Reese Hospital and Medical Center	2929 S. Ellis Ave. Chicago, IL 60616	(312) 791-2544

Indiana

Indiana University Medical Center	1120 South Dr. Indianapolis, IN 46202-5115	(317) 274-0265

Iowa

University of Iowa Department of Anesthesia Pain Clinic	Newton Rd. Iowa City, IA 52242	(319) 356-2320

Kansas

Kansas University Medical Center Department of Anesthesiology Pain Clinic	3900 Rainbow Blvd. Kansas City, KS 66103	(913) 588-3315

Kentucky

University Hospital Albert B. Chandler Medical Center	800 Rose St., Rm. N-202 Lexington, KY 40536-0084	(606) 233-5956

Louisiana

Touro Center for Chronic Pain and Disability Rehabilitation	1401 Fouchter St. New Orleans, LA 70115	(504) 897-8404

Maine

Mercy Hospital Pain Clinic	144 State St. Portland, ME	(207) 879-3668

Maryland

The Johns Hopkins Hospital Blaustein Pain Treatment Center	60 N. Wolfe St. Baltimore, MD 21205	(301) 955-3270
National Institutes of Health NIDR/NIH Pain Clinic	Bldg. 10, Rm. 3C-403 Bethesda, MD 20205	(301) 496-5483
University of Maryland Medical System	22 S. Greene St., Suite S11C Baltimore, MD 21201	(410) 328-5063

Massachusetts

Baystate Medical Center	759 Chestnut St. Springfield, MA 01199	(413) 784-3520

Beth Israel Hospital	330 Brookline Ave. Boston, MA 02215	(617) 732-6707
Brigham and Women's Hospital	75 Francis St. Boston, MA 02115	(617) 732-6707
Massachusetts General Hospital Pain Center	15 Parkman St., WAC-324 Boston, MA 02114-3139	(617) 726-8810

Michigan

Henry Ford Hospital	2799 W. Grand Blvd. Detroit, MI 48202	(313) 876-8078
University of Michigan Medical Center	C233 Med Inn Building Ann Arbor, MI 48109-0824	(313) 763-5459

Minnesota

Mayo Clinic, Rochester	200 First St., SW Rochester, MN 55905	(507) 255-4240
Mayo Pain Clinic and Pain Management Center	200 SW First St. Rochester, MN 55909	(507) 255-4240
University of Minnesota Hospitals Neurosurgery Department	420 Delaware Minneapolis, MN 55455	(612) 624-6666

Mississippi

University of Mississippi Medical Center	2500 N. State St. Jackson, MS 39216	(601) 984-5805

Missouri

Washington University • Barnes Hospital • St. Louis Children's Hospital	660 S. Euclid Ave. St. Louis, MO 63110-1093	(314) 362-8820

Nebraska

University of Nebraska Hospital and Clinic Nebraska Pain Management Center	42nd & Dewey Ave. Omaha, NE 68105	(402) 559-5868

Nevada

Pain Institute of Nevada	850 S. Rancho Dr., Suite D Las Vegas, NV 89106	(702) 878-8252

New Hampshire

Dartmouth-Hitchcock Medical Center	Hanover, NH 03755	(603) 650-6040
Dartmouth-Hitchcock Medical Center	One Medical Center Dr. Lebanon, NH 03756-0001	(603) 650-8690

New Jersey

UMDNJ-Robert Wood Johnson Medical Center	One Robert Wood Johnson Place, CN19 New Brunswick, NJ 08903	(908) 937-8751
UMDNJ-University Hospital	90 Bergen St., Suite 3400 Newark, NJ 07103	(201) 982-2080

New Mexico

University of New Mexico Hospital Veterans Affairs Medical Center, Albuquerque	Albuquerque, NM 87131-5216	(505) 272-2733

New York

Albany Medical Center Hospital	618 Central Avenue Albany, NY 12206	(518) 459-4117
Brookdale Hospital Medical Center	1275 Linden Blvd., 719 CHC Brooklyn, NY 11212	(718) 240-5356
Columbia–Presbyterian Medical Center Pain Treatment Center	622 W. 168 St. New York, NY 10032	(212) 305-7114
Memorial Sloan Kettering Cancer Center	1275 York Ave. New York, NY 10021	(212) 639-6594
Mount Sinai Medical Center	Box 1192 New York, NY 10029	(212) 241-6372
The New York Hospital	525 E. 68th St. New York, NY 10021	(212) 746-2960
North Shore University Hospital Center for Pain Management	300 Community Rd. Manhasset, NY 11030	(516) 562-4887
St. Joseph Hospital Health Center	5100 West Taft Rd., Suite 5D Liverpool, NY 13088	(315) 452-2054
St. Luke's Roosevelt Hospital	428 W. 59th St. New York, NY 10019	(212) 523-6137
SUNY Buffalo General Hospital	100 High St. Buffalo, NY 14203	(716) 845-2220
SUNY Health Science Center	450 Clarkson Ave. Brooklyn, NY 11203	(718) 270-1525
University Hospital-SUNY at Stony Brook	Health Sciences Center L4-060 Stonybrook, NY 11794-8480	(516) 444-2975
University of Rochester Medical Center	601 Elmwood Ave. Rochester, NY 14642	(716) 275-2141
Westchester County Medical Center	Grasslands Rd., Macy-W Valhalla, NY 10595	(914) 285-7692

North Carolina

Duke University Medical Center Duke Pain Clinic	Box 3094 Durham, NC 27710	(919) 684-6542
North Carolina Baptist Hospital Bowman Gray School of Medicine Pain Control Center	Medical Center Blvd. Winston-Salem, NC 27157-1077	(919) 716-5530
North Carolina Medical Hospital Pain Program	Box 532 Chapel Hill, NC 27514	(919) 966-1057

Ohio

The Cleveland Clinic Foundation	9500 Euclid Ave. Cleveland, OH 44195	(216) 444-3769
University of Cincinnati Medical Center Pain Relief Center	234 Goodman St. Cincinnati, OH 45267	(513) 558-5664

Oregon

Oregon Health Sciences University	3181 S.W. Sam Jackson Park Rd. Portland, OR 97201	(503) 494-7641

Pennsylvania

Albert Einstein Medical Center	5501 Old York Rd., Tower Bldg. Philadelphia, PA 19141	(215) 456-6950
Hershey Medical Center	P.O. Box 850 Hershey, PA 17033	(717) 531-8433
Hospital of the University of Pennsylvania	3400 Spruce St. Philadelphia, PA 19104-4283	(215) 662-3742
Temple University Hospital	Broad and Ontario Sts. Philadelphia, PA 19140	(215) 221-3326
Thomas Jefferson University Hospital	834 Chestnut St., Suite T-150 Philadelphia, PA 19107-5127	(215) 955-7246
University Health Center of Pittsburgh Presbyterian-University Hospital UPMC Pain Evaluation and Treatment Institute	Baum Blvd. at Craig St. Pittsburgh, PA 15213	(412) 578-3100

South Carolina

Richland Memorial Hospital	Five Richland Medical Park Columbia, SC 29203	(803) 434-6151

Tennessee

Vanderbilt University Medical Center	1211 21st Ave., S Medical Arts Building, Suite 324 Nashville, TN 37232	(615) 343-7072

Texas

MD Anderson Cancer Pain Center Department of Neuro-oncology	1515 Holcombe Blvd. Box 8 Houston, TX 77030	(713) 792-2824
Methodist Hospital Baylor College of Medicine	Smith Tower, Suite 1003 6550 Fannin Houston, TX 77030	(713) 798-7356
Texas Tech University Health Sciences Center	3601 4th St. Lubbock, TX 79430	(806) 743-3112
University of Texas Health Sciences Center at San Antonio	7703 Floyd Curl Dr. San Antonio, TX 78284-7838	(210) 567-4543
University of Texas Southwestern Dallas County Hospital District-Parkland Memorial Hospital Zale-Lipshy University Hospital Texas Scottish Rite Hospital for Children	5323 Harry Hines Blvd. Dallas, TX 75235-9068	(214) 648-5498
University of Texas Pain Clinic at Hermann Hospital	6431 Fannin, MSB 5-020 Houston, TX 77030	(615) 322-6683

Utah

University of Utah Medical Center Pain Clinic	50 N. Medical Dr. Salt Lake City, UT 84132	(801) 581-7246

Vermont

University of Vermont Fletcher Allen Health Care Pain Clinic	MCHV Campus 111 Colchester Ave. Burlington, VT 05401	(802) 656-2415

Virginia

Naval Medical Center, Portsmouth	Portsmouth, VA 23708-5100	(804) 398-7266
University of Virginia Pain Center	Box 293 Charlottesville, VA 22908	(804) 924-5581
Virginia Commonwealth University Pain Center	Box 516 Richmond, VA 23298	(804) 786-9162

Washington

University of Washington Pain Clinic	1959 NE Pacific St. Seattle, WA 98195	(206) 548-4282
Virginia Mason Medical Center	1100 Ninth Ave., B-2AN Seattle, WA 98111	(206) 223-6980

West Virginia

West Virginia University Health Sciences Center Pain Clinic, Department of Anesthesiology	Morgantown, WV 26505	(304) 293-2006, (304) 293-3279

Wisconsin

Medical College of Wisconsin Affiliated John L. Dohne Hospital	8700 W. Wisconsin Ave. Milwaukee, WI 53226	(414) 257-6257
University of Wisconsin Clinical Science Center (Pain Research Group)	600 Highland Ave. Madison, WI 53742	(608) 263-7660

Source: Adapted from American Society of Regional Anesthesia Pain Fellowships and American Pain Society Directory of Pain Centers.

Guidelines for the Use of Opioids in Pain Treatment

Guidelines for the Prescription of Controlled Substances Issued by the Drug Enforcement Agency

1. A prescription for a controlled substance is lawful only if issued for a legitimate medical purpose by an individual practitioner acting in the usual course of professional practice. Prescriptions under the law may not be issued for narcotic drugs for the purpose of detoxification or maintenance of narcotic addicts.
2. All prescriptions for controlled substances must bear the following information:
   a. Name of patient
   b. Home address of patient
   c. Name of practitioner
   d. Address of practitioner
   e. Registration number of practitioner
   f. Name of the drug, strength, and quantity of the medicine to be dispensed
   g. Directions for use
3. All prescriptions must be dated with the day when issued to the patient and must be signed manually on that day by the practitioner.
4. It is illegal under both Federal and State Law to issue a prescription for other than a legitimate bona fide medical need or to date a prescription other than the date when it is issued to the patient and signed by the practitioner.
5. Schedule II controlled substances require written prescriptions prior to dispensing. They may not be refilled. A Schedule II drug may be dispensed in an emergency by a pharmacist upon oral prescription of a practitioner if the quantity is limited to the emergency period, if the prescription is reduced immediately to writing by the pharmacist and contains all the information required of written prescriptions except the signature of the prescriber, if the pharmacist knows the prescriber, or makes a reasonable effort to verify the order's validity, and if the prescriber issues to the pharmacist a written prescription within 48 hours of the oral order. If the pharmacist does not receive a written prescription from the prescriber within 72 hours, he or she must by law notify the DEA regional office.
6. A controlled substance prescription must be for no more than 30 days of medicine.

Massachusetts General Hospital Pain Center Guidelines on Prescribing Controlled Substances for Patients with Nonmalignant Chronic Disease

1. Controlled substance prescriptions are not sent by mail.

2. Prescriptions are not written as "brand name medically necessary" or "no substitution."

3. When chronic opioid therapy is initiated, the primary referring physician must concur with this decision and continue to monitor the patient as well. If, as the patient is observed, there is no demonstrable benefit to the patient's function or quality of life, then the opioid should be tapered. Before starting to taper a drug, the Pain Center physician should discuss the plan in advance with the primary referring physician if one can be identified and if the patient has been seen by that physician during the past year. The concurrence of the primary referring physician with the decision to start or taper opioids must be documented in the chart.

4. Where there is no primary physician, the Pain Center provides the patient with the opportunity to secure such a physician. We do not become the primary source of general medical care for any patient.

5. Discovery that the patient has obtained concurrent prescriptions for controlled substances from multiple doctors results in termination of the Pain Center's relationship with the patient.

6. The second instance of a lost or otherwise early depletion of a prescription will result in no further controlled substances being dispensed to that patient from our unit. The need does not necessarily result, however, in cessation of the therapeutic relationship with our unit, nor in our ceasing to prescribe noncontrolled substances.

7. There are to be no prescription refills if a patient arrives without an appointment prior to the time of his or her next scheduled refill. Even when a medical follow-up visit is not necessary, the patient must still inform the center at least the day before picking up a prescription. Failure to do so disrupts the center's schedule and needlessly inconveniences those working in it or waiting to be seen.

8. Options for physician therapy, behavioral medicine treatment, or other consultations (e.g., psychiatry, orthopedics), as appropriate, should be offered to patients who are being tapered from chronic opioid use. These options may be offered through an inpatient rehabilitation program, providing insurance is available to cover it, or, if not, even through MGH outpatient departments (e.g., Addictions Service).

9. No longer than 1 month should elapse between scheduled follow-up appointments during the long-term follow-up of any

patient receiving controlled substances in the absence of malignant disease.

10. Apart from the regulatory dimension, our first role is to treat the patient. Thus it is essential that our notes document the history, physical and laboratory findings, diagnosis and plans for medical and other therapies (including specifics and timing of schedules for tapering opioids). Initiation or tapering controlled substances in the absence of a documented medical rationale is not acceptable.

IV

Standards of Treatment: The American Pain Society's Quality Assurance Standards for Relief of Acute and Cancer Pain

In the majority of patients with acute pain and chronic cancer pain, comfort can be achieved with the attentive use of analgesic medications. Historically, though, the outcomes of analgesic treatment have often not been satisfactory, largely because clinical care units have had no systems in place to ensure that the occurrence of pain is recognized and that when pain persists, there is rapid feedback to modify treatment. These suggested standards are offered as one approach to developing such a system. Individual facilities may wish to modify these standards to suit their particular needs.

The guidelines are intended for hospitals and chronic care facilities in which only conventional analgesic methods are used (e.g., intermittent parenteral or oral analgesics) as well as those using the most modern technology for pain management. In either case, the quality of pain control will be enhanced by a dedicated pain management team whose personnel acquire special training in pain relief. Newer, more aggressive methods of pain control, such as patient-controlled analgesia, epidural opiate administration, and regional anesthetic techniques, may provide better pain relief than intermittent parenteral analgesics in many patients, but carry their own risks. Should institutions choose to use these methods, they must be delivered by an organized team with frequent follow-up and titration and adequate briefing of the primary care givers. Such teams should be organized under one of the recognized medical departments of the facility. Specific standards for such methods, monitored by that department, might well augment the general guidelines articulated here.

I. RECOGNIZE AND TREAT PAIN PROMPTLY

Chart and Display Pain and Relief (Process)

A measure of pain intensity and a measure of pain relief are recorded on the bedside vital sign chart or a similar record that facilitates regular review by members of the health care team and is incorporated in the patient's permanent record.

1. The intensity of pain or discomfort is assessed and documented on admission, after any known pain-producing procedure, with each new report of pain, and at regular intervals that depend on the severity of pain. A simple, valid measure of intensity will be selected by each clinical unit. For children, age-appropriate pain intensity measures will be used.

2. The degree of pain relief is determined after each pain management intervention, once sufficient time has elapsed for the treatment to reach peak effect (e.g., 1 hour for parenteral analgesics and 2 hours oral analgesics). A simple, valid measure of pain relief will be selected by each clinical unit.

Define Pain and Relief Levels to Trigger Review (Process)

Each clinical unit will identify values for pain intensity rating and pain relief rating that will elicit a review of the current pain therapy, documentation of the proposed modifications in treatment, and subsequent review of its efficacy. This process of treatment review and follow-up should include participation by physicians and nurses involved in the patient's care. As the general quality of treatment improves, the clinical unit will upgrade this standard to encourage a continuous process of improvement.

Survey Patient Satisfaction (Outcome)

At regular intervals to be defined by the clinical unit and the quality assurance committee, each clinical unit will assess a randomly selected sample of patients who have had surgery in the past 72 hours, have another acute pain condition, or have a diagnosis of cancer. Patients will be asked whether they have had pain during the current admission. Those patients who have experienced pain will then be asked about the:

1. Current intensity of their pain
2. Intensity of the worst pain they experienced in the past 24 hours (or other interval selected by the clinical unit)
3. Degree of relief obtained from pain management interventions
4. Satisfaction with the staff's responsiveness to their reports of pain
5. Satisfaction with relief provided

II. MAKE INFORMATION ABOUT ANALGESIC READILY AVAILABLE (PROCESS)

Information about analgesics and other methods of pain management, including charts of relative potencies of analgesics, is situated on the unit in a way that facilitates writing and interpreting orders. Nurses and physicians can demonstrate the use of this material. Appropriate training to treat their patients' pain is available to health professionals and is included in continuing education activities.

III. PROMISE PATIENTS ATTENTIVE ANALGESIC CARE (PROCESS)

Patients are informed on admission, verbally and in written form, that effective pain relief is an important part of their treatment, that their communication of unrelieved pain is essential, and that health professionals will respond quickly to their reports of pain.

IV. DEFINE EXPLICIT POLICIES FOR USE OF ADVANCED ANALGESIC TECHNOLOGIES (PROCESS)

Advanced pain control techniques, including intraspinal opioids, systemic or intraspinal patient-controlled anesthesia or continuous opioid infusion, local anesthetic infusion, and inhalational analgesia, are governed by policy and standard procedures that define the acceptable level of monitoring of patients and define appropriate roles and limits of practice for all groups of health care providers involved. Such policy includes definitions of physician accountability, nurse responsibility to the patient and the physician, and the role of pharmacy.

V. MONITOR ADHERENCE TO STANDARDS (PROCESS)

1. An interdisciplinary committee, including representation from physicians, nurses, and other appropriate disciplines (e.g., pharmacy), monitors compliance with the above standards, considers issues relevant to improving pain treatment, and makes recommendations to improve outcomes and their monitoring. Where a comprehensive pain management team exists, its activities are monitoring through the parent department's quality assurance body, which may also serve as the facility's quality assurance committee for pain relief. In a nursing home or very small hospital where an interdisciplinary pain management committee is not feasible, one or several individuals may fulfill this role.

2. At least the chairperson of the committee has experience working with issues related to effective pain management.

3. The committee meets at least every 3 months to review the process and outcomes related to pain management.

4. The committee interacts with clinical units to establish procedures for improving pain management where necessary and reviews the results of these changes within 3 months of their implementation.

5. The committee provides regular reports to administration and to the medical, nursing, and pharmacy staffs.

Drug Doses

Table AV-1. Oral nonsteroidal anti-inflammatory drugs

Generic name	Trade name	Adult dosage	Pediatric dosage
Acetaminophen	Tylenol	650–975 mg q4h	10–15 mg/kg q4h
Acetylsalicylic acid	Aspirin	650–975 mg q4h	10–15 mg/kg q4h
Choline magnesium trisalicylate	Trilisate	500–750 mg q8–12h	10–25 mg/kg bid
Diclofenal sodium	Voltaren	25–75 mg q8–12h	
Diflunisal	Dolobid	250–500 mg q8–12h	
Etodolic acid	Lodine	200–400 mg q6–8h	
Fenoprofen calcium	Nalfon	200 mg q4–6h	
Flurbiprofen	Ansaid	100 mg q8–12h	
Ibuprofen	Motrin	400–800 mg q6–8h	4–10 mg/kg q6–8h
Indomethacin	Indocin	25–50 mg q8–12h	
Ketoprofen	Orudis	25–75 mg q6–8h	
Ketorolac	Toradol	10–50 mg q6–8h	1 mg/kg q6–8h
Meclofenamate sodium	Meclomen	50 mg q4–6h	
Naproxen	Naprosyn	250–500 mg q8–12h	5–7 mg/kg q12h
Naproxen sodium	Anaprox	250–550 mg q6–8h	
Phenylbutazone	Butazolidin	100 mg q6–8h	
Piroxicam	Feldene	10–20 mg every day	
Salsalate	Disalcid	500 mg q4h	
Sulindac	Clinoril	150–200 mg q12h	
Tolmetin	Tolectin	200–600 mg q8h	5–7 mg/kg q6–8h

Table AV-2. Pediatric pain management

Generic name	Trade name	Dosage
Nonnarcotic analgesics		
Acetaminophen	Tylenol	10–15 mg/kg PO q4h
		10–20 mg/kg PR q4h
Acetylsalicylic acid	Aspirin	10–20 mg/kg PO q4h
Choline magnesium salicylate	Trilisate	10–20 mg/kg PO q6–8h
Ibuprofen	Motrin	4–10 mg/kg PO q6–8h
Naproxen	Naprosyn	5–7 mg/kg PO q8–12h
Tolmetin	Tolectin	5–7 mg/kg PO q6–8h
Narcotic analgesics		
Codeine		0.5–1.5 mg/kg PO q4–6h
Fentanyl	Sublimaze	1.0–1.5 μg/kg IV q1–2h
Hydromorphone	Dilaudid	0.05–0.10 mg/kg PO q6h
Meperidine	Demerol	1.0–1.5 mg/kg PO, IM q4h
		0.5–1.0 mg/kg IV q4h
Methadone	Dolophine	0.2 mg/kg PO q6–12h
		0.1 mg/kg IV q6–12h
Morphine		0.3–0.5 mg/kg PO q4h
		0.1–0.2 mg/kg IM q3–4h
		0.02–0.05 mg/kg IV q2–4h
Oxycodone		0.05–0.15 mg/kg PO q4-6h

Table AV-3. Pediatric pain management

| Drug | Loading dose | Continuous intravenous analgesia[a] | | |
		Bolus[b]	Infusion	4 hours maximum
PCA morphine	0.5–0.10 mg/kg	0.02 mg/kg q8–10min	0.03–0.05 mg/kg per hr	0.35 mg/kg
Morphine infusion	0.5–0.1 mg/kg		0.01–0.05 mg/kg per hr	
Fentanyl infusion	0.5–1.5 μg/kg		2–4 μg/kg per hr	
Demerol	0.5–1.0 mg/kg		0.5 mg/kg per hr	

| Drug | Continuous epidural/caudal | | |
	Concentration	Bolus	Infusion
Morphine[a]	0.1 mg/ml	0.2–0.4 ml	0.1–0.3 ml/kg per hr
Bupivacaine plus Fentanyl[c]	0.1% 2–5 μg/ml	0.25–0.40 ml	0.2–0.35 ml/kg per hr

[a] ages 1 year and up.
[b] ages 7 years and up.
[c] bupivacaine only for age < 1 year.

Table AV-4. Commonly prescribed narcotic tablets

Drug name	Ingredient(s)	Dosage
Darvocet N-50	Propoxyphene 50 mg Acetaminophen 650 mg	1–2 PO q3–4h
Darvocet N-100	Propoxyphene 100 mg Acetaminophen 650 mg	1–2 PO q3–4h
Darvon with ASA	Propoxyphene 65 mg Acetylsalicylic acid 389 mg Caffeine 32 mg	1–2 PO q3–4h
Darvon Cmpd	Propoxyphene 32 mg Acetylsalicylic acid 389 mg Caffeine 32 mg	1–2 PO q3–4h
Lorcet	Hydrocodone 10 mg Acetaminophen 650 mg	1–2 PO q4–6h
MS Contin	Morphine (slow release) 15, 30, 45 mg	1 PO q8–12h
Percocet	Oxycodone 5 mg Acetaminophen 325 mg	1–2 PO q3–4h
Percodan	Oxycodone 5 mg Acetylsalicylic acid 325 mg	1–2 PO q3–4h
Tramadol	50 mg	1–2 PO q4–6h max 400 mg/d
Tylenol #1	Acetaminophen 300 mg Codeine 7.5 mg	1–2 PO q3–4h
Tylenol #2	Acetaminophen 300 mg Codeine 15 mg	1–2 PO q3–4h
Tylenol #3	Acetaminophen 300 mg Codeine 30 mg	1–2 PO q3–4h
Tylenol #4	Acetaminophen 300 mg Codeine 60 mg	1–2 PO q3–4h
Tylox	Oxycodone 5 mg Acetaminophen 500 mg	1–2 PO q3–4h
Vicodin	Hydrocodone 7.5 mg Acetaminophen 750 mg	1–2 PO q4–6h
Wygesic	Propoxyphene 65 mg Acetaminophen 650 mg	1–2 PO q3–4h

Table AV-5. Opioid analgesic doses in adult and pediatric patients

Generic name	Trade name	Equi-analgesic doses		Adult doses		Pediatric doses	
		Oral	Parenteral	Oral	Parenteral	Oral	Parenteral
		Opioid agonist analgesics					
Codeine		30 mg q3–4h	10 mg q3–4h	30 mg q3–4h	10 mg q3–4h	0.3 mg/kg q3–4h	0.1 mg/kg q3–4h
Hydrocodone	Vicodin, Lorcet	30 mg q3–4h		10 mg q3–4h		0.2 mg/kg q3–4h	
Hydromorphone	Dilaudid	7.5 mg q3–4h	1.5 mg q3–4h	6 mg q3–4h	1.5 mg q3–4h	0.06 mg/kg q3–4h	0.015 mg/kg q3–4h
Levorphanol	Levo-Dromoran	4 mg q6–8h	2 mg q6–8h	4 mg q6–8h	2 mg q6–8h	0.04 mg/kg q6–8h	0.02 mg/kg q6–8h
Meperidine	Demerol	300 mg q2–3h	100 mg q3h		100 mg q3h		0.75 mg/kg q2–3h
Methadone	Dolophine	20 mg q6–8h	10 mg q6–8h	20 mg q6–8h	10 mg q6–8h	0.2 mg/kg q6–8h	0.1 mg/kg q6–8h
Morphine		30 mg q3–4h	10 mg q3–4h	30 mg q3–4h	10 mg q3–4h	0.3 mg/kg q3–4h	0.1 mg/kg q3–4h
Oxycodone	Percocet, Tylox, Percodan	30 mg q3–4h		10 mg q3–4h		0.2 mg/kg q3–4h	
Oxymorphone	Numorphan		1 mg q3–4h		1 mg q3–4h		
		Opioid agonist–antagonist and partial agonist analgesics					
Buprenorphine	Buprenex		0.3–0.4 mg q6–8h		0.4 mg q6–8h		0.004 mg/kg q6–8h
Butorphanol	Stadol		2 mg q3–4h		2 mg q3–4h		
Nalbuphine	Nubain		10 mg q3–4h		10 mg q3–4h		0.1 mg/kg q3–4h
Pentazocine	Talwin	150 mg q3–4h	60 mg q3–4h	50 mg q4–6h	10 mg q3–4h		

Food and Drug Administration State Drug Schedules

Table AVI-1. Schedules for controlled substances prescribed for patients in pain

Schedule 1

None

Schedule 2

Opioids: morphine, codeine, fentanyl, hydromorphone, meperidine, levorphanol, oxycodone

Stimulants: amphetamine, methylphenidate

Marihuana: dronabinol

Schedule 3

Opioids: nalorphine; mixtures of limited specified quantities of codeine, dihydrocodeine, hydrocodone, morphine or opioid with noncontrolled medicinal ingredients

Schedule 4

Opioids: pentazocine

Benzodiazepines: valium, clonazepam, flurazepam, midazolam, triazolam

Schedule 5

Opioids: cough suppressant preparations

Dermatomes and Nerve Distribution

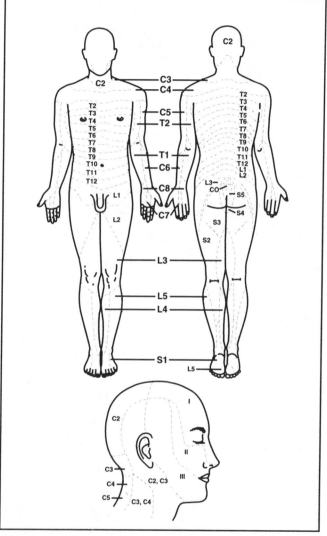

Fig. AVII-1. Sensory dermatones. Note that cranial nerves I, II, and III are the sensory division of the trigeminal nerve (V). (Adapted from Devinsky O, Feldman E, Examination of the Cranial and Peripheral Nerves. London: Churchill, 1988.)

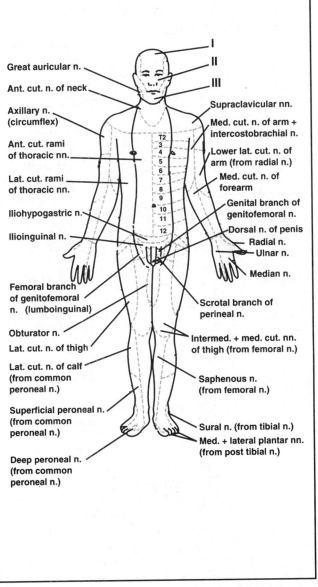

Great auricular n.

Ant. cut. n. of neck

Axillary n.
(circumflex)

Ant. cut. rami
of thoracic nn.

Lat. cut. rami
of thoracic nn.

Iliohypogastric n.

Ilioinguinal n.

Femoral branch
of genitofemoral
n. (lumboinguinal)

Obturator n.
Lat. cut. n. of thigh

Lat. cut. n. of calf
(from common
peroneal n.)

Superficial peroneal n.
(from common
peroneal n.)

Deep peroneal n.
(from common
peroneal n.)

I

II

III

Supraclavicular nn.

Med. cut. n. of arm +
intercostobrachial n.

Lower lat. cut. n. of
arm (from radial n.)

Med. cut. n. of
forearm

Genital branch of
genitofemoral n.

Dorsal n. of penis

Radial n.

Ulnar n.

Median n.

Scrotal branch of
perineal n.

Intermed. + med. cut. nn.
of thigh (from femoral n.)

Saphenous n.
(from femoral n.)

Sural n. (from tibial n.)
Med. + lateral plantar nn.
(from post tibial n.)

T2
3
4
5
6
7
8
9
10
11
12
L1

Fig. AVII-2. Sensory innervation of the skin—frontal view (A) and posterior view (B). The figures are a schematic of the distribution of the sensory nerves.

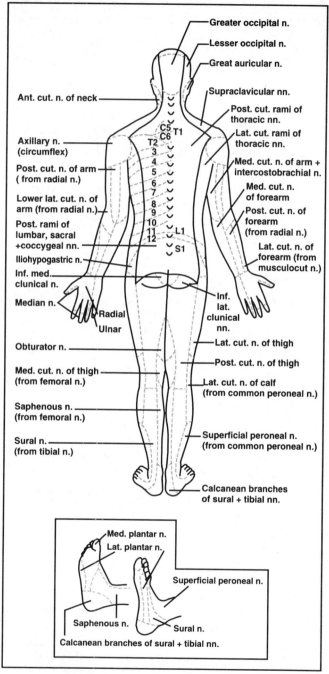

Greater occipital n.

Lesser occipital n.

Great auricular n.

Ant. cut. n. of neck

Supraclavicular nn.

Post. cut. rami of thoracic nn.

Axillary n. (circumflex)

Lat. cut. rami of thoracic nn.

Post. cut. n. of arm (from radial n.)

Med. cut. n. of arm + intercostobrachial n.

Lower lat. cut. n. of arm (from radial n.)

Med. cut. n. of forearm

Post. cut. n. of forearm (from radial n.)

Post. rami of lumbar, sacral +coccygeal nn.

Lat. cut. n. of forearm (from musculocut n.)

Iliohypogastric n.

Inf. med. clunical n.

Median n.

Radial

Ulnar

Inf. lat. clunical nn.

Obturator n.

Lat. cut. n. of thigh

Post. cut. n. of thigh

Med. cut. n. of thigh (from femoral n.)

Lat. cut. n. of calf (from common peroneal n.)

Saphenous n. (from femoral n.)

Sural n. (from tibial n.)

Superficial peroneal n. (from common peroneal n.)

Calcanean branches of sural + tibial nn.

C5 T1
C6
T2
3
4
5
6
7
8
9
10
11
12
L1
S1

Med. plantar n.

Lat. plantar n.

Superficial peroneal n.

Saphenous n.

Sural n.

Calcanean branches of sural + tibial nn.

Fig. AVII-2. Continued.

446

Index

Index